It has been the con... ... ... St. Andrew's Ambulance Association that ambulance work should keep pace with the advances of the science and art of healing. To fulfil this aim it has been decided to publish a new hand-book to replace the former one, which has served such a useful and educational purpose for many years. Only by reason of the former hand-book being out of date has the expediency of this new publication been considered.

The St. Andrew's Ambulance Association still adheres to the principle that, in order to practise ambulance work, a knowledge of the human frame and of the nature of life is fundamental. For this reason anatomy and physiology are dealt with in considerable detail so that the advanced ambulance pupil may be able to understand the principles which govern the practice of first-aid. It is hoped that the practical application of this knowledge will be the means of alleviating suffering and of saving life. Junior pupils, under the guidance of their instructors, will be able to extract from the pages of the book that which is necessary for an elementary course.

From the authors' point of view it would have been desirable to deal separately with anatomy, physiology and first-aid, but the reader has been indulged to a certain extent by an intermingling of these subjects in the hope that continuous reading may not be tedious.

The authors desire to place on record their indebtedness to the Controller of His Majesty's Stationery Office for his kind permission to publish portions of the stretcher drill of the Royal Army Medical Corps, and to the Order of St. John and the St. John Ambulance Association for their courtesy in permitting their text-book, *Protection of the*

Civil Population in Chemical Warfare, by Major F. K. Humphreys, T.D., to be reprinted in the Appendix of this hand-book; to Dr. R. Scott Frew, Dr. John Gracie, Mr. Wellwood R. Ferguson and Mr. James H. H. Henderson for assistance in technical matters and for their constructive criticism of manuscripts and proofs; to Mr. William J. McLean, of the Glasgow School of Art, whose original anatomical drawings greatly enhance the value of this book; and to the printers, Messrs. Robert MacLehose & Co. Limited, who have given that care and attention which has earned them their well-deserved reputation.

We desire to pay tribute to the late Sir George Thomas Beatson, whose classical *Ambulance Handbook* has been our guide and inspiration; advances in the sciences and the advent of new methods of treatment alone justify its replacement.

GLASGOW, *August*, 1933.

PREFACE TO THE SECOND EDITION.

THE exhaustion of the first edition within the past two years has necessitated the publication of this edition. The authors have taken the opportunity of effecting slight alteration and addition to the text and index of the first edition. They desire to thank those who have offered kind and constructive criticism by which they have been guided wherever practicable.

GLASGOW, *August* 1935.

PREFACE TO THE THIRD EDITION.

THE rapid sale of the second edition has necessitated the publication of a third edition of the Ambulance Hand-book. The authors have again availed themselves of the opportunity of effecting slight alterations and additions to the previous text. Their thanks are once more due to those who by their valuable criticism have added to the usefulness of the book.

GLASGOW, *August* 1937.

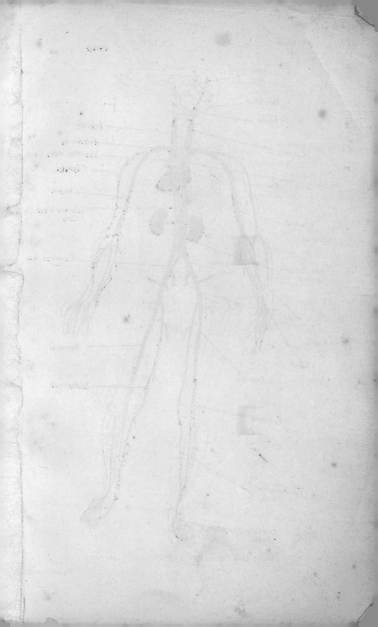

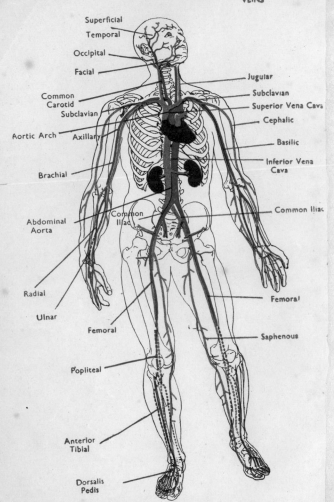

THE SKELETON AND BLOOD-VESSELS.

AMBULANCE HAND-BOOK

ON THE PRINCIPLES OF

FIRST-AID TO THE INJURED

BY

ERIC G. GERSTENBERG
M.B., Ch.B., F.R.C.S.E., F.R.F.P.S.G.

JOHN B. GAYLOR
M.A., B.Sc., M.B., Ch.B., F.R.F.P.S.G.

WILLIAM C. GUNN
T.D., M.D., D.P.H., LT.-COL. R.A.M.C.(T.)

Nineteenth Edition

GLASGOW
ST. ANDREW'S AMBULANCE ASSOCIATION
(*Incorporated by Royal Charter*)
1954

COPYRIGHT

1st Edition	September 1933.	
2nd	,,	November 1934.
3rd	,,	(with alts.) October 1935.
4th	,,	October 1937.
5th	,,	October 1938.
6th	,,	November 1938.
7th	,,	April 1939.
8th	,,	May 1939.
9th	,,	September 1939.
10th	,,	October 1939.
11th	,,	March 1940.
12th	,,	November 1940.
13th	,,	May 1941.
14th	,,	October 1942.
15th	,,	November 1943.
16th	,,	March 1946.
17th	,,	December 1948.
18th	,,	January 1950.
19th	,,	June 1954.

Artificial Respiration
by the
Holger Nielsen Method
see Supplement at end of Book.

PRINTED IN GREAT BRITAIN

CONTENTS.

LIST OF ILLUSTRATIONS.

PLATES IN COLOUR.

PLATES.

vii

FIGURES.

SYLLABUS OF AMBULANCE LECTURES

WITH

CORRESPONDING CHAPTERS OF HAND-BOOK.

FIRST LECTURE.

A. Introductory remarks, explaining clearly the scope and object of lay help in ambulance work, special attention being drawn to the need for it, as well as the usefulness and simplicity of it.

(Chaps. I. and II.)

B. Short sketch of the general anatomy and physiology of the human body, including a brief description of the functions of digestion, absorption, circulation, respiration, excretion, secretion, and innervation.

(Chap. III.)

C. Uses of a bandage—The two kinds of bandage, the triangular and roller—Description of Esmarch's triangular bandage, pointing out (1) its advantages, (2) method of folding and fastening it, (3) its application in different ways—The roller bandage—General rules for applying and fixing. Special forms of roller bandage used in first-aid work.

(Chap. IV.)

SECOND LECTURE.

A. Short account of the skeleton, with brief description of the structure and varieties of the joints and muscles, and surgical shock.

(Chaps. V. and VI.)

B. (1) *Fractures*—Their varieties, causes, symptoms, and dangers—Their temporary treatment and the apparatus necessary for it. (2) *Dislocations*—How they differ from

xiii

fractures, and the first-aid in such cases—Sprains and strains, their symptoms and treatment.

(Chaps. VII. and VIII.)

C. Illustrations of the temporary treatment of the following *simple* fractures—(1) collar bone, (2) upper arm, (3) fore arm, (4) hand, (5) thigh, (6) leg, (7) foot, (8) lower jaw.

(Chap. VII.)

THIRD LECTURE.

To be devoted to practical work, when the members of the class will exercise themselves in the use of the triangular and roller bandage and the temporary treatment of the different fractures mentioned in the previous lecture.

FOURTH LECTURE.

A. (1) General description of the circulation of the blood, and the mechanism by which it is carried on—(2) Distinction between arterial, venous, and capillary haemorrhage—(3) Names of the main arteries of the body, with their situation—(4) Points where arterial circulation may be arrested by pressure—(5) Dangers of hæmorrhage.

(Chaps. IX. and X.)

B. General treatment of haemorrhage :—I. *Internal haemorrhage*—First-aid in cases of (1) bleeding from the nose, (2) spitting of blood, (3) vomiting of blood. II. *External haemorrhage*—(1) Application of cold, either by water or exposure to air, (2) Elevation of part, (3) Local pressure, (4) Distant pressure on main artery supplying wound, either by hand or tourniquet, (5) Two kinds of tourniquet : elastic and improvised.

(Chap. X.;

C. Show mode of applying elastic tourniquet, and of making an improvised one—Give illustrations of arrest of haemorrhage from (1) scalp, (2) neck, (3) armpit, (4) upper arm, (5) fore arm, (6) hand, (7) thigh—Give illustrations of temporary treatment of a *compound* fracture, with haemorrhage in upper or lower extremity..

(Chaps. X. and XI.)

FIFTH LECTURE.

To be devoted to practical work, when the members of the class will exercise themselves in the arrest of haemorrhage in various situations, including ruptured varicose veins, and in the treatment of wounds.

SIXTH LECTURE.

A. Short account of respiration, its objects and mechanism.
(Chap. XII.)

B. Asphyxia, its causes, symptoms, and treatment—Immediate treatment of those apparently drowned, or suffocated by (1) hanging, (2) poisonous gases, (3) choking, etc., etc.
(Chap. XIII.)

C. Show mode of performing artificial respiration (Schäfer's method), and also the treatment of cases of asphyxia.
(Chap. XIII.)

SEVENTH LECTURE.

To be devoted to practical work generally, when the members will exercise themselves in performing artificial respiration, and in the treatment of fractures, wounds, etc.

EIGHTH LECTURE.

A. Short account of the alimentary and excretory systems.
(Chaps. XIV. and XV.)

B. Poisons—their classification, symptoms, and treatment.
(Chap. XVI.)

NINTH LECTURE.

A. Short account of the nervous system, giving various states of insensibility, their symptoms and treatment.
(Chaps. XVII. and XVIII.)

B. Burns, scalds, frost-bites, and electric shock.
(Chaps. XIX.)

C. Foreign bodies in the eye, nose, and ear. Acute abdomen.
   Hernia. Childbirth. Determination of death and signs
   of death.

(Chap. XX.)

TENTH LECTURE.

Removal of the injured by means of stretchers, special attention being directed to (1) the proper carriage of the
   stretcher, (2) the manner of placing it, (3) the loading
   and unloading it, (4) the position of the patient on it,
   (5) suggestions as to overcoming difficulties on the
   road, (6) hints as to the conveyance of stretchers by
   rail, road, steamer, etc. and short account of some of
   the improvised methods of removing injured persons
   when no stretchers or regular conveyances are available,
   as by the two-handed, three-handed, and four-handed
   seats.

(Chap. XXI.)

CHAPTER I.

INTRODUCTION.

THE condition of modern civilization demands that everyone should have some knowledge of how to deal with an emergency of sudden illness. It is not simply a pursuit for the few, but all members of the community should know the elements of first-aid. The acquisition of the necessary knowledge is not difficult ; its interest far outweighs any consideration of the inconvenience of learning and its general usefulness is incalculable. To be an efficient first-aid man or woman is a quality of highest citizenship and sooner or later is bound to be part of the equipment of every responsible person in a civilized community. No apology, therefore, is necessary for the production of a Handbook of Ambulance which will bring this knowledge within the reach of everyone.

To avoid any misconception of terms, it is well to point out here that the words Ambulance and First-aid have practically the same significance. There is no essential difference between an ambulance man and a first-aid man. *First-aid may be defined as being the immediate assistance rendered to a person suddenly taken ill, whether as the result of an accident or as the result of some disease.* First-aid is essentially a form of treatment, and treatment is always carried out with a view to aiding the patient towards recovery. The measures adopted are of a temporary character, because the first-aid man has no pretensions to becoming a practitioner of medicine. He is ever aware that qualified medical opinion is always to be sought as early as possible, and out of respect for qualified medical opinion he always makes himself subservient to it whenever

A

the doctor arrives. The treatment furthermore is immediate. The condition of the patient is an emergency and
demands attention at once before a doctor can possibly
arrive. Immediate attention may mean actually saving a
life, or it may mean that the course of recovery will be
shortened and be attended with much less suffering. These
happy issues are dependent upon efficiency; should there be
carelessness in administering the emergency treatment, life
may be lost, or the patient may have much more suffering
and subsequent deformities may be rendered more cripp-
ling. The first-aid man must also observe the condition of
his patient as closely as possible, since great weight may be
placed on his word by the doctor who has subsequent care
of the case. The practice of first-aid gives scope for ingenuity, since any suitable material at hand has to be
utilized in providing the means of treatment.

The practice of first-aid is honoured in antiquity ; it is
as ancient as the history of man. Primitive people had
recourse to emergency treatment in the accidents of the
hunt and of war. References can be found to such practice
throughout ancient and modern literature. The greatest
doctors, writers and philosophers of ancient times were the
Greeks, and it may be permitted to refer to their literature
for an example. In the *Iliad* Homer tells of Machâon, that
god-like man, plucking arrows from wounds, squeezing out
the blood and pouring in assuaging drugs. The parable of
the Good Samaritan needs no exposition, such is his hon-
ourable repute. It is interesting to note that the Good
Samaritan used wine to pour into the wounds, unwittingly
in accordance with the best antiseptic measures of modern
surgery. Since those ancient times several factors have
been at work to advance the practice of first-aid. An increasing humanitarian philosophy has aroused greater
solicitude for those who are ill. This implies an increasing
preparedness for emergency illness and consequently urges
the more general knowledge of first-aid. The enlightenment
of medical science, which has been growing rapidly within

the past century, has pointed out the absolute necessity for efficient emergency treatment on the part of the layman. This again means training all people to have an appreciation of the nature and treatment of sudden illness. Two other influences must be mentioned, the influence of war and of modern developments in industry. During the Napoleonic campaigns, Baron Larrey was responsible for the development of much first-aid practice, and the work of Florence Nightingale is so well known that her name is immediately associated with the good offices of ambulance organization. The South African War of 1899-1902 and the Great War of 1914-1918 have both contributed to the more efficient organization of military first-aid, and the lessons of war are not inapplicable to the needs of civilian life. In this age of complicated machinery and lofty structure the occupations of men have become more hazardous and, as a consequence, the further development of first-aid service has been rendered necessary. Only organized service can hope to meet the daily needs of civil life. As a result of humanitarian opinion, medical enlightenment and public demand, the St. John Ambulance Association was founded in London in 1878. Its sphere speedily became national and now extends to India and the Dominions overseas. Four years later, in 1882, the St. Andrew's Ambulance Association was formed in Glasgow. Like the older Association, no limit was placed upon its sphere of work within the Empire, but, for the most part, it has confined its activities to Scotland. In 1908 an agreement was made between the Venerable Order of St. John of Jerusalem and the St. Andrew's Ambulance Association whereby the former undertook that its Ambulance Department should abstain from work in Scotland and the latter similarly undertook to abstain from work in England. The two societies thus work side by side and render incalculable service in their respective spheres of labour.

CHAPTER II.

GENERAL PRINCIPLES OF FIRST-AID.

THIS chapter is intended to give a survey of the qualities which ought to characterise the first-class ambulance man, and to state the general principles of tending the injured.

Qualities, beyond those manifest in the everyday man pursuing mundane tasks, are expected to be evident in the ambulance man while performing his duty. This does not mean that the ambulance worker has exceptional qualities unattainable by most, because many, who have never been called upon to exercise those superior qualities, will rise to an occasion which demands the exercise of more than ordinary resource.

Ambulance work may demand courage amounting to bravery, sacrifice in varying degree, and infinite patience. Admittedly, on most occasions, there is no great strain associated with ordinary emergencies, but there may be one occasion in the life of any man which calls out the highest attributes of humanity and to which meritorious response has come from the most unexpected quarters.

The ambulance man, while exercising almost heroic qualities on certain occasions, must possess under all circumstances characteristics which do not excite so much approbation and yet, owing to the necessity of their constant exercise, are more important than heroics. The first of these is avoidance of alarm. Emergencies of sudden illness may be attended by so much stress and strain on those who witness them that it is not unnatural for panic to arise. Such panic must be avoided at all costs. In some cases, such as fire in crowded places, lack of discipline will reap disaster. If the ambulance man has no control over himself he cannot be expected to have any control over others nor to be able to treat the injured efficiently. This brings out the second constant quality, that of being able to command. It is an attribute of personality and, in proportion as the personality is strong and amiable, so will the ambulance man exercise control over a crowd provided his efficiency merits the respect of those with whom he has to deal. Idle curiosity on the part of those who have little else to do and the desire to interfere on the part of the officious will cause a number of people to gather round any accident. These people must be kept at a distance and they must not be allowed to interfere with the discharge of efficient emergency treatment. These rules of personal comportment and of general attitude towards those who are witnesses of an accident are to be observed in all accidents.

Having dealt with the behaviour of the ambulance man and his exercise of control upon those around him while he is about to perform his work, we will now proceed to a few generalities with regard to his conduct towards his patient. There is nothing more distressing to the sick than an unsympathetic attendant. In disease much benefit is derived from the exercise of sympathy on the part of the medical attendant and from the patient's confidence in his ability. What is true of medical practice is equally true of first-aid practice. Sympathy towards the patient and the power of inspiring confidence are two essential attributes of the first-aid worker ; the former will depend upon his general character, the latter will be the result of knowledge, resource, manipulative dexterity and personal confidence in the efficacy of the measures about to be applied.

In the interest of any injured person skilled medical opinion must be obtained at once. First-aid is merely a form of treatment to be carried out before a doctor can possibly come to see the case. An ambulance man who takes it upon himself to act as a practitioner of medicine

by applying a course of treatment other than first-aid, or
who neglects to summon a doctor, is accepting a responsibility which he is totally unable to bear and is adopting a
policy which will inevitably cause him regret. The golden
rule of first-aid work is to send for a doctor or have the
patient conveyed in an ambulance to a hospital where
medical assistance is readily available.

Whenever possible it is advisable to send the doctor
some details with regard to the circumstances of the accident. As a general rule the more obvious the condition
the less detail need be sent. For instance, it is sufficient to
convey the message " severe internal hæmorrhage " or
" compound fracture of the femur " with directions as to
where the patient may be found, but where a person is
found insensible it will be necessary to venture some
details as to the circumstances of the case together with
some information as to the history of the patient in so far
as it can be obtained from those who are with him.

A patient must not be left in such a position after an
accident as to render him liable to receive further injury.
The removal of the patient to a place of safety is one of
the first considerations in treating an emergency. Thus it
follows that a gassed man must be taken out of the atmosphere which has been responsible for his condition ; a man
injured in the middle of a busy thoroughfare should be
removed to a place where he can be better treated and
where there is less chance of further calamity. It does not
follow that this measure should be adopted in all cases
before any ameliorative procedure is adopted, because there
are conditions, with which the reader will become familiar,
where life depends on the rapidity with which these can be
treated. In such conditions removal of the patient, sending immediately for a doctor and keeping back a crowd are
purely secondary to the primary objective of instituting
immediate first-aid measures.

In most emergencies the patient should be lying in the
recumbent position. If the condition be serious there is

no other option, but if the patient is able to stand it will often be found disadvantageous to treat him while in the erect posture. Even in cases of fracture or wound of the arm, where bandages have only to encircle the limb, the patient should be seated. In many of the emergencies with which we shall have to deal, special directions are given as to the position of the patient and the position of the ambulance man relative to the patient.

There is seldom an accident of any degree of severity where it is unnecessary to remove some of the patient's clothing, or at least to loosen clothing. This procedure. particularly in the case of treating female patients, has to be tempered with a discretion which no handbook on ambulance can instil into the unreceptive mind. It is well to remember that a false sense of modesty may work disaster ; in severe bleeding from a woman's thigh no consideration of indignity must stand in the way of obtaining sufficient exposure of the injury in order to treat it properly. Ruthless exposure is naturally to be condemned, but refraining from any necessary exposure is even more culpable since it is conceivable that such negligence may cost the patient her life. Frequently it is necessary to loosen tight clothing about the neck and trunk. The manner in which this should be done will depend upon the urgency of the case. Sometimes it may be necessary to tear or cut a man's collar, but usually a collar can be loosened in the ordinary way. Seldom does men's clothing interfere with the movements of the chest, but unfortunately some women persist in the practice of wearing tight corsets. In any case of embarrassment to breathing in women wearing tight corsets these garments must be loosened, laces may be cut with a knife or scissors ; tight belts have to be similarly dealt with. The necessity for such practice in the first-aid treatment of women is becoming less common because the " hour glass " waist, for which there was not one iota of justification, is not fashionable and because women are learning to keep their figures within aesthetic limits by exercise rather than by compressing their abdomens inside absurd stays.

One further point of general interest remains. Many laymen are under the impression that all cases of sudden illness, whether due to an accident or to the manifestations of disease, should be treated by administering some stimulant. Some indication is given later of those conditions where stimulation is necessary. The method of stimulation usually adopted in first-aid practice is to apply smelling salts to the nostrils. Other methods of general stimulation are the application of heat to the body, rubbing the limbs and giving hot drinks. Later on some detail is given about the action of alcohol on the human being. Alcohol should never be administered by anyone other than a qualified practitioner in cases of sudden illness, with the single exception of carbolic acid or lysol poisoning. The reason for such a statement is that only a doctor can decide when alcohol will do good in an emergency and that in many emergencies of sudden illness the administration of alcohol is harmful.

CHAPTER III.

GENERAL ANATOMY AND PHYSIOLOGY.

(A) CELLULAR NATURE OF THE LIVING BODY.

It is common knowledge that living material is made up of cells. A cell is the unit of living substance; it possesses a limiting membrane bounding the cell, a nucleus

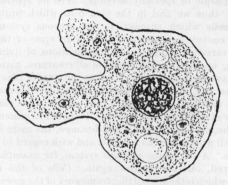

FIG. 1.—A CELL.

which is situated centrally and is made up of concentrated living matter, and a ground substance, cytoplasm, which fills up the whole cell and in which the nucleus is embedded (Fig. 1). On the integrity of the nucleus the vitality of the cell depends, but the functions of the cell depend mainly on the changes which occur in the cytoplasm. Here we find stores of food in minute particles; in the cytoplasm, waste products gather, and from the cytoplasm these waste products are discharged.

The conception of a living cell must include some idea of interchange between the contents of the cell and the surroundings in which the cell finds itself. There is a free passage of material from outside the cell membrane into the cytoplasm and free discharge from the interior to the exterior. The simplest of creatures consists of a single cell only ; this cell carries out all the functions of vital activity.

When we ascend higher in the evolutionary scale we find that creatures become more and more complex and that they are made up of an increasing number of cells. According to the complexity of the creature there is a setting aside of specially developed cells for special func- tions ; thus we find in the skin cells which protect, in bone cells which support, in the nervous system cells which convey messages and so on. In spite of the very great variation in the types and functions of living cells making up that most complex of all creatures, man, these cells have their source in one cell at the start of life. From this first cell, which is formed by the union of a male and female element, all cells spring no matter what the com- plexity of their function may be. It should be remembered that the more specialised a cell becomes, the more fixed is that cell with regard to function and with regard to regen- eration. A cell of the nervous system, for example, once destroyed, can never grow again. Cells of the fibrous tissue, which is the supporting framework of the more active tissues, are not highly specialised ; consequently fibrous elements, which are situated everywhere throughout the body, are adaptable and can subserve the function of over- growth for the purpose of replacing more highly specialised cells. More will be said of this later, when the healing of wounds is being considered, but the examples of fibrous tissue elements growing to replace loss of substance in the liver or in the skin may be quoted at the moment. It must not be imagined that all specialised cells have lost the power of multiplication ; far from it, the deeper cells of the skin are constantly replacing those more superficial layers which are always being rubbed off. The foregoing is not calculated to give the reader a limited or restricted view of living matter or of the cell. He should at once realize that the word cell, although it conveys the conception of something which is limited and something the contents of which have no interchange with the outside, has been applied to the unit of living substance merely for want of a better simple term.

(B) THE BODY FROM AN ANATOMICAL POINT OF VIEW.

We shall commence the study of the human body with a consideration of its structural composition or anatomy and at a later stage we shall find ourselves in a better position to explain its functions or physiology.

To become acquainted with the structural composition of the body is to learn its anatomy, for anatomy is the science of structure. For our purpose we shall study descriptive anatomy, which deals with the structure, form and relations of the organs and parts comprising the human body.

EXTERNAL CONFIGURATION OF THE BODY.—When we look at a human being we see that the body is naturally divisable into the head, neck, trunk and limbs. Grouped together, the head, neck and trunk form what is sometimes called the axial portion of the body in which are found the organs essential to life. The limbs form the appendicular portion of the body; the arms are concerned with prehension or grasping; the legs with locomotion or walking.

INTERNAL STRUCTURE OF THE BODY.—Let us imagine that we are about to dissect the human body. No matter where we commence we must first cut through the skin which forms a protective covering on the external surface generally. When the skin is removed there is found immediately below it a layer of fat which varies in thickness in different regions and in different people. Below the fat are found distinct masses of red flesh which can be separated from one another and are known as the muscles. Each muscle has its own sheath of tough fibrous tissue which

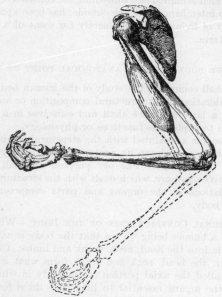

FIG. 2.—ACTION OF MUSCLE.

makes it a separate anatomical structure. This fibrous sheath has a silvery appearance and is called fascia. As a general rule muscles are elongated structures, the ends of which are attached firmly to bone directly or indirectly. The attachment nearer the axis of the body is known as the origin, while the other attachment is its insertion. As a rule each muscle arises from a definite area in one bone, expands into a fleshy belly and is inserted into some other bone. Under the muscles are found rigid structures, the bones, to which the muscles are attached. The bones form the strong framework of the body, giving strength to limbs and protection to vital organs. Bones are attached to one another so as to form hinges or joints of various types. Since muscles possess the power of shortening themselves, and since there is usually one or more joints between the areas of muscular origin and insertion, movement about the joints is possible (Fig. 2).

Running through the fat and between the muscles are observed tubular structures, the blood vessels and solid cords, the nerves (Plate II.). At various points both blood vessels and nerves can be seen entering the muscles and branching through their substance. There are other structures, slender and delicate tubes, the lymph vessels which form a network in the tissues throughout the body. Lymph vessels are so minute that they cannot be recognized by the unaided eye, but they communicate at many places with small bean-shaped bodies, the lymphatic glands. These are quite apparent in the vicinity of the blood vessels near the joints.

AXIAL PORTION.—The superficial structures of the axial portion of the anatomy are essentially similar to those of the limbs, but when we come to the bones a different arrangement is found. In the mid line of the back there is a column of bones, the vertebral column, supporting the skull on its upper end, giving attachment to the ribs in the region of the chest and resting below upon the pelvis. The pelvis is a basin-like formation formed by a girdle of bones. This girdle is made up of the lowest part of the vertebral column wedged between a pair of large flattened bones which have prolongations meeting in front to complete the circle. When the body is in the erect position the thigh bones support the pelvis. As already mentioned, the ribs arise from the vertebral column behind in the chest region and, being curved, they extend partially round the chest to

assist in the formation of the thorax. This is completed in
front by the breast bone, which is joined to the ribs by
gristle-like structures known as the costal cartilages.

The arms are slung on a girdle of bones called the pectoral girdle. This is formed in front by the collar bones,
which are separated by the upper end of the breast bone,
and behind by two wing-like bones, the shoulder blades,
which are attached to the outer ends of the collar
bones.

The trunk is divided into two main compartments by a
dome-shaped sheet of muscle called the diaphragm. Above,
there is the cavity of the thorax containing the heart, the
lungs and the great blood vessels of the body at their commencement. Below, there is the cavity of the abdomen,
the walls of which are composed of sheets of muscle. It
contains the stomach and intestines, the liver, the spleen,
the pancreas, the kidneys and the urinary bladder.

In the thorax the lungs are separated from one another
by the tissues which support the heart and the great blood
vessels in the middle of the chest. Surrounding the lungs
and the heart are special membranes, moist and glistening,
termed serous membranes. In the case of the lung the
membrane is called the pleura, which has two layers
enclosing a cavity, the pleural cavity; the layers of the
pleura are in contact with one another and glide over each
other with the movements of the chest in breathing. Each
pleural cavity forms a complete closed sac and the membrane lining it is a continuous sheet; that part of the
membrane covering the organ is termed the visceral layer,
while that part of the membrane which is outermost and
against which the visceral layer rubs is termed the parietal
layer. This description suffices for all serous membranes.
An idea of the precise relationship of such a structure may
be obtained by the following analogy. Take a balloon and
partially inflate it; hold the balloon in the hollow of the
left hand, with the fist of the right hand indent the surface
of the balloon and press the fist of the right hand towards

the palm of the left hand. In this position we have a continuous sheet of balloon wall representing a continuous sheet of serous membrane ; the right hand represents the organ covered by a visceral layer of serous membrane, the left hand lined by the parietal layer represents the wall of the chest or abdomen. There is a serous membrane covering the heart and the great vessels at their commencement ; it is termed the pericardium. The peritoneum is a serous membrane lining the peritoneal cavity and investing the stomach and intestines, the liver and the spleen ; the kidneys and the pancreas are situated on the posterior abdominal wall and are separated from the parietal peritoneum by fat (Plate III.).

The head is divided into a cranial and a facial portion— the former is that part of the head which contains the brain ; the latter comprises the bones and other structures forming the face. The cranial cavity is continuous with a canal in the vertebral column. This canal is occupied by a prolongation of the brain called the spinal cord. Through certain openings in the floor of the skull and sides of the vertebral column nerves arising from the brain and spinal cord emerge to go to all parts of the body. In the bones of the face are recesses for the organs of special sense, the eyes, the nose, the ears and the tongue.

APPENDICULAR PORTION—STRUCTURE OF THE LIMBS.— To apply this general knowledge to the appendicular portion of the anatomy we find that a limb is covered by skin and underlying fat. When these structures have been removed there are revealed the muscles clothing the several bones and joints of the limb. The blood vessels, nerves and lymphatics pursue their course as already described according to the general rule.

In the foregoing description we have briefly outlined the general conformation of the body and the arrangement of the tissues. We shall now proceed to investigate the functions, or physiology, of the body and see how the tissues are grouped together to form the various systems. Later we shall describe the more intricate structure of the systems and their special organs.

(C) THE BODY FROM A PHYSIOLOGICAL POINT OF VIEW.

The term physiology literally means a discourse on nature : we may express its significance better by calling physiology that study which investigates life. When we speak of human physiology we refer to the study of natural processes as they occur in the healthy human being.

The nature of life has been a problem which has concerned the minds of scientists and philosophers of all ages, but it would be fruitless, for our present purposes, to consider either the philosophic or the strictly scientific conceptions of life. Let us satisfy ourselves with an examination of those ideas which arise in our own minds when we think of life generally. Immediately the word "life" is mentioned, a definite picture presents itself. We see mentally some creature, a man, possessing certain attributes by which we recognize that he is alive. He moves, he is warm, he breathes, he eats, he thinks and speaks. Death is the cessation of these functions without the capability of resuscitation. We may set ourselves the task of finding an analogy, something to which we can compare the living creature. Possibly the first thing we think of as being like a living creature is an engine. The analogy is well-worn, but it is sufficiently good to fix in our minds some of the conceptions of life. Considering, then, the human body as a mere machine, which has to maintain itself in the struggle for existence, there are certain things which are essential to its life. Like the engine, the body has to develop energy, and that energy in the case of both comes from the burning of fuel. The fuel in the case of the engine is coal or oil ; in the case of the body it is food.

Food is burned in the body in much the same way as coal is burned in the furnace of the locomotive. The human being is set the task of acquiring his own fuel. He

PLATE II.

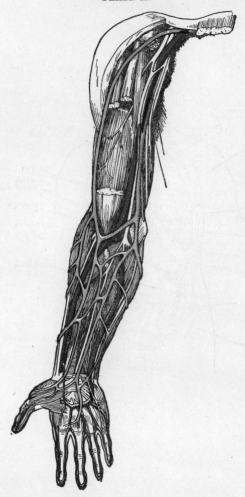

INTERNAL STRUCTURE OF A LIMB.

PLATE III.

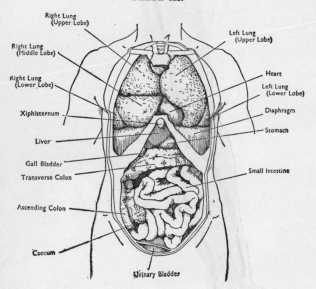

Right Lung (Upper Lobe)
Right Lung (Middle Lobe)
Right Lung (Lower Lobe)
Xiphisternum
Liver
Gall Bladder
Transverse Colon
Ascending Colon
Caecum

Left Lung (Upper Lobe)
Heart
Left Lung (Lower Lobe)
Diaphragm
Stomach
Small Intestine

Urinary Bladder

must have some means of feeling that fuel is required and some means of obtaining food by directing the energy which he develops. He knows that he requires food because he is hungry, an idea which arises because he has a nervous system. This same nervous system enables him to direct his energy to hunt for food or to do work in order to buy food. The nervous system is like the headquarters of some great army. Messages arrive to announce the state of the stores, to tell the position of any of its various members, to indicate the nature of its surroundings; in these headquarters, all the incoming messages are taken into consideration; then messages go out to direct movements to find food or to make some impression on the environment. Let us now dismiss the analogy of the army to consider once more the body as a machine. The fuel or food has been acquired by means of a locomotor system, which is that system whereby we perform movements, under the direction of the great centres of control in that part of the nervous system called the brain.

The fuel as obtained at first is in the crude state and cannot be utilized by the body. There has, of necessity, to be a digestive system in which the fuel will be broken up and put into a suitable form for burning. This system consists of the mouth, gullet, stomach and intestines. In the mouth, the fuel is broken up into small masses which pass on by way of the gullet to the stomach, where certain juices act on the fuel and convert it into simpler substances. These are passed on further into the intestines, where other juices act to present the fuel in its ultimate form. Here, fuel is now available for combustion or burning to supply the energy necessary for the functions of life. We have next to consider how this fuel is taken up and distributed to all parts of the body. As a matter of mere mechanical design, convenience would indicate that this fuel should be of such a nature as to be easily dissolved in some fluid; further, this fluid should be driven round the body through a system of pipes, by means of a pump. These conditions are met by the state of affairs in the human body. The fluid carrying round fuel which is soluble is the blood; the pump driving the blood through the body is the heart; the pipes are the blood vessels, and this whole system is referred to as the circulatory system. From the heart blood is at first driven through large tubes—the main arteries of the body. These vessels go to all parts of the body. They branch again and again until very minute vessels called capillaries are formed. The thinness of the capillary wall permits the interchange of materials from blood to tissue or *vice versa*. In the wall of the intestine fine capillaries lying very near the inside surface are capable of allowing fuel to be absorbed by the blood. The blood from the intestinal capillaries as well as from the capillaries in all other parts of the body finds its way back to the heart by travelling through a system of veins.

Having reached the heart, blood rich in fuel and poor in oxygen is next pumped through the lungs in order to pick up oxygen which is necessary for the burning of the fuel. This gas, oxygen, is contained in the atmosphere; at each breath air is drawn through the nose and windpipe into the lungs in order to give the blood a ready supply of oxygen.

On its way through the capillaries of the lungs blood becomes, as it were, refreshed; it is then taken back to the heart, which organ pumps it again through the whole body. The above scheme is a review of the nature of the circulatory system.

The mechanism whereby oxygen is made available to the blood is termed the respiratory system.

Let us review briefly the foregoing systems which render the human body an efficient machine. It has a nervous system, ruling its locomotor system, thus enabling it to obtain crude fuel; it has a digestive system to refine fuel so that it is easily taken in the blood to all parts of the body. By this means any organ in the body can have fuel to burn for the production of energy; the fuel would not burn if oxygen were not available and therefore the respiratory system exists to meet this requirement. It will be readily understood, however, just as there is ash and steam exhaust from a locomotive, that there are some waste products from the human engine.

Food is refined by the digestive system, but every food has its ash which the body cannot use, and consequently this ash must be expelled from the body. The refinery called the digestive system has its by-products for which it has no use and these it simply passes on to the exterior. The waste gas of burning, carbon dioxide, is passed out by the respiratory system, to make room for oxygen coming in. Some other waste products may be eliminated in the sweat, but the main channel for the elimination of waste is through the kidneys and the vehicle for such waste is the urine.

The body is much too complicated a mechanism to compare to any machine and the above summary of its physiology is all too inadequate, but it may suffice to give the reader a general idea of the subject. There are some things for which no analogy can be found. Human beings have the power of reproducing their kind. The reproductive system consists of those organs which stamp the individual as belonging to one or other sex. The conception of the nervous system simply as a control house is inadequate and tawdry, for the brain harbours the highest faculties of the intellect. Furthermore, there are associated with the great systems certain complementary organs necessary for the proper functioning of these systems. In the digestive system there are present a great variety of chemical substances of a very complex nature. These are essential for the breaking up of food into simpler materials which will be easily absorbed. The manufacture of these chemical substances is carried on in certain glands which are supplied with pipes or ducts to allow their products to escape into the digestive tract. The body is supplied with a storehouse for the fuel so that it is possible to be deprived of food for a considerable period of time without the efficiency of the human machine being much impaired. The main storehouses in the body are the liver, the muscles and the fat. Fuel stored in any of these situations can be used when the occasion demands. It is interesting to note that all the fuel coming from the digestive tract, with the exception of fuel in the form of fat, has to pass through the liver before it can reach any other organ. Fuel in the form of fat is taken into the blood by lymph vessels ; this is but one of the functions of the lymphatic system.

There is another system of glands which bear a most important part in the human economy and these are called the ductless glands. They are very highly specialized organs which secrete fluids of very potent action, not through a duct, but directly into the blood stream. These may be referred to later, but attention is drawn to them just now because they play not only a most important part in the growth of the human body, but also in the regulation of the utilization of certain fuel, and in the general behaviour of the individual such organs cannot but be important. The more information we have of them, the more does the human organism appear to be the plaything of their products.

There are certain features about human life in general which might be mentioned. The great essentials to the human machine are food, water and oxygen. The nature of the food requirements will be discussed later but water is in demand everywhere in the body and a large proportion of the body's composition is made up of water. It is a convenient vehicle for the excretion of waste products which are taken away in solution. As there is a constant loss of water by the kidneys, by the skin and by the lungs, it does not surprise us to find that a large part of our everyday diet is composed of water. To eat a salad is simply a very pleasant way of taking a drink of water. Blood, although thicker than water, is largely water, and consequently a great many different substances in solution can be carried about the body. Oxygen is as essential to life as either water or food since energy comes from burning of fuel. Lack of oxygen spells disaster to life ; just as the candle flame is extinguished when it is deprived of air, so does the flame of life flicker out when respiration ceases.

A natural consequence of the burning processes going o.. in the body is the production of heat. This heat production maintains the whole body at a definite temperature which, in the normal individual, is 98·4 degrees Fahrenheit. This temperature is disturbed by a great variety of causes, of which the most important are the majority of diseases attacking man. There is a perfect mechanism to keep the body at a constant temperature. When exercise is being performed the temperature of the body rises with the increased chemical activity ; then the heat-regulating mechanism of the body operates so that the excessive heat produced may be dissipated. This is accomplished by a complicated nervous control of the blood vessels in the skin and of the sweat glands. The vessels of the skin become engorged with blood, thus permitting the general temperature of the body to be lowered ; further, evapora- tion of sweat is always attended by the loss of heat. It may be mentioned in passing that alcohol produces the same effect on the blood vessels of the skin and conse- quently heat is lost to the body. There is, however, no increase of heat production, and exposure to cold may have disastrous consequences for the alcoholic through too great a diminution in the temperature. Again, the opposite may occur when an individual is exposed to an abnormally high temperature for some time. The heat-regulating mechan- ism of the body becomes paralysed and life may be brought to an end from too great an accumulation of heat, as in heatstroke.

We have given the reader a glimpse of the things which are essential to life and have attempted to aid him in under- standing the elements of physiology by presenting him with certain mechanical analogies. It cannot be over-emphasized that any mechanical view of human life is far too simple and in no way approaches an adequate conception of vital phenomena. Nature is jealous of her secrets ; only from time to time does she yield some truth to an occasional scientist who by dint of constant striving makes some discovery and adds to the store of human knowledge.

CHAPTER IV.

BANDAGES, THEIR USES AND APPLICATION.

BANDAGES are pieces of cloth used for various purposes in first-aid and in surgical practice.

THE USES OF BANDAGES ARE :

(1) To give support to injured limbs.
(2) To fix and retain dressings in position.
(3) To fix splints and retain them in position.
(4) To apply pressure for the arrest of bleeding.
(5) To stop the circulation in a limb as in cases of snake-bite.

The form of a bandage varies and, according to the shape of the cloth, several different types of bandage are described. The ideal material for a bandage is a soft and strong fabric, such as calico, gauze or flannel, but any available fabric or cloth material will suffice in emergency ; thus one can make use of strips of linen or cotton sheets, handkerchiefs, towels or even shirts.

VARIETIES OF BANDAGE :

1. The triangular bandage.
2. The roller bandage.
3. Special forms of bandage such as the T bandage and the four-tailed bandage.

1. THE TRIANGULAR BANDAGE.—This bandage was introduced by Professor Esmarch, and it is the one most commonly used in first-aid work. The triangular bandage has the advantages of being efficient and simple, is quickly and easily applied, and can readily be improvised from

any available cloth or fabric. A piece of cloth about 38″ square, when cut diagonally into two portions, gives a pair of triangular bandages. Such a bandage is described as having a point, two ends, a lower border or base, and two

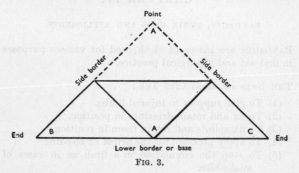

FIG. 3.

side borders or sides. The point is the right angle, the ends are the two acute angles, the base is the long side opposite the right angle, and the sides are the two short sides opposite the ends. (Fig. 3.)

METHODS FOR FOLDING THE BANDAGE:

(1) FOR STORAGE.—Spread the bandage out flat and fold it down the middle by placing one end on the top of the other. In this way a new triangle, half the size of the original, is formed ; the next procedure consists of bringing the acute angles of the fresh triangle towards the right angle, thus forming a square. The square thus formed is folded into two so as to give an oblong half the size of the square ; the two narrow ends of the oblong are folded towards one another in the middle line so as to form a second square, which is again folded about the middle line formed by the opposed free ends. This small oblong package is the form in which the triangular bandage is conveniently stored. (Fig. 4.)

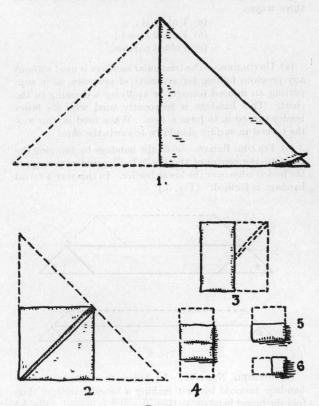

FIG. 4.

(2) FOR USE.—The triangular bandage may be used in three ways :

<blockquote>
(*a*) Unfolded ;
(*b*) Folded broad ;
(*c*) Folded narrow.
</blockquote>

(*a*) UNFOLDED.—The triangular bandage is used without any previous folding for a variety of purposes, as in supporting an injured forearm or applying a dressing to the chest. This bandage is frequently used with its lower border turned in to form a hem. When used in this way the turned-in surface should be towards the skin.

(*b*) FOLDED BROAD.—Fold the bandage by bringing the point to the centre of the lower border and superimpose the folded edge over the lower border. In this way a broad bandage is formed. (Fig. 5.)

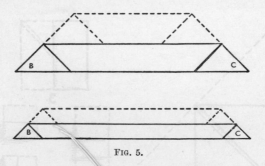

FIG. 5.

(*c*) FOLDED NARROW.—In order to make a narrow bandage proceed by first making a broad bandage, then fold the broad bandage so that its width is halved. (Fig. 5.)

METHOD OF FASTENING THE ENDS OF THE TRIANGULAR BANDAGE.—This may be done by the use of a safety-pin or by tying a knot. In the latter case the knot should always be a reef knot, never a granny knot.

THE USE OF A SAFETY-PIN.—When inserting a safety-pin its point should be made to penetrate both layers of cloth at least four times before fixing the point in the catch. The manoeuvre of insertion is carried out by performing a kind of darning motion. The safety-pin is used principally to fix the point of the unfolded bandage.

THE REEF KNOT.—To tie a reef knot hold one end of the bandage in each hand. Twist the end held in the right hand over, round and under the end held in the left hand. In this way a simple half knot is tied and the ends of the

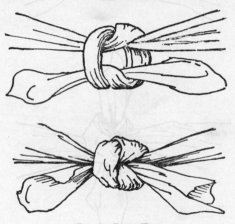

FIG. 6.—REEF KNOT.

bandage change hands. Now twist the end held in the left hand over, round and under the end held in the right hand. Once more the ends change hands, and this time a loop is formed in such a manner that the free ends lie in line with the bandage, and on one side the loop passes over both the bandage and its corresponding end while on the other side the loop passes under both the bandage

and its corresponding end. When tightened, the reef knot
locks the ends securely, does not slip and yet is easily
untied (Fig. 6). In the granny knot the ends lie at

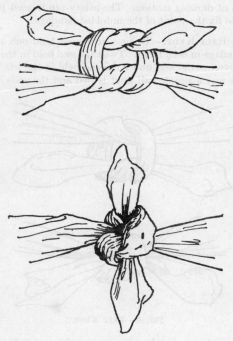

FIG. 7.—GRANNY KNOT.

right angles to the line of the bandage and the loop passes
between the bandage and its corresponding end on each
side. A granny knot is less secure and should never
be used when tying the ends of a triangular bandage.
(Fig. 7.)

THE USES OF THE TRIANGULAR BANDAGE:

1. FOR SUPPORT OF THE UPPER LIMB.—This is effected by using the bandage in the form of one of the three varieties of sling :

> (a) Large arm sling.
> (b) Small arm sling.
> (c) Sling for support of the elbow.

(a) LARGE ARM SLING.—The unfolded triangular bandage is placed over the front of the chest, the point towards the side of the injured arm, one end over the shoulder of the uninjured side and the other end hanging free. The lower border of the bandage should be perpendicular and the point at a level just above the elbow of the injured side. Carry the free end over the shoulder of the injured side and round the neck, and tie the ends in a reef knot. The knot should rest in the hollow just above the clavicle on the uninjured side, and should be tied with the sling in such a position that it supports and will continue to support the forearm horizontally. The point is brought round in front of the elbow and pinned to that part of the sling which covers the front of the forearm. This type of sling may be used in cases of injury of the arm and forearm except where there is a fracture of the humerus or of the elbow joint. (Plate IV., B and C.)

(b) SMALL ARM SLING.—The triangular bandage folded broad is placed with one end over the shoulder of the injured side and the rest of the bandage hanging vertically downwards over the front of the chest. With the elbow joint of the affected limb bent to a right angle the lower end of the bandage is brought up in front of the forearm over the shoulder of the uninjured side and tied to the other end so that the knot rests in the hollow above the clavicle of the affected side. Thus the horizontal position of the arm is maintained. This sling is useful in fractures of the humerus and of the elbow joint. (Plate V.)

(c) SLING FOR SUPPORT OF THE ELBOW JOINT.—In the application of this type of sling the unfolded triangular bandage is applied with the point towards the *uninjured side*, the upper end over the shoulder of the injured side and the lower end hanging vertically downwards. The elbow of the injured side is flexed across the chest so that the fingers rest upon the clavicle of the uninjured side. Thus the bandage lies between the chest and the flexed upper limb, the lower border running vertically downwards beyond the point of the elbow. While supporting the point of the bandage with one hand, carry the lower end upwards and forwards over the elbow and forearm to meet the other end, which has been brought round the back of the neck over the shoulder of the unaffected side ; here a reef knot is tied in the hollow just above the clavicle, thus providing a partial support for the elbow of the injured limb. The lower border of the triangular bandage, if the sling be properly applied, passes round the arm at a short distance above the elbow. The final step is to carry the point of the bandage forwards and over the forearm towards the shoulder of the affected side, where it is pinned to the sling in such a way that adequate support is given to the forearm in order to maintain the attitude of flexion. This sling is useful when it is desired to give support to and to maintain elevation of a severely wounded hand or forearm. (Plate VI.)

2. TO FIX AND RETAIN DRESSINGS IN POSITION.—In every case of wounding a pad of clean dressing material must be placed over the wound before the bandage is applied. The directions given for the first dressing of wounds (see Chapter XI) should be carried out, and whenever possible the first dressing should be antiseptic or aseptic.

WOUNDS OF THE SCALP.—Fold the lower border of the triangular bandage so as to form a hem about an inch and a half wide ; standing behind the patient place the bandage upon the head in such a way that the centre of the hem

folded inwards lies on the middle of the forehead just above
the nose and that the point is directed backwards towards
the nape of the neck. Carry the ends round either side of the
head just above the ears, cross them over the point of
the bandage immediately below the occipital protuberance,
bring them back to the front of the forehead and tie them
securely in a reef knot. Now pull down the point so as to
stretch the bandage firmly over the head. Finally the point
is turned upwards and pinned on to the bandage on the
top of the head. (Plate VII.)

WOUNDS OF THE TEMPLE, THE FOREHEAD OR THE BACK
OF THE HEAD.—Take a triangular bandage folded narrow,
place its centre over the dressing covering the wound, carry
the two ends round the head so that the bandage encircles
the cranium twice above the level of the ears and tie the
ends in a reef knot over the dressing.

An alternative method for wounds of the temple is to
place the centre of the triangular bandage folded narrow
over the temple of the uninjured side. The ends are then
carried round the head and crossed over the wounded
temple and tied off above the level of the ears in a reef
knot as before. (Plates VIII. and IX.)

WOUNDS OF THE CHIN, EARS AND SIDE OF FACE.—The
centre of a triangular bandage folded narrow is placed under
the chin and the ends are tied on the crown of the head.
Such a bandage is convenient since it covers an area which
includes the side of the face, ears and chin ; it may be
used in an emergency for a wound of any of these parts.
(Plate X.)

WOUNDS OF THE EYES.—The application of the bandage
is similar to that described for a wound of the forehead,
but the bandage is applied with its centre over the bridge
of the nose and the ends are carried round the head over
the ears and under the occipital protuberance. The ends
are brought forward and tied over the bridge of the nose.
If only one eye is affected the bandage is made to pass

obliquely so that on the affected side the lower part of the ear is covered and on the unaffected side the bandage passes above the ear and the sound eye.   (Plate X.)

WOUNDS OF THE NECK.—In this situation the centre of the bandage folded narrow is placed over the dressing and is made to encircle the neck twice before tying.   For a wound high up in the back of the neck place the centre of the bandage over the front of the neck, carry the ends backwards, cross them over the wound and bring them forwards and upwards over the forehead, where they are tied.

WOUNDS OF THE SHOULDER.—A triangular bandage is folded with a hem along its lower border.   The bandage is placed on the shoulder so that the point reaches up towards the ear on the affected side and the hem is at the level of the middle of the humerus.   Carry the ends round the arm to encircle it twice and tie them over the outer aspect of the limb.   Support the forearm in a narrow arm sling which will cover the first bandage a little below its point.   Bring the point over the sling and pin it in position over the prominence of the shoulder.   (Plate XI.)

WOUNDS OF THE CHEST.—Take an unfolded triangular bandage, fold the lower border so as to form a hem, and place the centre of the hem over the front or back of the chest to one or either side according to the position of the wound.   In the application of the bandage the folded hem should be towards the chest wall.   The point is carried over the shoulder of the affected side, and the ends are carried round to the back in the case of wounds of the front of the chest and to the front in wounds of the back.   Tie the ends towards the affected side so that a long free end is left ; this free end is brought vertically upwards and tied to the point.   The method is also applicable to wounds of the side of the chest, but alternatively one may use a triangular bandage folded broad with its centre over the dressing and its ends tied on the opposite side.   (Plates VIII. and IX.)

WOUNDS OF THE ABDOMEN.—The method of application is the same as that for wounds of the side of the chest, where a triangular bandage folded broad is used.   (Plate XI.)

WOUNDS OF THE ARM.—A triangular bandage folded narrow is applied with its centre over the dressing on the wound ; the ends are carried round the arm so as to encircle it twice and tied in a reef knot over the outer aspect of the limb.   The forearm is then supported in a small arm sling.

WOUNDS OF THE ELBOW.—In this case one of two methods may be used :

(a) Bend the elbow almost to a right angle.   Take a triangular bandage and turn in a broad hem along the lower border.   Place the centre of the hem over the back of the forearm with the point of the bandage directed upwards.   Carry the ends forward, cross them in front of the elbow joint, then bring them backwards round the lower part of the arm and tie off in a reef knot above the point of the elbow.   Now pull the point of the bandage taut, fold it downwards over the knot and pin it in this position. (Plate XI.)

(b) Bend the joint and place the centre of a triangular bandage folded broad over the point of the elbow, cross the ends over the front of the joint, carry them backwards round the upper part of the forearm, cross them behind the elbow so as to secure the lower edge of the broad bandage, bring the ends forward again and after crossing in front of the joint once more carry the ends backwards round the lower part of the arm.   Tie off the ends in a reef knot on the outer aspect of the limb, and in this way secure the upper edge of the broad bandage.

In either method of bandaging the elbow the forearm should be supported in a large arm sling.

WOUNDS OF THE FOREARM OR WRIST.—The triangular bandage should be folded narrow and applied in the

B

same manner as described for wounds of the arm. Thereafter the forearm should be supported in a large arm sling.

WOUNDS OF THE HAND.—I. *To bandage the open hand.*— Take an unfolded triangular bandage, fold a hem along the lower border, place the centre of the hem over the palmar aspect of the wrist and the point beyond the tips of the fingers. Now fold the point over the back of the fingers and hand so that it rests on the forearm just above the wrist. Draw the ends of the bandage downwards on each side and carry them backwards so as to cross on the back of the wrist over the point. Then carry the ends round the wrist, cross them in front, and finally tie them over the point on the back of the wrist. Fold the point over the knot towards the fingers and pin it in this position. (Plate X.)

II. *To bandage the palm.*—(*a*) Take a triangular bandage and fold it narrow, place the centre over the dressing in the palm, carry the ends round the back of the hand leaving the thumb free, and cross them obliquely ; return the ends to the front, cross them once again, and finally tie over the back of the wrist. To bandage the back of the hand the centre of the bandage is placed over the dressing and the process is reversed.   (Plate X.)

(*b*) Place a firm pad over the dressing in the palm and bend the fingers over the pad so as to make a fist. Place the centre of a triangular bandage folded broad across the back of the wrist ; take the end on the thumb side and carry it obliquely over the front of the fist across the knuckles and back again to the thumb side behind the wrist ; now bring the other end obliquely across the fist in the opposite direction. Finally, bring both ends to the front of the wrist, cross them and tie over the back of the wrist.   (Plates X. and XII.)

After the application of a bandage to the hand it is usual to support the upper limb in a sling.

Wounds of the Hip.—Tie a triangular bandage folded narrow round the waist like a belt with the knot on the injured side. Take a second bandage and fold its lower border ; with the point upwards apply the centre of the hem to the outer aspect of the thigh well below the wound. Wind the ends round the limb, cross them on its inner aspect and tie them on the outer aspect of the thigh. Pass the point under the first bandage, turn it down over the knot and pin it in position. (Plates VIII. and IX.)

Wounds of the Thigh or Leg.—Apply the triangular bandage folded *broad* in the same manner as was described for wounds of the arm.

Wounds of the Knee.—Fold a hem along the lower border of a triangular bandage and place it over the knee joint with the centre of the hem just below the knee-cap and with the point directed upwards over the knee. Carry the ends round the back of the joint, cross them and bring them forwards over the point of the bandage above the knee-cap, where they are tied. Fold the point down over the knot and pin it to the hem. (Plate XI.)

Wounds of the Sole of the Foot.—Place the centre of a triangular bandage folded narrow over the dressing ; cross the ends over the instep and carry them behind the heel in a figure-of-eight fashion ; bring the ends forward and cross them again over the instep. Cross the ends once again on the sole and tie them over the top of the foot. For a wound on the top of the foot the centre of the triangular bandage folded narrow is placed over the wound and thereafter the ends are carried twice round the heel and foot in a figure-of-eight fashion as in the last case.

To cover the Foot. Place centre of an unfolded triangular bandage on the sole of the foot with the point directed beyond the toes and the centre of the lower border behind the heel. Fold the point over the toes and top of the foot so that it rests on the front of the lower part of the leg. Now carry the ends forward round the ankle over the point, cross them over the instep, pass them under the sole, cross them again and tie them over the top of the foot near the toes ; bring the point down and pin it in position. (Plate XII.)

WOUNDS OF THE LOWER ABDOMEN OR PERINAEUM.— Take a triangular bandage unfolded and place the lower border uppermost about the level of the waist with the centre over the middle line of the body and the point hanging down. Carry the ends backwards and tie them behind, leaving one end longer than the other. Now draw the point downward, pass it backward between the legs and then upward and tie it to the longer free end of the lower border. (Plate XI.)

WOUNDS IN THE GROIN.—Fold the bandage narrow and place its centre just below the buttock on the back of the thigh ; bring the ends forward and cross them over the dressing pad in the groin. Now make firm tension on the ends and carry them backwards above the hip bones and tie behind or to one side. If one triangular bandage is not long enough, two may be tied together end to end. (Plate XII.)

LIMB TORN OFF.—To bandage the stump of an amputated limb. After stopping the bleeding and dressing the wound, fold a hem along the lower border of a triangular bandage and place the centre of this border under the limb at a convenient distance from the end of the stump. Now carry the ends round the limb and tie them together so as to fix the point.

THE ROLLER BANDAGE.

A ROLLER BANDAGE is a strip of some material rolled upon itself. The length of such a bandage varies from four to six yards, and the width from one to four inches. The narrow and short bandages are used for such parts as the fingers; bandages of an intermediate size are used for the head and limbs, while the longest and broadest are used for the trunk. The free end of the bandage is called the *tail*, and the part still unwound is known as the *head*. The material from which the bandage is made varies with the purpose for which it is intended. If pressure is to be applied to the bandaged part, a stretchable material, such as flannel or butter-cloth, is used; for fixing dressings or splints the bandage is made from unbleached calico, or from linen. Bandages suitable for each purpose may be bought already rolled, but as one of these may not be at hand, the method of preparing a make-shift roller bandage will be shortly described.

Whatever material is chosen, it should have been washed, for new fabrics are stiff and difficult to apply. The width of bandage required is then marked out by two short parallel cuts with a pair of scissors, and the strip is torn from the main piece. The selvage (threads which are apt to project from the edges) is then removed with the scissors, and the bandage is ready to be rolled. To do this, one or two short folds are made in one end of the bandage; the remainder is then laid upon a table, or along the thigh, and held straight and taut with the left hand, while the right hand rolls the first folds along the strip toward the tail.

GENERAL RULES FOR APPLYING THE ROLLER BANDAGE:

(1) Always fix the bandage by laying the tail obliquely on the limb, and covering it by two or three turns over each other.

(2) Keep the head of the bandage a finger's length from the limb—do not simply roll the bandage around it. By following this rule the pressure on the limb may be kept uniform.

(3) In the case of a limb, bandage from below upward, and from within outward over the front of the limb.

(4) Apply each turn with the same pressure.

(5) Each turn should overlap two-thirds of the turn below it.

(6) Do not bandage a fractured limb below the splints.

(7) When the bandage is finished fix the end by a safety pin; or tear it up the middle for a few inches, then tie the two ends in the first half of a reef knot, pass them in opposite directions around the limb, and tie them together.

A. THE SPIRAL BANDAGE.—This may be applied to the upper arm, but on account of the varying girth of the leg, thigh, and forearm at different levels, it is not possible to apply a bandage to them as a continuous spiral. In order that the bandage may fit these parts it is used as a *Spiral Bandage with Reverses*. To apply such a bandage, for example to the leg, it is first fixed at the ankle. It then ascends the leg rather steeply, and on reaching the front of

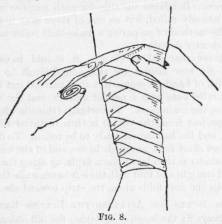

FIG. 8.

the limb a " reverse " is made. To do this, the last turn is fixed by the thumb of the disengaged hand, while the hand carrying the head is allowed to drop and is turned over, so that the bandage forms a fold with the edge against the fixing thumb and the inner surface of the bandage becomes the outer. Care must be taken that the bandage falls over in a natural fold, and is not simply twisted. The bandage then descends steeply to the back of the limb, ascends to the front, and is again reversed, and so on up the limb. A neatly applied reversed spiral bandage will have all the reverses in the same line. (Fig. 8.)

B. The Figure-of-8 Bandage.—This method is used for bandaging the ankle, knee, and elbow joints, and is useful in first aid for limiting the swelling which follows a sprain of one of these joints, particularly if the bandage is of some stretchable material such as flannel. Starting with a turn round the joint, the bandage is applied in ever-widening loops around the limb, alternately, above and below the joint. For the elbow and ankle the "waist" of the 8 is in front of the joint; for the knee the "waist" is behind the joint. (Fig. 9.)

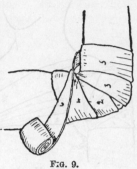

Fig. 9.

C. The Spica Bandage.—This is a modified figure-of-8 bandage, and is specially used to cover in the neighbourhood of the hip and shoulder joints. The bandage is first fixed to the limb as described. In the case of the hip the bandage is then carried over the front of the thigh, around the pelvis, back over the front of the thigh, and then around behind the thigh to its starting point. It is continued in the same way, each loop being a little

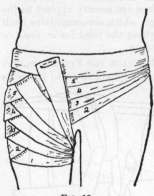

Fig. 10.

higher up the thigh and pelvis, until the bandage is ended. (Fig. 10.)

In the case of the shoulder, after the bandage has been

fixed to the upper arm it is carried from behind forward through the arm-pit, then over the shoulder and back

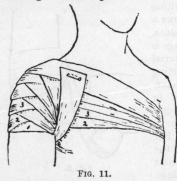

of the chest under the opposite arm-pit, across the chest and over the shoulder to its starting-point. These loops are continued, each a little higher up the arm and opposite arm-pit, till the bandage is ended. (Fig. 11.)

FIG. 11.

D. Somewhat intricate methods of applying a roller bandage to the head are used, but for first-aid purposes the triangular bandage will be found as effective and more comfortable.

In hospital practice dressings are usually applied to the head by a soft gauze bandage, which accommodates itself to the shape of the skull without the need for reverses or any special method of bandaging.

E. To Use the Roller Bandage for Fixing Splints a length of bandage is torn off, folded so as to halve its

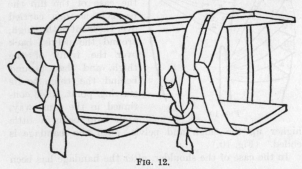

FIG. 12.

length, and passed with suitable precautions under the splinted limb. One of the free ends is passed through the loop, and is then tightened and tied to the other free end, in such a way that the knot lies on the splint and does not press upon the injured limb. (Fig. 12.)

SPECIAL FORMS OF BANDAGE USED IN FIRST-AID WORK.

These are (1) the T bandage and (2) the Four-Tailed bandage.

(1) THE T BANDAGE.—This bandage is principally used for the application of dressings to the perinaeum, which is that part of the body situated in front of the anus and

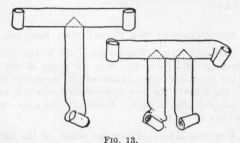

FIG. 13.

between the thighs. The T bandage is so called because it consists of two strips of cloth fastened to each other like the letter T (Fig. 13). This bandage may be made from a piece of roller bandage about three inches wide : the horizontal portion, about five feet long, is tied round the waist like a belt ; the vertical portion, about three feet long, is fastened to the centre of the horizontal portion behind, passed forward between the thighs and tied in front to the horizontal portion. In practice the vertical portion is commonly split or made double, in which case the split tails or both ends are tied at some distance apart to the belt in front.

(2) THE FOUR-TAILED BANDAGE.—This bandage may be used for the treatment of a fractured lower jaw or for the fixation of dressings on the chin or the scalp. To make

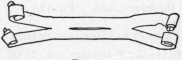

FIG. 14.

a four-tailed bandage take a strip of calico roller bandage about four inches wide and three feet long, and divide each end lengthwise to within two inches of the centre. (Fig. 14.)

APPLICATION OF THE FOUR-TAILED BANDAGE.

(a) FOR THE JAW.—Make a small slit in the centre of the bandage and place this over the point of the chin : carry the two lower ends upwards and tie them over the top of the head, carry the two upper ends backwards and tie them off under the occiput. Finally tie the ends together at the back of the head.

(b) FOR THE HEAD.—Place the centre of the bandage over the wound and carry the ends round the head so as to cross each other at right angles. When the bandage is used for the forehead the lower two ends are tied under the occiput and the upper ends are crossed over the lower ones and tied off under the chin. When the bandage is used for the back of the head the upper ends are tied under the chin while the lower ends are crossed over the upper ends and tied on the forehead.

CHAPTER V.

THE general bony framework of the human body is known as the skeleton. It is constituted by a series of bones supplemented in certain regions by cartilage or pieces of gristle and connected together by strong bands of fibrous tissue called ligaments. In the human skeleton some two hundred individual bones are present, and as we have seen they vary in form, structure and arrangement, according to their function.

Owing to the symmetrical arrangement of the body many of the bones are paired or double, as in the limbs, while single bones occur in the axial portion of the body : each unpaired bone is divisible into two similar halves, which are fused in the middle line to form a single mass. Thus it is apparent that the skeleton plays an important part in the general conformation of the body.

The skeleton may be divided into an axial part which includes the bones of the head and trunk and an appendicular part which comprises the bones of the limbs. (Figs. 15 and 16.)

According to their shape, bones are spoken of as being long, flat, short and irregular.

LONG BONES are found in the limbs. Each has a cylindrical shaft or body of compact bone and two extremities formed by expansions at its ends. Running through the centre of the shaft there is a cavity called the medullary canal and in the living body this space is occupied by a small quantity of spongy bone and yellow marrow. The extremities are mainly composed of cancellous bone and

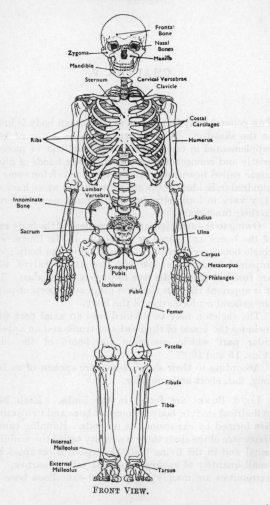

FRONT VIEW.

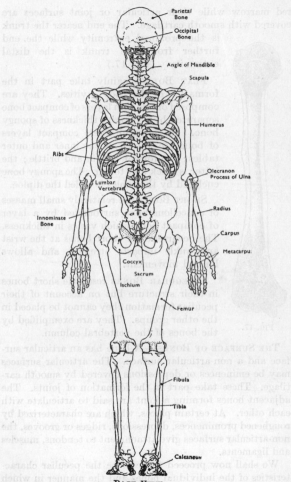

Parietal Bone
Occipital Bone
Angle of Mandible
Scapula
Humerus
Ribs
Olecranon Process of Ulna
Lumbar Vertebrae
Radius
Innominate Bone
Carpus
Metacarpus
Coccyx
Sacrum
Ischium
Femur
Fibula
Tibia
Calcaneus

BACK VIEW.

red marrow while their articular or joint surfaces are covered with smooth cartilage. The end nearer the trunk is the proximal extremity while the end further from the trunk is the distal extremity. (Fig. 17.)

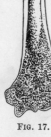

FLAT BONES mainly take part in the formation of the body cavities. They are composed of two thin layers of compact bone separated by a variable thickness of spongy bone. In the skull these compact layers of bone are known as the inner and outer tables : the former is thin and brittle ; the latter is thick and tough. The spongy bone enclosed by the tables is called the diploë.

SHORT BONES are relatively small masses of cancellous bone surrounded by a layer of compact bone which varies in thickness. The occurrence of short bones at the wrist and ankle imparts strength and allows limited movement.

IRREGULAR BONES resemble short bones in their structure but on account of their peculiar formation they cannot be placed in the other groups. They are exemplified by the bones of the vertebral column.

FIG. 17.

THE SURFACE OF BONES.—A bone has an articular surface and a non-articular surface. The articular surfaces may be eminences or depressions covered by smooth cartilage. These take part in the formation of joints. The adjacent bones forming a joint are said to articulate with each other. At certain places, which are characterized by roughened prominences, depressions, ridges or grooves, the non-articular surfaces give attachment to tendons, muscles and ligaments.

We shall now proceed to describe the peculiar characteristics of the individual bones and the manner in which

THE FACE or the front portion of the skull is formed by fourteen separate bones which are rigidly joined together with one exception. They have essentially the structure of flat bones, but are somewhat irregular in shape to provide protection for the organs of smell, sight and taste.

The bones of the face are :

Two maxillae or upper jaw bones.
One mandible or lower jaw bone.
Two nasal.
Two lachrymal.
Two palate.
Two turbinate.
One vomer.
Two malar or zygomatic.

THE MAXILLARY BONES unite in the middle line to form the upper jaw. They form the central portion of the face and take part in the formation of the mouth, the nose and the orbits or eye sockets. Each maxilla contains a large air-filled cavity or sinus communicating with the cavity of the nose, and each has eight conical sockets in its lower border for the upper row of teeth.

THE MANDIBLE or the lower jaw bone resembles a flattened arch and has sixteen sockets in its upper border for the lower row of teeth. It consists of a front part or body and two side portions. These extend backwards and then upwards at right angles to carry rounded knobs or condyles articulating on either side with the base of the skull in the glenoid fossae.

These parts of the jaw bones which carry the teeth are called the alveolar margins. In the adult there are sixteen teeth usually present in the upper jaw and a similar number the lower jaw. On each side of the middle line above and w there are, from before backwards, the following teeth:

One middle incisor.   Two premolars.
One lateral incisor.   Three molars.
One canine.

of these ridges on each side are the a
them are the middle fossae. Two
the petrous parts of the temporal
backwards separating the middle
which lie behind. (Fig. 19.)

THE ANTERIOR FOSSAE are m
bone on each side of a median
the ethmoid. Thus they form
nasal cavities.

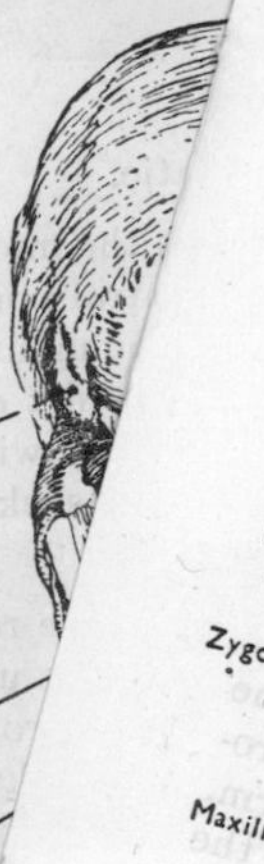

they are connected togethe
the reader should be able to
of each bone in the skelet
quently required in ambul
with the names of the bon
to recall many of the arter

THE AXIAL SKELETON.-
cludes the series of bones
(1) The skull.
(2) The vertebra
(3) The ribs and

THE SKULL is a hollow
front and supported up

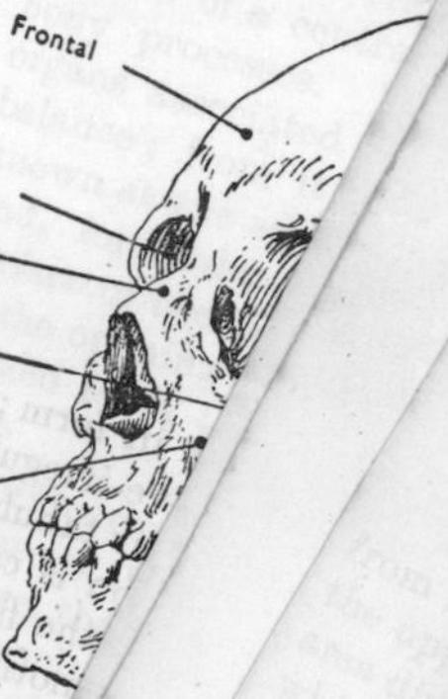

External O

Frontal

Orbit

Nasal Bone

Zygoma

Maxilla

Mastoid
Process of
Temporal Bone

Posterior
Nares

Palate

FIG. 2

THE MIDDL
are formed by
bones behind

THE POS
pressions i
sphenoid
The foram
the front

column. Wh
of two diffe
hollow ovoi
there are th

THE NASAL BONES form the bridge of the nose and are joined together in the middle line of the face.

THE LACHRYMAL BONES are very delicate and form part of the inner walls of the orbits.

THE PALATE BONES mainly form the back part of the roof of the mouth or hard palate.

THE VOMER forms the dividing partition or septum of the nose between the nostrils. It is shaped somewhat like a ploughshare.

THE TURBINATE BONES are small curved structures on the side walls of the nasal cavity. They increase the area of mucous membrane lining this cavity.

THE MALAR BONES form the prominences of the cheeks and the outer parts of the orbits. Each is joined to the frontal, temporal and maxillary bones by processes bearing corresponding names.

THE VERTEBRAL COLUMN, SPINE OR BACKBONE.—The vertebral column is composed of a series of bones called vertebrae. These are connected together by cartilage and ligaments to form a flexible column or central axis about which the trunk turns. Movement between the individual bones is slight, but the combined mobility of the column is considerable and allows rotation as well as bending backwards and forwards and from side to side. (Fig. 21.)

There are five different regions described in this series of bones. From above downwards they are called the

Cervical or neck region		7 bones.
Dorsal or thoracic region		12 ,,
Lumbar or loin region -		5 ,,
Sacral } pelvic region {		1 bone.
Coccygeal } {		1 ,,

Viewed from the side the spine is seen to have four natural curves. It arches forwards in the cervical and lumbar regions and backwards in the dorsal and sacro-

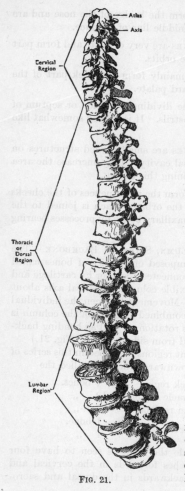

Atlas

Axis

Cervical Region

Thoracic or Dorsal Region

Lumbar Region

FIG. 21.

coccygeal regions. The vertebrae are irregular bones but are symmetrical in form. In childhood there are thirty-three vertebrae, but during adolescence the nine of the lowest fuse to form the two bones known as the sacrum and the coccyx, five bones in the former and four in the latter. The vertebrae which undergo fusion are referred to as false vertebrae while the true vertebrae are those which remain as separate bones. Thus we find that in adult man the vertebral column comprises twenty-six separate bones in all.

There are certain features common to all true vertebrae. Each typical vertebra consists of a body in front and an arch behind; these enclose a foramen, the vertebral foramen. The body is composed mainly of spongy bone and is cylindrical in form, having flattened upper and lower surfaces which are bound to corresponding surfaces of adjacent bodies by discs of fibrocartilage, the intervertebral discs. These discs act as buffers which reduce the effect of any jolting of the spine. (Fig. 22.)

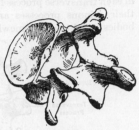

FIG 22.

The vertebral arch arises from the back of the body and gives origin to several bony processes: one transverse process projects laterally from each side, and from the back of the arch a spinous process extends backwards and downwards. The portion of the arch between the body and the transverse process on each side is termed the pedicle; the part behind the transverse process on each side is known as the lamina. From the junction of the pedicle with the lamina on either side spring two articular processes, two superior projecting upwards, with their articular surfaces directed backwards, and two inferior projecting downwards, with their articular surfaces directed forwards. There are therefore four articular processes, two upper and two lower. By means of these articular processes the arches of the adjacent vertebrae articulate with each other. In the vertebral column the bodies form a pillar in front for the support of the head and trunk while the arches constitute a canal behind for the protection of the spinal cord. Further, the pedicles of the arches are notched on their upper and lower aspects and the notches of contiguous vertebrae form the intervertebral foramina, one on either side, for the transmission of the spinal nerves. The above description embodies all the essential features of a vertebra but we find the following variations in the bones of different regions.

THE CERVICAL VERTEBRAE are the smallest of the true vertebrae. They have the features of a typical vertebra with its canal for the passage of the spinal cord : in addition, they are characterised by the presence of a foramen in each transverse process for the passage of a blood vessel ; their spinous processes are forked or bifurcated ; their bodies are thin and somewhat flattened.

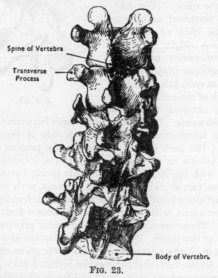

Spine of Vertebra

Transverse Process

Body of Vertebra

FIG. 23.

THE DORSAL VERTEBRAE are larger and increase in size from above downwards. They are distinguished by the presence of articular facets on the sides of their bodies and on their transverse processes for articulation with the heads and tubercles of the ribs respectively. Their bodies are somewhat triangular or heart-shaped and their spinous processes are long and oblique. (Fig. 23.)

THE LUMBAR VERTEBRAE are the largest of the series. They are characterised by their strong kidney-shaped bodies and long transverse processes.

THE SACRUM, the larger of the false vertebrae, is a large triangular mass of bone formed by the fusion of five vertebral segments, the intervertebral foramina persisting to transmit certain of the lower spinal nerves. It is concave

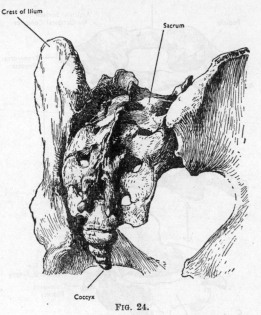

Crest of Ilium

Sacrum

Coccyx

FIG. 24.

forwards from above downwards; has its apex pointing downwards and is wedged between the hip bones. This bone, in common with the other vertebrae, has a central canal continuous with the spinal canal. (Fig. 24.)

THE COCCYX is the rudimentary remnant of the tail. It consists of four vertebral segments fused together to form a small cone-shaped bone articulating with the lower end of the sacrum.

Two vertebrae call for special description; these are referred to as the peculiar vertebrae. The first cervical vertebra is called the atlas. It is a ring-shaped bone having

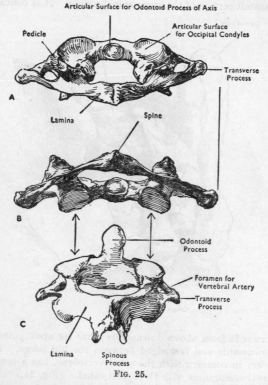

Articular Surface for Odontoid Process of Axis

Pedicle

Articular Surface for Occipital Condyles

Transverse Process

A

Lamina

Spine

B

Odontoid Process

Foramen for Vertebral Artery

Transverse Process

C

Lamina

Spinous Process

FIG. 25.

no proper body. A strong ligament traverses the circle of bone to form two compartments. The anterior compartment receives an upward projection from the body of the vertebra below; the posterior compartment forms its vertebral foramen. On the upper surface of its sides are two concave articular facets on which rest the condyles of the occipital bone.

The second cervical vertebra is named the axis. From the upper surface of its body arises a projection of bone known as the odontoid process which fits into the anterior compartment of the atlas. This forms a special pivot about which the atlas, carrying the head, rotates. (Fig. 25.)

THE THORACIC OR CHEST WALL is supported by twelve ribs on either side, the dorsal region of the vertebral column behind and the sternum or breast bone in front. In addition to these bones are pieces of cartilage, the costal cartilages, joining the ribs to the sternum.

There is the same number of ribs in the male as in the female. The ribs are numbered one to twelve from above downwards. The upper seven are the true ribs and have attachment to the sides of the breastbone directly through costal cartilages. The lower five are the false ribs; of these,

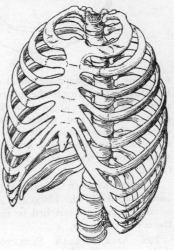

FIG. 26.

numbers eight, nine and ten have their appropriate cartilage attached to the cartilage immediately above. Ribs eleven and twelve have their cartilage-tipped ends free and are spoken of as the floating ribs. (Fig. 26.)

A TYPICAL rib has a head, a neck, a tubercle and a body.

The head is situated behind and articulates with the bodies of two adjacent vertebrae. The neck is roughly cylindrical and is that constricted part between the head and the tubercle. The tubercle articulates with the transverse process of the lower of the two adjacent vertebrae. The body is long, curved and band-like and its anterior

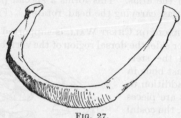

FIG. 27.

end joins the appropriate costal cartilage. That part of the body just anterior to the tubercle, where the rib is most curved, is called the angle of the rib. All the ribs, with the exception of the first, which is flat and horizontal, curve downwards and forwards like the hoops of a barrel. The conformation of the ribs as a whole impart a funnel shape to the thorax, which is narrow above and broad below. (Fig. 27.)

THE STERNUM OR BREAST BONE is an elongated flat bone, shaped like the blade of a short broad sword. Its lateral margins are notched to receive the clavicles and the costal cartilages.

THE APPENDICULAR SKELETON.—The appendicular skeleton comprises the bones of the upper and lower limbs. In these portions of the skeleton there is a similarity in the general form and structure of the bones although functional differences exist between the upper and lower groups. The bones of the upper extremities are comparatively lighter than those of the lower extremities, since the former subserve mainly the function of grasping or prehension while the latter are intended for support and locomotion.

THE UPPER LIMB is divided into definite anatomical regions—the shoulder, the arm, the forearm, and the hand. In each upper limb there are thirty-two separate bones. They are named :

The clavicle or collar bone ⎫ shoulder.
The scapula or shoulder blade ⎭

The humerus—arm.

The radius ⎫ forearm.
The ulna ⎭

Eight carpal bones ⎫
Five metacarpal bones ⎬ hand and wrist.
Fourteen phalangeal bones ⎭

THE SHOULDER has two bones, the clavicle in front and the scapula behind.

THE CLAVICLE OR COLLAR BONE is a slender long bone curved like the italic letter '*f*'. It is placed horizontally in front of the thorax and extends from the sternum to the scapula above and in front of the first rib. Its inner

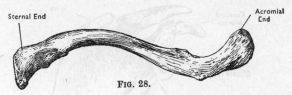

Sternal End   Acromial End

FIG. 28.

end articulates with the sternum, its outer end with the acromion process of the scapula. Viewed from the front the inner half appears convex and the outer half concave. This bone acts as a special fulcrum or prop, keeping the arm out from the side and allowing the muscles to give lateral motion to the arm. The clavicle is exposed to sudden shocks affecting any part of the arm and, on this account, it is frequently broken. (Fig. 28.)

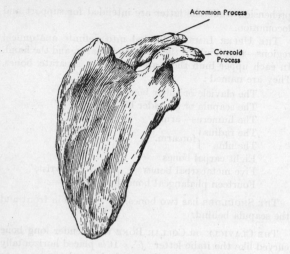

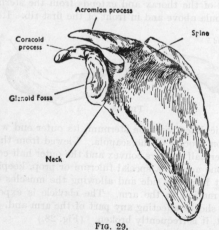

Fig. 29.

THE SCAPULA OR SHOULDER BLADE is a flat triangular bone lying on the back of the thorax over the upper ribs. Its upper and outer angle is thick and has an oval cup-shaped depression called the glenoid cavity which provides an articular surface for the head of the humerus. On the posterior surface of the blade an oblique ridge of bone, the spine of the scapula, runs upwards and outwards to terminate in a curved bony process called the acromion. This process arches forward over the shoulder joint, forms the point of the shoulder and articulates, as we have seen, with the outer end of the clavicle. The coracoid process is another bony projection arching forward, upwards and outwards from the upper end of the glenoid region. The scapula is thickly clothed with muscles which provide its only attachment to the chest wall and protect its outer surface. Accordingly this bone enjoys a wide range of movement and is seldom broken. (Fig. 29.)

The scapulae and clavicles take part in the formation of the pectoral or shoulder girdle by which the arms are attached to the trunk. This upper girdle is an incomplete ring characterised by its lightness and mobility.

THE ARM has only one bone, the humerus.

THE HUMERUS is a typical long bone with a globular head at its upper end and a flattened expansion for its lower extremity. On the posterior surface of the lower end there is a deep depression, the olecranon fossa, for the reception of the olecranon process of the ulna. The head rotates in the glenoid cavity and with it forms the shoulder joint, a ball and socket joint. The lower extremity articulates with the upper end of the ulna and, to a lesser extent, with the head of the radius to form the elbow joint. This is a perfect example of the hinge type of joint. (Fig. 30.)

THE FOREARM has two bones, the radius and the ulna.

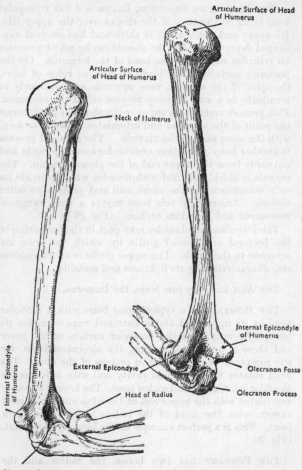

Articular Surface of Head of Humerus

Articular Surface of Head of Humerus

Neck of Humerus

Internal Epicondyle of Humerus

Internal Epicondyle of Humerus

External Epicondyle

Head of Radius

Olecranon Fossa

Olecranon Process

Olecranon Process of Ulna

FIG. 30.

'THE RADIUS lies along the outer or thumb side of the forearm. Its upper end or head is small and cylindrical: its lower end is expanded and has a wide articular surface for the proximal row of carpal bones. A pointed process, the styloid process of the radius, may be felt under the skin on the thumb side of the wrist. (Fig. 31.)

THE ULNA is situated along the inner side of the forearm. Its upper end is large and deeply grooved in front by the sigmoid notch to articulate with the lower end of the humerus: posteriorly, its upper end forms the olecranon process. The lower end is small, terminates in a pointed or styloid process and takes little part in the formation of the wrist joint. Thus it is apparent that the ulna provides the major articular surface for the humerus, and the radius is principally concerned with the formation of the wrist joint.

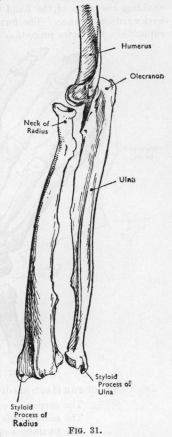

FIG. 31.

We find also that the radius rotates on the ulna above while the ulna revolves round the radius below

C

In this way a rolling movement is imparted to the forearm enabling the palm of the hand to be turned forwards or backwards with ease. The former movement is termed supination, the latter pronation.

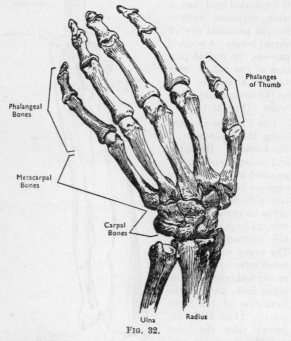

Phalanges of Thumb

Phalangeal Bones

Metacarpal Bones

Carpal Bones

Ulna   Radius

FIG. 32.

THE BONES OF THE HAND are divisible into three regions:

The carpus or wrist.
The metacarpus or palm.
The phalanges or fingers.

THE CARPUS OR WRIST is a compound joint composed of eight short bones which are arranged in two rows. As the

enumeration of these bones serves no useful purpose to
the ambulance pupil their names are omitted. The carpal
bones are firmly joined together by strong ligaments but
have only a limited range of movement. They endow the
hand with additional strength and elasticity. (Fig. 32.)

The palm of the hand contains five metacarpal bones.
These and the phalanges are described as the " short-long "
bones. Their structure is characteristic of the long bones
but they are comparatively small and short and their
rounded heads are placed distally.

THE METACARPAL BONES articulate proximally with the
carpus and distally the knuckles are formed by their heads,
which articulate with the proximal bone of each finger.
The fingers have fourteen phalanges, there being three
in each except in the thumb which has two. They are
arranged in three rows and in each finger they are
numbered one to three in order from knuckle to nail.

THE LOWER LIMB is divided into four regions, the hip,
the thigh, the leg and the foot.

In each lower limb there are thirty-one separate bones.
They are named :

> The os innominatum or hip bone—haunch.
> The femur—thigh.
> The patella—knee-cap.
> The tibia or shin bone ⎫
> The fibula or brooch bone ⎬ leg.
> Seven tarsal bones ⎫
> Five metatarsal bones ⎬ ankle and foot.
> Fourteen phalangeal bones ⎭

THE OS INNOMINATUM or hip bone is a large flattened
irregularly shaped bone with its central part thickened and
somewhat constricted. Above, it expands into a broad
flat portion, THE ILIUM ; below, it forms a sort of arch which
consists of an anterior upper portion, THE PUBIS, and a
posterior lower portion called THE ISCHIUM. On the outer
aspect of the central part there is a deep cup-shaped

depression, the acetabulum or wine cup. This provides a secure articular socket for the globular head of the femur with which it forms the hip joint—another ball-and-socket

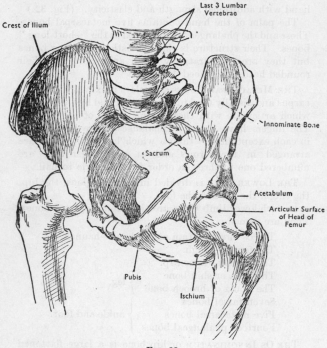

Crest of Ilium

Last 3 Lumbar Vertebrae

Innominate Bone

Sacrum

Acetabulum

Articular Surface of Head of Femur

Pubis

Ischium

FIG. 33.

joint. The ilium supports the flank of the lower abdomen: the pubis protects the bladder, the ischium supports the buttock and together the ischia are the bones on which we sit. The two hip bones are joined in front by their pubic portions, which, but for an intervening layer of car-

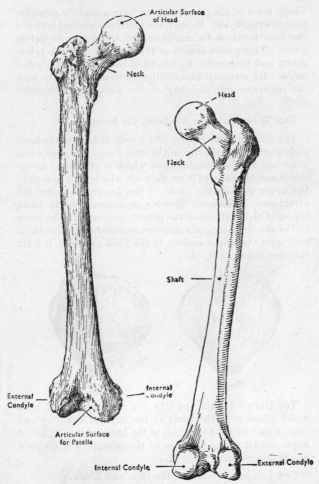

FIG. 34.

tilage, meet in the middle line to form a slightly movable joint or symphysis. Behind, the sacrum is wedged between the iliac portions to complete the bony ring or pelvic girdle. This girdle assists in the formation of the pelvic cavity and transmits the weight of the body to the lower limbs. Its strength and rigidity contrast markedly with the lightness and mobility of the pectoral or shoulder girdle. (Fig. 33.)

THE THIGH has only one bone, the femur.

THE FEMUR is the longest and strongest bone in the body and extends from the hip to the knee joint. The upper end is formed by the globular head which is prolonged downwards and laterally to form the neck which joins obliquely the upper end of the shaft of the femur. Opposite the attachment of the neck there is a prominence on the outer aspect of the shaft called the greater trochanter. The lower end of the shaft expands into two rounded condyles which rest upon the upper surface of the tibia and with it form the knee joint. (Fig. 34.)

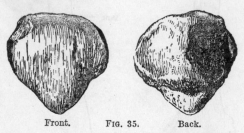

Front.   FIG. 35.   Back.

THE PATELLA OR KNEE CAP is a small triangular bone which glides over the front of the femoral condyles and takes a part in the formation of the knee joint. Its broad upper border forms the base of the triangle and its apex points downwards. (Fig. 35.)

THE LEG has two bones, the tibia and fibula.

THE TIBIA OR SHIN BONE lies along the inner side and towards the front of the leg. Its upper end is enlarged to form the head which provides a broad flat articular surface

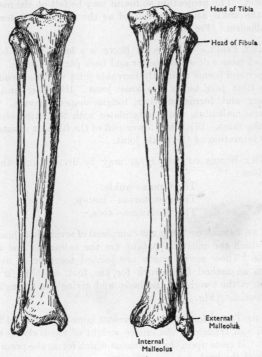

Head of Tibia

Head of Fibula

External Malleolus

Internal Malleolus

FIG. 36.

for the condyles of the femur. The shaft is somewhat triangular in section and its front border, in its entire length, can be felt under the skin of the leg. This prominent ridge is known as the shin. The lower end of the tibia is enlarged and forms an articular surface to rest upon the

upper surface of the talus, the uppermost of the seven
tarsal bones. In addition, a terminal tongue-shaped process of the tibia embraces the talus on its internal or medial
aspect. The projection so found may be felt on the inside
of the ankle and is spoken of as the medial or internal
malleolus. (Fig. 36.)

THE FIBULA OR BROOCH BONE is a long slender bone
which passes down the outer and back part of the leg. Its
upper end forms a slightly movable joint with the head of
the tibia just below the knee joint. Its lower end is
larger and forms another tongue-shaped process, the
lateral malleolus, which articulates with the outer aspect
of the talus. With the lower end of the tibia, it assists in
the formation of the ankle joint.

THE BONES OF THE FOOT may be divided into three
regions:

> The tarsus—ankle.
> The metatarsus—instep.
> The phalanges—toes.

THE TARSUS OR ANKLE is composed of seven short bones,
of which the most important are the calcaneus and the
talus. These seven bones are jointed together so as to
form an arched framework for the foot, enabling it to
support the weight of the body and giving it a springlike
resilience. (Fig. 37.)

THE TALUS forms the uppermost bone or summit of the
arch and transmits the entire weight of the body to the
foot. It rests upon the calcaneus which forms the prominence of the heel.

THE INSTEP has five metatarsal bones which lie parallel
to one another articulating behind with the tarsal bones
and in front with the first row of phalanges. They are
longer than the metacarpals of the hand but similar in
other respects.

The Toes have fourteen phalanges, there being three in
each digit except in the case of the great toe, which has
two. These phalanges are somewhat smaller than the
corresponding bones of the hand.

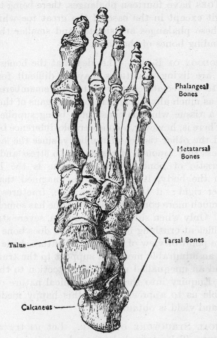

Phalangeal
Bones

Metatarsal
Bones

Tarsal Bones

Talus

Calcaneus

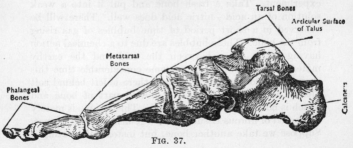

Tarsal Bones

Articular Surface
of Talus

Metatarsal
Bones

Calcaneus

Phalangeal
Bones

Fig. 37.

THE TOES have fourteen phalanges, there being three in each digit except in the case of the great toe which has two. These phalanges are shorter and smaller than the corresponding bones of the hand.

PHYSIOLOGY OF BONE.—The idea that the bones of the skeleton are living structures may be difficult for some readers to appreciate, but it is to be remembered that they are as much alive as are the other organs of the body. Bone is a tissue which is constantly being supplied with blood. There is, however, a considerable difference between bone and the other tissues of the body, since the latter do not possess that amount of resistance to stress and strain characteristic of bone. Although bone is the hardest tissue in the body, it must not be imagined that it is altogether rigid ; if this were the case, fractures would be very much more common. Every bone has some degree of yield. Only when subjected to sudden, severe stress, or when sufficient crushing force is applied, does bone break. From the point of view of its physical nature, bone forms, at once, an admirable means of support to the trunk and limbs and an unequalled means of protection to the vital organs. Enquiry into the gross chemical nature of bone will enable us to appreciate how this happy medium of rigidity and yield is obtained.

CHEMICAL STRUCTURE OF BONE. Let us try a little experiment. Take a fresh bone and put it into a weak solution of an acid—nitric acid does well. There will be observed in a short period of time bubbles of gas rising from the bone. These bubbles are due to a chemical action having taken place between the acid and the earthy material in the bone. After some considerable time this chemical action is completed and there is left behind soft pliable material, which is the animal part of bone and which is not destroyed by the acid. This residue is mainly composed of fibrous tissue rich in a gelatine-like substance. Suppose we take another bone, but instead of treating it with acid we roast it. The animal constituents are destroyed and brittle earthy material is left behind. This earthy material is made up of phosphate of calcium and other salts of calcium or lime. From these experiments we observe that bony material from the chemical point of view is partly of earthy and partly of animal origin. The earthy elements impart strength and resistance to bone while the animal elements give it that necessary yield.

THE PHYSICAL FEATURES OF BONE.—The strength of bone varies according to its intimate structure. Two types of bone are described depending upon the compact or loose build of the tissue : (1) Ivory or compact bone, and (2) Cancellous or spongy bone.

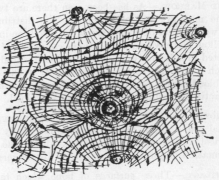

FIG. 38.—MICROSCOPIC SECTION OF IVORY BONE.

(1) IVORY BONE forms the hard, resistant outer shell of the bones of the skeleton. In structure, the elements composing this type of bone are closely packed together, but even although this close aggregation occurs, minute spaces for blood vessels and nerves exist. When living compact bone is cut across blood oozes from the cut surface. If the blood be wiped off, the surface presents an ivory appearance. (Fig. 38.)

(2) CANCELLOUS OR SPONGY BONE is continuous with, but is enclosed in the shell of ivory bone. It is to be found in all the bones of the body, but in the long bones of the limbs it is more or less confined to the ends. Spongy bone in bulk is soft and is formed by an interlacing network of strands of bony material.

From what has been said it will be seen that there is a considerable amount of space inside the ivory shell. Some of this space is filled by cancellous bone, which is, in itself, an empty substance. The spaces between the strands of cancellous bone are filled by red bone marrow, and the space inside the shaft of a long bone contains yellow marrow.

BONE MARROW.—As has been seen there are two kinds of bone marrow—red and yellow. The distribution of these two varieties of bone marrow has also been indicated. The yellow marrow is merely a tissue composed of fat cells supported in a fine network of fibrous tissue. Red marrow is much more active than the yellow, it has a much richer blood supply and it fulfils the important function of manufacturing certain constituents of the blood.

PERIOSTEUM.—This material, as its name suggests, is wrapped round about bone. All bone is entirely covered by periosteum except in those areas which take part in the formation of joints. It is a tough fibrous membrane.

CARTILAGE.—Those surfaces of bone which take part in the formation of movable joints are covered by cartilage or gristle which is smooth, tough and yielding. This material also exists in the front of the chest, extending between the free ends of the ribs and the sternum or breast bone, and thus facilitates the movements of respiration.

BONE AT DIFFERENT AGES.—It is to be borne in mind that the nature of bone varies considerably with the age of the individual. As a person grows older the proportion of earthy material in bone increases and consequently the

There are three types of muscle :

Skeletal - - Voluntary.
Cardiac ⎫
Visceral ⎬ - - Involuntary.

From this classification it is seen that the skeletal muscles, which are primarily concerned with the movements of skeletal structures, are voluntary or directly under control of the will, while the cardiac and visceral muscles are involuntary and not under control of the will.

SKELETAL MUSCLE.—The skeletal musculature, the flesh of the body, is responsible for a large proportion of the body weight. It is mainly concerned with the movements of the skeleton as a whole or in its individual parts. The fibres which go to make up a single voluntary muscle have definite distinguishing characteristics when viewed under a microscope. The individual skeletal muscle fibres are seen to have very fine stripes which run at right angles to the longitudinal axis of the fibre, and therefore the name " striped muscle " is sometimes applied to this type. When a voluntary muscle is attached to bone it may be attached directly by its muscle fibres or through the medium of a strong fibrous tissue which may take the form of a cord-like structure, in which case it is termed a tendon, or a sheet-like formation, in which case it is called an aponeurosis.

CARDIAC MUSCLE.—Cardiac muscle composes the walls of the heart. It is not controlled by the will and has the characteristic of rhythmic contraction and relaxation. This characteristic renders it at once one of the most remarkable tissues in the body, since these movements occur more frequently than once a second throughout the threescore and ten years of life.

The individual cardiac muscle fibres resemble skeletal muscle, both types being striped, but differ from it in that the fibres of heart muscle branch while the fibres of skeletal muscle are unbranched.

liability to fracture is much greater in the aged. In young people animal matter is in greater quantity and incomplete fractures often occur. These fractures are associated with bending of the intact part of the bone and are spoken of as " greenstick " fractures. In the early years of life the ends of the long bones are separated from the shafts by a layer of cartilage. These separate ends are spoken of as epiphyses and only become firmly united to the shaft when the intervening cartilage is replaced by bone in adolescence.

THE GROWTH OF BONE.—In the early stages of development of the human being there is no bone in the body ; where bones are to be formed there is an antecedent laying down of cartilage or membrane. In this mass of cartilage there appears a bony centre, which is termed a centre of ossification, and, from it, the process of the laying down of bone takes place until the whole mass is replaced by true bone. It is usual for a single bone to have more than one centre of ossification. The long bones of the body, for example, usually have a centre for the shaft, a centre for each epiphysis and a centre for any important process.

The development of bone is much too complicated and controversial a subject to consider in detail here. It may be remarked, however, that the deep layer of periosteum seems to be active while the centre of ossification is active, and that ossification not only extends from the centre, outwards, but also from the periosteum, inwards. In the growing child and in the adolescent the ends of the long bones are concerned with the process of growth. In the neighbourhood of the epiphyseal cartilage new bone is constantly being laid down. This process is completed when the bones stop growing. It follows that any severe injury to the end of a long bone, if inflicted early in life, may seriously impair its growth, with the result that the limb will be stunted.

THE SKELETON FROM THE MECHANICAL POINT OF VIEW.

The bones of the body have to be efficient mechanically. This efficiency depends upon two different factors:

(1) The intimate structure of individual bones.

(2) The general arrangement of the bones.

(1) That the bones of the limbs are well adapted for the purposes of support and of imparting rigidity is easily understood from the form of the ivory shell of the shaft, but there is, in addition to this, an arrangement of cancellous bone which is designed to bear stress and strain. To quote one example, in the head and neck of the femur there is an interlocking network of strands of cancellous bone resembling the arrangement of interlacing iron girders on great cantilever bridges. This arrangement is calculated to take the stresses of the weight of the body and the adaptation to this end is perfect.

(2) The general arrangement of the bones.

Let us take into account firstly those bones which are concerned with the protection of vital organs. They are flat in the case of the skull and form a hard, resistant box to contain the brain. In the chest wall a great number of bones exist to give protection to the organs of circulation and respiration. Here it is desirable, however, that in addition to protection there should also be a considerable freedom of movement. The lungs and heart are therefore protected by the movable cage formed by the ribs. Comparing the protection of the organs in the chest with the protection of the brain, the former are efficiently guarded in virtue of the elasticity and yield of the ribs, and the latter, in virtue of the hardness of the skull. The very movements which the bones have to make should be in accordance with sound mechanical principle. This, of course, depends on the efficiency of joints, of bones, of muscle and of tendon. The mechanical principles are merely those of the lever and the pulley. The lever action

is demonstrated when a load in the hand is raised by bending the elbow, and the pulley action is observed when the lower limb is straightened at the knee.

JOINTS.

A joint is that combination of structures met with when two or more bones come into contact. A joint may be referred to as an articulation.

Classification of joints:

1. Movable joints—
   (a) Ball and socket.
   (b) Hinge.
   (c) Gliding.
   (d) Pivot.

2. Slightly movable joints.

3. Immovable joints.

1. THE MOVABLE JOINTS are formed by the junction of the articular ends of bones. The articular ends are covered by smooth cartilage and are held in contact by strong fibrous bands. These ligaments are specially strengthened by the fibrous sheath of the joint termed the capsule, with its ligaments, joins the ends of the bones which take part in the joint. Lining the interior of the joint, except over the articular cartilage, is the synovial membrane, which secretes a clear, thick fluid of the nature of the synovial fluid. The articular cartilage is smooth and uniform. Inside the joint intervening pads of cartilage, which are covered by synovial membrane, depends upon the synovial fluid together with the...

VISCERAL MUSCLE.—This is the simplest type of muscle and has a very wide distribution throughout the body. Its individual fibres are spindle-shaped and non-striped, hence they are termed plain muscle fibres. Plain muscle is not under control of the will. Reference will be made to the distribution and function of this type of muscle when such subjects as digestion, respiration and circulation are being considered.

It is a point worthy of note that, when plain muscle is stretched or contracts violently, pain results, as in colic.

ANATOMY OF THE SKELETAL MUSCLES.—The skeletal muscles form the great bulk of the muscular tissue or flesh of the body. In addition to their essential function of contractility they clothe the bones, support and strengthen the joints and form a protective covering for the cavities of the trunk. They are exposed to injury in all kinds of accidents and it is therefore necessary for the ambulance pupil to become acquainted with the form, situation and arrangement of the more important muscles and even with the names of some of them. It will be found that muscles may be named according to certain of their characteristics, such as their action, their shape, their position or the direction of their fibres.

Since several muscles act in unison to carry out one particular movement we find that the muscles are arranged in definite groups. For example, in " flexion " of the elbow joint the movement is effected by the flexor group of muscles in the front of the arm. In this act of flexion the flexor muscles are referred to as agonists while the muscles on the back of the arm, the extensors, which relax during flexion, are spoken of as antagonists or opponents. Similarly, muscles which produce abduction are called abductors and their opponents are named adductors ; again, the pronator muscles have the supinators as their opponents.

At the natural orifices of the body there are circular

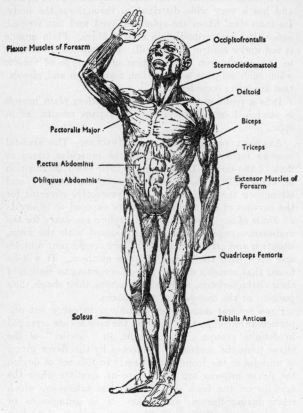

Flexor Muscles of Forearm

Occipitofrontalis

Sternocleidomastoid

Deltoid

Biceps

Triceps

Pectoralis Major

Rectus Abdominis

Obliquus Abdominis

Extensor Muscles of Forearm

Quadriceps Femoris

Soleus

Tibialis Anticus

FIG. 42.—SKELETAL MUSCLES.

'THE RADIUS lies along the outer or thumb side of the forearm. Its upper end or head is small and cylindrical: its lower end is expanded and has a wide articular surface for the proximal row of carpal bones. A pointed process, the styloid process of the radius, may be felt under the skin on the thumb side of the wrist. (Fig. 31.)

THE ULNA is situated along the inner side of the forearm. Its upper end is large and deeply grooved in front by the sigmoid notch to articulate with the lower end of the humerus: posteriorly, its upper end forms the olecranon process. The lower end is small, terminates in a pointed or styloid process and takes little part in the formation of the wrist joint. Thus it is apparent that the ulna provides the major articular surface for the humerus, and the radius is principally concerned with the formation of the

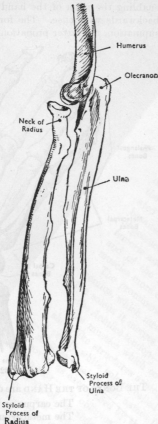

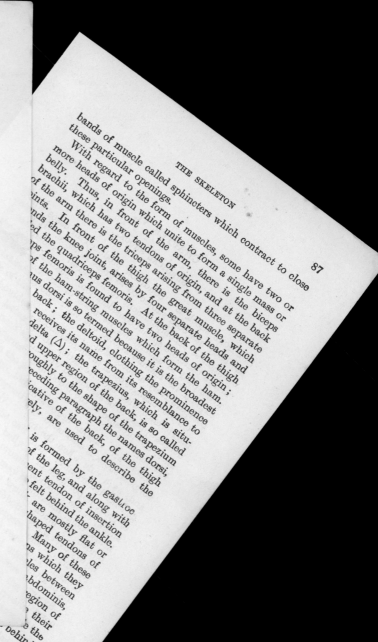

Humerus

Olecranon

Neck of Radius

Ulna

Styloid Process of Ulna

Styloid Process of Radius

FIG. 31.

wrist joint. We find also that the radius rotates on the ulna above while the ulna revolves round the radius below

C

bands of muscle called sphincters which contract to close these particular openings.

With regard to the form of muscles, some have two or more heads of origin which unite to form a single mass or belly. Thus, in front of the arm, there is the biceps brachii, which has two tendons of origin, and at the back of the arm there is the triceps arising from three separate points. In front of the thigh the great muscle, which extends the knee joint, arises by four separate heads and is called the quadriceps femoris. At the back of the thigh the biceps femoris is found to have two heads of origin: one of the ham-string muscles which form the ham.

The latissimus dorsi is so termed because it is the broadest of the back: the deltoid, clothing the prominence of the shoulder, receives its name from its resemblance to the Greek delta ($\triangle$): the trapezius, which is situated over the back and upper region of the back, is so called owing roughly to the shape of the trapezium ...

... In the preceding paragraph the names dorsi, delta, indicative of the shape, of the thigh, respectively, are used to describe the ...

... is formed by the gastroc... ... of the leg, and along with ... prominent tendon of insertion ... felt behind the ankle. ... are mostly flat or ... shaped tendons of ...

Many of these ... tendons which they ... muscles between ... abdominis, ... region of ... their ... the ... behind ...

In this way a rolling movement is imparted to the forearm enabling the palm of the hand to be turned forwards or backwards with ease. The former movement is termed supination, the latter pronation.

Phalanges of Thumb

...dius

...three regions:

...sed of

...as the

CHAPTER VI

SURGICAL SHOCK.

SURGICAL shock is a condition produced in cases where the body has been subjected to gross violence. It is the commonest accompaniment to industrial accidents and merits therefore special consideration. Medical men have attempted to understand its mode of causation and to explain its manifestations but their efforts have been comparatively unsuccessful.

Curious changes occur in surgical shock; there is marked interference with the circulation and the attendant evidences appear to be associated with this particular disturbance, the pressure of the blood in the blood vessels being lowered.

There are various degrees of surgical shock. Severe surgical shock is associated with severe injury to the body and, as a rule when the injury is slight, there is little general disturbance. Another factor, which appears to be of great importance in determining the degree of surgical shock, is the situation of the injury. An injury over the heart, lung, intestine or other internal organ will be attended by much greater surgical shock than a similar injury over a less vital part. Breaking of bone is attended by surgical shock which varies with the size of the bone broken. Thus profound surgical shock occurs in the breaking of a thigh bone.

SYMPTOMS OF SURGICAL SHOCK.—Symptoms are abnormalities which are observed by the patient.

(1) PROSTRATION.—The patient feels limp and exhausted. He says he is tired and that he is incapable of ...al exertion.

(2) NAUSEA AND SICKNESS.—There is actually a feeling of discomfort in the abdomen. This may be associated with vomiting.

(3) HEADACHE, GIDDINESS AND RINGING IN THE EARS.— These are quite characteristic. The patient feels giddy, the head aches and frequently there is a buzzing noise heard in the ears.

(4) SHIVERING.—The patient is cold, a condition asso-ciated with circulatory embarrassment.

SIGNS OF SURGICAL SHOCK.—Signs are objective phenomena and are observed by persons other than the patient.

(1) INCREASE IN THE PULSE RATE.—The pulse in surgi-cal shock is feeble and frequent ; the degree to which this is manifest is proportional to the severity of the surgical shock.

(2) FREQUENT AND SHALLOW BREATHING.—Simultane-ously with the increase in the pulse rate there is an in-crease in the number of breaths per minute.

(3) PALLOR.—Every shocked patient is pale. This feature is dependent upon the depression of the circulation.

(4) COLD SWEATING.—Frequently beads of cold sweat are visible on the forehead. Cold sweat on a pallid face is extremely characteristic of shock.

(5) LOW BODY TEMPERATURE.—The temperature of the body is lowered well below the normal of 98·4 degrees Fahrenheit. This is dependent upon the sweating, the lowering of vital activity and the circulatory disturbance.

(6) FLACCIDITY OF THE BODY.—Flaccidity is a techni-cal term used to denote looseness or laxity when applied to the voluntary muscles. If the limbs of a shocked person are raised or moved there is marked absence of resistance.

(7) MENTAL SYMPTOMS.—It is easy to understand that, in such a condition as surgical shock, the mentality of the

individual is impaired along with the other functions of the body. This sign may manifest itself in varying degrees, from simple slowing of the mental processes to their complete suspension resulting in unconsciousness.

(8) DILATION OF THE PUPILS.—If the eyes be examined it will be found that the pupils are wide or dilated.

TREATMENT OF SURGICAL SHOCK.

Surgical shock is a morbid condition, and in severe degrees it is the responsible factor in causing death. Surgical shock is aggravated by manipulative interference, a point of extreme importance in the treatment of any injury. Take, for example, a broken thigh. This injury is attended by intense surgical shock ; any movement of the injured limb will increase the degree of shock ; thus the ambulance man must cut down manipulation to the absolute minimum when applying splints. The first law in the treatment of surgical shock is to avoid unnecessary handling.

Surgical shock is often aggravated by bleeding and, as will be seen later, the condition of many an injured person is the result of the manifestations of surgical shock and loss of blood combined. Of paramount importance in the treatment of shock is the treatment of any evident hæmorrhage. When bleeding has been controlled the ambulance man is in a position to proceed with the other measures which will counter shock.

Bearing in mind these first two points, the treatment of surgical shock falls under the headings postural treatment and stimulant treatment.

POSTURAL TREATMENT.—The patient should be laid flat on his back and the head should be kept low. A patient suffering from shock will faint when in a semi-recumbent position because of the general depression of the circulation ; the heart is totally unable to cope with the demands made upon it when the patient is in any position other than that of complete rest. It is very valuable to lower the head below the general level of the body ; this procedure increases the blood supply to the brain and raises the blood pressure.

STIMULANT TREATMENT.—The application of warmth is the first of the measures to be applied in the general stimulation of the body. Cover the patient with blankets ; place hot-water bottles round him, taking care not to burn the skin. Exposure of the patient to cold enhances the effects of surgical shock. Rubbing or chafing the limbs from the hands and feet towards the heart is an effective procedure since it is calculated to aid the return of blood to the heart ; by this means the failure of the circulation is counteracted to a certain extent. The function of breathing is helped by the application of smelling salts to the nostrils ; the breathing becomes deeper and less frequent. Smelling salts should be applied for a second or two at intervals and not held constantly up against the nose. General stimulation of vital functions is effected by the administration of hot coffee or tea by the mouth, always provided the patient is able to swallow. To attempt to administer such fluids by the mouth in the unconscious patient is to court disaster.

CHAPTER VII.

FRACTURES.

A FRACTURED bone is a broken bone, and the word "fracture" may be defined as a solution in the continuity of bone.

Fractures may be divided into several different classes, according to the type and extent of the injury. From the first-aid point of view all fractures without exception are either simple or compound.

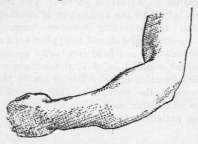

FIG. 43.

A SIMPLE FRACTURE is a solution in the continuity of a bone unattended by a wound communicating between the site of fracture and broken skin or mucous membrane. (Fig. 43).

A COMPOUND FRACTURE is a solution in the continuity of a bone attended by a wound of the adjacent tissues, of such a nature as to cause a communication between broken skin or mucous membrane and the actual site of fracture.

To exemplify the two varieties of fracture, let us consider a fractured rib. If the rib is broken without the end of either fragment penetrating the skin of the chest or the air-containing tissues of the lung, then the fracture is simple ; if there is a wound, either from the skin surface or from the air-containing tissue of the lung down to the site of the fracture, then the injury is a compound fracture.

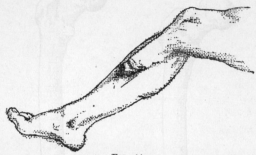

FIG. 44.

It should be clearly understood that a surface wound may occur in close proximity to a fracture without the fracture being compound ; only when the wound communicates with the actual break in the bone does the fracture become compound. Further, it happens frequently that the surface wound is inconspicuous, and the fact that it may communicate with the fracture is overlooked. Such an oversight might cause the loss of a limb or even death from general blood poisoning, since this communicating wound forms a path of entrance for microbes of septic disease. (Fig. 44.)

A COMPLICATED FRACTURE may be either simple or compound, but, in addition, is associated with injury to some important adjacent structure. The more important adjacent structures which may be injured by the break are nerves, blood-vessels and the body cavities. For example, a simple or a compound fracture of the humerus may tear the radial nerve (*see* Fracture of Humerus).

Any simple or compound fracture may be classified further according to the particular manner in which the bone is broken.

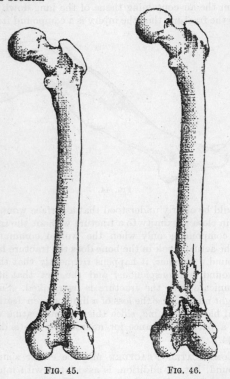

FIG. 45.   FIG. 46.

AN IMPACTED FRACTURE is one where the end of one fragment is driven into the end of the other fragment. For example, an impacted fracture is seen where the shaft of the femur is telescoped inside the broader head. (Fig. 45.)

A COMMINUTED FRACTURE occurs where there is splintering of bone at the site of fracture. This requires no example. (Fig. 46.)

According to the line of fracture in a bone, adjectives such as transverse, oblique and spiral may also be applied in naming a fracture. (Fig. 47.)

A MULTIPLE FRACTURE occurs when a bone is broken in two or more places with an appreciable distance between the sites of fracture.

A GREENSTICK FRACTURE is one in which there is an incomplete break across the shaft of a bone. It is always associated with bending of the unbroken portion and with longitudinal splitting of the shaft. This type of fracture only occurs in the relatively soft bones of children, and is simulated by the incomplete breaking of a green twig. (Fig. 48.)

A SEPARATED EPIPHYSIS is a special variety of fracture which may occur at either end of a long bone in children

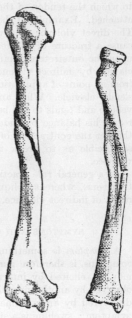

FIG. 47.   FIG. 48.

and in young people before the bony union of the epiphysis with the shaft (*see* Physiology of Bone).

CAUSES OF FRACTURES.—A fracture is always caused by violence. Three different types of violence are recognized —direct, indirect and muscular. A fracture is said to be caused by direct violence when the fracture occurs at the site of the violence. A fracture due to indirect violence occurs at a distance from the point of application of the violence. A fracture by muscular violence occurs when muscular contraction is strong enough to break the bone to which the tendon of the strongly contracting muscle is attached. Examples of these various causes are as follow : The direct violence of a wheel passing over a thigh will cause a fracture of the femur of the first type. Falling upon the outstretched hand may cause a fracture of the clavicle by indirect violence ; the violence is transmitted from its point of application, the hand, up the limb to the slender clavicle. When an individual jumps off a moving vehicle and tends to fall backwards, he may endeavour to regain his balance by suddenly straightening his legs ; in this act the contraction of the quadriceps muscle may be so forcible as to break the patella by sheer muscular violence.

As a general rule fractures due to direct violence are transverse, whereas oblique and spiral fractures are the result of indirect violence.

SYMPTOMS AND SIGNS OF FRACTURES.

A *symptom* is something of which the patient himself complains, is therefore purely subjective in character and may be elicited by interrogation. A *sign* is something observed by another individual, is purely objective, and is discovered by an examination of the patient. Pain is a symptom ; swelling is a sign.

SYMPTOMS OF A FRACTURE.

1. Pain.
2. Disability (loss of function).
3. The sensation of actual breaking of bone.
4. General symptoms of shock—faintness, shivering and weakness.

SIGNS OF A FRACTURE.

1. Tenderness.
2. Unnatural Mobility.
3. Swelling.
4. Deformity (angular).
5. Shortening.
6. Crepitus.

SYMPTOMS.—1. PAIN, with rare exceptions, is present in all fractures, and is felt most severely at the site of the fracture. It is the most urgent of the patient's complaints and is aggravated by any movement of the part.

2. DISABILITY varies according to the importance of the function of the fractured bone. It is great when such a bone as the femur, the humerus, the clavicle or the skull is broken. The disability may be comparatively slight in a fracture of the fibula, where the main support of the leg is still intact.

Disability is due to loss of rigidity and to pain.

3. THE SENSATION OF BREAKING OF BONE is an occasional symptom and is self-explanatory.

4. GENERAL SYMPTOMS OF SHOCK vary in proportion to the extent of the injury. In a fracture of the femur, where there is much tissue damage, the degree of surgical shock may be extreme.

SIGNS.—1. TENDERNESS is demonstrated by the evidences of pain when the fractured part is moved or pressed upon by the examiner. Tenderness is greatest when pressure is applied over the site of fracture.

2. UNNATURAL MOBILITY is revealed by the presence of movements where rigidity normally obtains. It may be observed when the patient moves or during the application of splints, but on no account should a first-aid man set out intentionally to discover its presence by manipulation. When unnatural mobility is discovered it is a certain sign of fracture, but a fracture may exist without unnatural mobility, as in an impacted fracture.

D

3. SWELLING is due to the effusion of blood and serum, which always occurs in the vicinity of a fracture, although it may not be immediately apparent. Swelling may increase for some considerable time after a fracture, and this has to be remembered during the application of temporary splints.

4. DEFORMITY is due to the displacement of fragments of a bone. It is partly accounted for by the original violence, partly by the distorting action of unopposed muscles, and partly by the weight of the limb. Deformity may be evidenced by angular displacement or by over-riding of the fragments : it may be modified by the presence of swelling. Injudicious handling may increase deformity. Deformity is not necessarily apparent where a fracture exists.

5. SHORTENING of a fractured bone occurs when the fragments override at the site of fracture. This shortening is due to muscular pull to which there is no stable resistance. It does not occur where one alone of the two parallel bones of the forearm or leg is broken, or when there is no displacement of the fragments. Some degree of shortening also occurs with impacted fractures.

6. CREPITUS is a grating sensation elicited when the broken ends of bone rub together. It is a certain sign of fracture, if felt, but may well be absent, as when there is impaction, wide separation of the fragments, or the inter-vention of some soft tissue between the broken ends. There are few occasions on which a doctor is justified in attempting to elicit crepitus, but there is never an occa-sion when it is permissible for a first-aid man to attempt deliberately to elicit crepitus. Great harm may be done and unnecessary suffering caused by attempting to rub the broken ends of bone together in order to elicit this sign.

The diagnosis of fracture depends upon the recognition of certain symptoms and signs rather than on any one single piece of evidence. When, as happens rarely, all the above signs are present, the diagnosis is easy, but, more often, when only a few suspicious signs are observed, making the diagnosis doubtful, the injury should be treated as one of fracture.

THE EXAMINATION OF AN INJURED PERSON WHEN A FRACTURE IS SUSPECTED.

There are certain precautions which a first-aid man should observe, and certain rules which he should follow, when called upon to examine an injured person suspected of having a fracture. The injured person must not be removed from the site of accident until the question of fracture has been decided, or until the treatment necessary to render removal safe has been applied. In all cases the patient, if not already in a reclining position, should be placed in such a posture and made as comfortable as possible. With a fracture of the upper extremity it is enough that the patient should be sitting, but with all other fractures the patient must be lying down. Before proceeding to examine the injured part, attention should be paid to the general condition of the patient. It is always wise to reassure the injured person, since he is invariably anxious and alarmed. Surgical shock must be looked for and treated at the very outset before any other examination is carried out. The injured person may then be briefly questioned as to the nature of the accident and the presence of any symptoms of fracture. It is essential to have the site of suspected fracture exposed, and for this purpose it is usually sufficient to slit up the outer seams of a garment or very gently to draw aside the clothes covering the injured part. It is rarely ever necessary to remove completely even a single garment, and in every case the utmost care should be exercised to obviate any unnecessary exposure of the patient's body. The greatest care and gentleness must be observed in handling every fracture. Having exposed the injured part, look for any abnormality, such as swelling, deformity or wounding of the surface. If a wound is present, cover it with a dressing, antiseptic if possible (see chapter on Wounds). When the above-mentioned signs are sufficiently well marked to leave the examiner in no doubt as to the presence of a fracture, no further examination should be carried out. If, after looking at the site of injury, doubt exists, further examination is permissible ; the examiner's hand may now be gently passed over the site of injury. This procedure may reveal further evidence of fracture, such as tenderness, unnatural mobility or even crepitus. Once again the reader is warned that he is never permitted to seek for the last two signs deliberately. The injured person must always be examined systematically in the order given above, and should never be subjected to repeated examinations, which only cause unnecessary pain, delay and, perhaps, further injury. Whenever the first-aid man has sufficient evidence of the presence of fracture no further confirmatory examination should be carried out, but he should proceed to apply the necessary first-aid measures. If, after carrying out the examination already indicated, there is still any doubt as to the presence of a fracture as opposed to any less serious condition, the case must be treated as one of fracture.

THE DANGERS AND COMPLICATIONS OF FRACTURES.

It is highly important that anyone who attempts to render first-aid treatment to a case of fracture should be well acquainted with the immediate dangers and complications which may result from such an injury. A knowledge of these dangers is especially necessary when the question of treatment arises. The following facts should be borne in mind by the first-aid man during his examination of the injured person. A simple fracture may in itself be a relatively slight injury, but such an injury may be complicated by most serious damage to the adjacent structures. A fractured skull may be associated with grave damage to the brain ; with a fracture of a long bone the main artery to a limb may be torn ; a fractured rib may penetrate the pleura and the lung, while a fractured pelvic bone may rupture the urinary bladder. Further, a simple fracture may easily become a compound fracture if the injured person is roughly or carelessly handled. This may occur during initial examination by the inexperienced person, or during removal before appropriate treatment has been applied. In the case of a compound fracture two other dangers may arise, infection with the organisms or microbes of disease and haemorrhage. Of these the former is by far the greater danger, but either may seriously jeopardize the patient's chances of recovery or even bring about a fatal result. Finally, any case of fracture may be complicated by some degree of surgical shock, which may have a serious effect upon the patient's recovery, and which requires immediate and appropriate treatment. The more common complications of individual fractures are described later in their appropriate connection with these special fractures.

HEALING OR REPAIR OF FRACTURED BONE.

When a simple fracture occurs some of the surrounding soft tissues and small blood-vessels are torn, a collection of blood forms, and the part becomes swollen. The bleeding soon stops, and the effused blood becomes clotted around the broken ends of the bone. The blood clot then undergoes certain changes, and is ultimately replaced by a soft spongy form of bone known as callus. It will be seen that the process is similar in certain respects to the healing of a wound elsewhere and the following changes occur. First of all leucocytes (white blood cells) emigrate from the adjacent vessels and invade the blood clot ; in this way the clot is partly absorbed. Later, minute blood vessels bud off from the neighbouring capillaries and grow into the clot, thus forming a new mass of actively growing tissue called granulation tissue. Finally, young bone cells or osteoblasts arise from similar cells in the bone ends and pass into the granulation tissue, converting it into a mass of soft spongy bone or callus. At a still later stage the

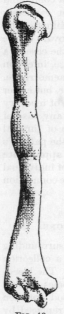

callus is transformed into hard bone by the deposition of lime salts. In the early stages of repair the softer callus forms in considerable excess, surrounds the ends of the bone, fills in the gap between the ends of the fragments and closes the medullary canal. After firm union has been established and as function returns, the excess of bone cement is absorbed, and only sufficient remains to unite the fragments firmly and restore their former rigidity : even the original form and length of the bone may be restored. This satisfactory issue depends upon the accuracy with which the fracture has been set, and the care with which apposition and alignment are maintained. (Fig. 49.)

It is to be noted that a compound fracture heals exactly in the same manner as a simple fracture, but there is added the grave danger of infection from the wounding of the soft parts. If organisms of disease gain access to the region of the fracture, healing of bone will be interfered with to an even greater extent than will be the healing of the soft tissues.

FIG. 49.

THE TREATMENT OF FRACTURES.

There are certain principles which are applicable to the first-aid treatment of fractures in general, but there are many variations in the treatment of individual fractures, according to the particular bone fractured, the variety of fracture and the circumstances of the accident. The principles of the first-aid treatment of a fracture aim at :

(1) THE PREVENTION OF FURTHER INJURY—for example, the prevention of a simple fracture becoming compound.

(2) THE TREATMENT OF THE MORE URGENT ASSOCIATED CONDITIONS : shock, severe haemorrhage at the site of fracture or wounds.

(3) THE FIXATION OF THE INJURED PART BY MECHANICAL MEANS in accordance with the first of these principles, and in order to restore the former rigidity of the part.

(4) THE TRANSPORT OF THE INJURED PERSON FROM THE SITE OF THE ACCIDENT TO A PLACE OF SAFETY.

(1) THE PREVENTION OF FURTHER INJURY.—This in itself should be quite obvious, and is so important as to warrant reiteration of the extreme dangers which may result from the careless handling of a fracture. A simple fracture may so easily become compound that want of care may greatly aggravate the injury or even cause death. Further injury is often caused by interference from ignorant spectators, and therefore it is the duty of every first-aid man to make himself master of the situation until such time as the patient is placed under medical care. The patient must on no account be moved from the place of accident until the appropriate treatment has been applied. As has already been mentioned, the examination must be carried out with as little disturbance as possible to the affected part.

(2) THE TREATMENT OF THE MORE URGENT ASSOCIATED CONDITIONS.

(a) *Surgical Shock* : the application of warmth, etc. (*see* Chapter VI.).

(b) *Haemorrhage.*—Some degree of haemorrhage accompanies every compound fracture : in the majority of cases it is slight and need not be treated specifically ; occasionally it is excessive, and it is absolutely necessary to stop the bleeding by digital pressure or the application of a tourniquet before any other measure is considered (*see* Chapter X.).

(*c*) *Wounds.*—The application of an antiseptic dressing is called for (*see* Chapter XI.).

(3) THE FIXATION OF THE INJURED PART BY MECH-ANICAL MEANS.—This is primarily to prevent an increase in the deformity, further damage to adjacent structures and increase in surgical shock. Rigid structures called splints may be applied, or immobility may be attained in certain instances by the application of bandages.

(4) THE TRANSPORT OF THE INJURED PERSON FROM THE SITE OF ACCIDENT TO A PLACE OF SAFETY.—This is only to be done when the fracture has been securely fixed in splints and when other urgent symptoms have been treated. In all fractures, except those of the upper extremity, the injured person must be placed upon a stretcher, which may have to be improvised. In fractures of the spine and pelvis the stretcher should be rigid. Even the loading of the injured person on the stretcher must be carried out systematically and according to the instructions under " Transport."

Those suffering from fracture of the upper limb, even if able to walk, should be assisted as faintness is apt to supervene in such cases.

COMPOUND FRACTURES.

In virtue of their special danger great care must be taken with compound fractures. It is advisable to clean the surrounding skin and to pour some antiseptic solution, as of iodine or weak lysol, over the wound and cover it with a dressing soaked in such an antiseptic lotion. In the absence of antiseptics it is permissible to cover the wound with a clean rag or with boracic lint. If gross angular deformity is present an attempt may be made to reduce this, but no attempt should be made to replace a fragment of bone which is protruding through the skin. A tourniquet should be placed in position proximal to the wound ; it is only to be tightened if bleeding becomes excessive. Splints may then be applied and treatment carried out as in the case of a simple fracture.

SPLINTS AND THEIR APPLICATION.

Splints are rigid structures which are applied to fractured limbs in order to give support, to restore the rigidity of the part and to prevent movement of the fragments. Some splints are specially constructed for ambulance work : others are improvised from any material which possesses the necessary strength and stiffness. While it is necessary that the ambulance pupil should understand the use of these specially made splints, it is to be remembered that such splints are only occasionally at hand when required. Therefore it is of even greater importance that every pupil should know also how to improvise splints.

IMPROVISATION OF SPLINTS.—No definite rules can be given to guide the ambulance pupil in the improvisation of splints, since no two fractures are the same and the circumstances of individual accidents vary. In these contingencies the ingenuity of the ambulance pupil is exercised to use any suitable material at hand. In improvised splints certain qualities are desirable : rigidity, strength and lightness, and appropriate size and form. With regard to the size and form, it is to be understood that too long splints are better than too short ones. Their minimum length should be such that the joint above and below the site of fracture may be fixed. If practicable the width of the splint should as nearly as possible approach that of the limb : in the case of the forearm it should be slightly wider than the thickest part of the limb. No limitation is placed upon the choice of materials which may be used, but mention must be made of those articles commonly employed for the improvisation of splints. Strips of box-wood, walking sticks, broom handles, folded newspapers, card-board sheets, metal strips, etc.

APPLICATION OF SPLINTS.—All splints should be padded before application with some soft material such as cotton wool, folded cloth or the like. The patient's clothes which have been cut or drawn aside may be replaced and used as padding. Before the application of splints it is also necessary to dress any wound, and in such cases a tourni-quet may be placed loosely in position for emergency use in case of subsequent haemorrhage.

In order to fix the splints in position triangular or roller bandages or simple strips of cloth may be used ; again the means of fixation may have to be improvised. When the splinting materials have been prepared and any necessary dressings have been applied, only gross de-formity, if present, should be reduced, but no attempt should be made to " set the fracture " or to restore the limb to its original length.

While the splints are being applied, the fragments of the broken limb must be supported and steadied in such a manner that the original alignment of the limb is restored as nearly as is possible. The procedure is most easily accomplished by firmly grasping the limb above and below the seat of fracture, and with the least possible disturbance gently pulling the fragments apart in the long axis of the limb. When this method is used extension is said to be applied to the part distal to the fracture ; while counter-extension is applied to the proximal part. Such a method involves the employment of one or more assist-ants, who must act under the instructions of the individual in charge of the case ; in a fracture of the lower limb two assistants are necessary, but in the case of the upper limb a single assistant is usually sufficient. When the limb has been straightened traction is maintained by the first-

aid assistants in the manner described above, while the ambulance man, with his hands free, adjusts the padding and splints in position and, later, fixes them by means of the improvised ties. The ties are made up of simple strips of cloth or other material, or of triangular bandages folded narrow, each tie being doubled upon itself. These are carefully slipped under the limb or the trunk before the splints are placed in position. If the injured person be lying upon a flat surface, it may be found convenient to pass the ties under the limb with the aid of a flat strip of wood : each tie is doubled over the end of such a stick or other similar article, and is thus more easily placed in position. When the splints have been ad-justed the ambulance man directs the assis-tant to transfer his grasp from the limb to the splints in such a manner that the limb

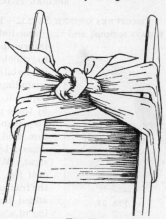

FIG. 50.

is steadied and held securely between the splints. One of the free ends of each tie is then passed over the limb, through the loop, and finally tied to the other free end (Fig. 50). In fracture of the leg and thigh, splints are applied to the inner and outer aspects of the limb which is extended ; in fracture of the forearm they are to be applied to the back and front, the limb being flexed at the elbow joint. Again, in a fracture of the lower limb, after splinting, the limbs should be tied together. After the application of splints to the arm the ambulance man must ascertain that the circulation distal to the fracture is satisfactory, as evidenced by the blanching produced by pressure on the finger-nails and the blushing on the release of pressure. In the case of the lower extremity the necessity for this test is hardly likely to arise, but whenever it is possible, without causing any undue disturbance, the pulse at the ankle should be felt.

SPECIAL FRACTURES.

FRACTURES OF THE SKULL.—Fractures of the skull are always serious, and the immediate danger from such head injury depends upon the extent to which the brain is damaged, its liability to infection and the wounding of associated soft parts. Injury to the head may be followed by three principal states of cerebral disturbance—concussion, laceration and compression—each evidenced by definite symptoms and signs. Wounding of the soft parts over the broken bone may render the fracture compound, with all the added dangers of infection. Tearing of a vessel beneath the broken bone (*e.g.* the middle meningeal artery) may cause haemorrhage and further damage to the brain; these effects may be evidenced immediately or after the lapse of some hours (Fig. 51). The knowledge of these facts should enable the ambulance pupil to realize that the symptoms, signs and treatment of a fractured skull are concerned more with the effects of injury to the brain and wounding of the soft parts than with the broken bone. In every case of severe head injury, fracture of the skull should be suspected. It should be fully understood that in some cases injury to the brain may be present without the occurrence of a fractured skull; in other

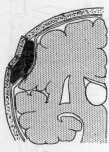

FIG. 51.

cases a fracture of the skull may be present in the absence of any immediate evidence of brain injury ; in still other cases a vessel may be torn inside the skull, when neither evidence of local head injury nor the immediate effects of brain disturbance are apparent. Fractures of the skull are conveniently divided into three groups—fractures of the vault, fractures of the base and fractures of the face. It is to be remembered, however, that each of these varieties of fracture may be associated with the effects of brain injury, concussion, laceration or compression.

CEREBRAL CONCUSSION is a condition which develops immediately after any sudden and violent shaking up of the brain ; it is most commonly seen after blows or falls upon the head, but any accident in which violence has been applied to the head may be followed by some degree of concussion. The condition is popularly referred to as " stunning," and, in some respects, it resembles surgical shock. The symptoms and signs of concussion vary in degree according to the severity of the blow, which may be quite trivial or so severe that the skull is fractured. In a mild case of concussion the injured person is momentarily dazed, or suffers from mental confusion for a few seconds or minutes ; in a severe case the symptoms of disordered cerebral function become more evident, and the injured person falls to the ground completely unconscious, in which state he may remain for several minutes or hours. In an uncomplicated case of concussion there is no gross damage to the brain. The patient may occasionally be roused by shouting at him, but, even if he can be roused, he appears shaken and dazed, and soon relapses into a state of insensibility. He is cold, pale and clammy, the temperature becomes subnormal, the pulse usually small and quick (occasionally irregular or varying in rate), and the breathing shallow. The pupils are usually equal and react to light. There is no paralysis, but the urine and faeces are often passed involuntarily. Recovery is heralded by the onset of vomiting, and in uncomplicated cases this generally occurs quite soon after the accident. The body then becomes warmer and, as the pulse and breathing improve, consciousness gradually returns.

CEREBRAL LACERATION is a condition in which the brain tissue is lacerated, bruised or contused. There is necessarily always some degree of concussion associated with cerebral laceration, because violence has been applied to the skull. In most cases the skull is fractured. The characteristic signs of cerebral laceration are seldom seen just at the time of injury, when, as a rule, concussion is much more in evidence. After a period of time the signs of concussion may be replaced by those of cerebral irritation, the direct result of cerebral laceration. As its name implies, the state of cerebral irritation is a condition of general irritability and restlessness dependent on brain injury. The patient may react to cerebral irritation in different ways ; he may be lying curled up, resisting any attention or interference ; on the other hand, he may be obstreperous, difficult to control, noisy and incoherent. He is always irrational. Further evidences of cerebral laceration depend upon the region of the brain damaged. These signs are manifested either by convulsive twitchings or paralysis. Effects such as the twitchings of one side of the body or of a single limb, or again the paralysis of one side of the body or of a single limb, indicate damage to the motor area of the opposite side of the brain. In cerebral laceration the pupils may be unequal, and one or both may fail to react to light. The careful observation and accurate recording of these signs may render invaluable assistance to the doctor who is called upon to localize the injury in the brain. From the state of cerebral irritation the patient may slowly recover within an indefinite period of time, or he may pass into a more serious condition— cerebral compression.

CEREBRAL COMPRESSION occurs when the pressure within the cranium rises suddenly and excessively ; it causes a disturbance of the brain functions which can be recognized by certain signs. Such a condition may develop after any head injury, and in this type of case the increased pressure is most commonly due to bleeding, either internal or external to the membranes of the brain. In nearly every case of cerebral compression there has been a preliminary stage of concussion, and, as a general rule, an appreciable period of time elapses between the injury and the onset of compression. In some cases the intervening period is one of perfect lucidity, and the injured person may appear to have made a complete recovery ; in other cases a transient period of cerebral irritation precedes the onset of compression without consciousness having been fully regained. In the early stage of compression there is an increase in the pressure at the point of haemorrhage. During this early stage there is a tendency for the spread of localized irritative symptoms ; the localized muscular twitching due to limited irritation may assume the proportions of a convulsion of a whole limb or of half the body as the cause of compression increases. When the pressure is sufficiently great the compressed area is no longer irritable but thrown out of action, and the convulsive twitchings are replaced by paralysis. Such a sequence of events is exemplified in the case of a blow on the head causing haemorrhage from the middle meningeal artery of one side ; as a result of the blow the patient has concussion at first, a period of lucidity may follow and then be replaced by the onset of irritative phenomena, which may be succeeded by paralysis of the opposite side of the body. The initial concussion is obviously explained by the blow ; during this time the pulse is soft, and, owing to this fact, little cr no haemorrhage has taken place from the site of rupture. Recovery from concussion is possible without the immediate occurrence of symptoms of compression, because the clotting has stopped the initial bleeding. Provided the patient remains at rest, no further haemorrhage may occur, but any exertion may result in a sudden recurrence of haemorrhage owing to the loosening of the clot as the pulse becomes stronger.

From this explanation it will be seen that one of the first precepts of first-aid is to keep every case of head injury quiet and at rest until the patient is seen by a doctor. When recurrence of haemorrhage commences, that area of the cerebral cortex at the site of the haemorrhage will be irritated ; in the case of the middle meningeal artery this area will be the motor cortex, hence the muscular twitching of an opposite limb or limbs. As blood accumulates locally the corresponding area of the motor cortex is thrown out of action, with the consequent paralysis of the opposite side of the body. It is to be remembered that unconsciousness may be present from the start, but on the other hand the patient may be conscious until after the onset of irritative signs. Consciousness is invariably lost once paralytic phenomena have appeared. In the late and fully developed stage of compression there is an increase in the general pressure inside the skull sufficient to affect the entire brain ; the earlier valuable localizing signs disappear and a state of deep unconsciousness supervenes. The patient cannot be roused, and he lies motionless upon his back. The pulse becomes slow and full ; at times the pulse rate may fall to between thirty and forty beats per minute, although its volume and force are intensified. The breathing becomes deep, slow and stertorous, so that the cheeks and lips are puffed in and out with each respiration. The limbs are flaccid and all the reflexes disappear. The pupils become dilated and do not react to light. The urine may be passed involuntarily or it may be retained. The face becomes flushed or cyanosed and the body temperature rises steadily ; in severe cases the temperature may reach 108° Fahrenheit. The heat of the body and the flushed face in compression contrast strongly with the cold and pallor of concussion and surgical shock.

FRACTURES OF THE VAULT OF THE SKULL.

CAUSES.—In most cases these fractures are due to direct violence, such as a blow or a fall upon the head.

SYMPTOMS AND SIGNS.—If the patient is conscious he will probably complain of pain in the head. The pain may be localized to the site where the violence was applied, or it may be generalized and be referred to as a " headache." Giddiness may also be complained of, especially if the patient attempts to rise. When concussion of any severity has occurred, it is usually found that the patient if conscious cannot remember either the accident itself or even the events which for a variable period of time preceded the accident.

There may only be a bruise or a contusion of the scalp, but more often there is an open wound rendering the fracture compound. There may be no immediate evidence of brain injury, but in most cases a fracture of the vault is accompanied by signs of cerebral concussion and later perhaps by signs of laceration or of compression.

FRACTURES OF THE BASE OF THE SKULL.

CAUSES.—These fractures are mainly due to indirect violence, such as falls from a height upon the top of the head or upon the feet or buttocks.

SYMPTOMS AND SIGNS.—Symptoms are present only when the patient is conscious, in which case they are similar to those of fracture of the vault. There may only be the signs of cerebral concussion, laceration or compression, but quite often the head injury will be evidenced in addition by a bruise mark or a wound of the scalp. Frequently there is bleeding from the nose, from the ears, and, occasionally, from the mouth, according to the site of the fracture. If the bones forming the orbital cavity nave been fractured, a blood-shot eye will appear and some protrusion of the eye-ball may rapidly develop. In some cases blood passes from the mouth to the stomach, and this may account for the appearance of blood in the vomit at a later period. These fractures are generally compound, because the line of the fracture very often communicates with the nose, the ear or the mouth.

TREATMENT OF HEAD INJURIES, INCLUDING FRACTURES OF THE BASE AND VAULT OF THE SKULL.

1. Examine for insensibility : if unconscious give no fluid by the mouth, and remove false teeth if these are present ; do not allow stimulants or spirits to be given to the patient even if perfectly conscious.

2. Examine the body generally, and if severe haemorrhage or any fracture of limbs, spine or pelvis is present treat accordingly.

3. Remove to a place of safety.

4. Send for medical assistance.

5. Cover up the body and keep the patient as warm as possible.

6. Examine the head for wounds or haemorrhage, arrest any active bleeding from a wound of the face or scalp and apply dressings. Do not attempt to stop bleeding from the nose or ears, but loosely plug the bleeding orifice with some antiseptic wool or gauze.

7. Make a careful note of any special signs such as twitching or paralysis of a limb or of one side of the body and note the side affected ; also note the condition of the pupils, the breathing and pulse rate, since these observations may be of invaluable aid to the surgeon in the later treatment of the case.

8. Remove the patient on a stretcher to his home or to hospital.

9. On arrival at the house place the patient in bed in a quiet and darkened room. Let the head be turned to one side and keep the air passages clear, since vomiting

often occurs in such cases, especially during the process of recovery. Keep the body and limbs warm by carefully arranged hot-water bottles, and apply iced water or cold cloths to the head. Never apply hot-water bottles directly to the skin. Watch and make a note of any particular change in the patient's condition until the doctor arrives. If cerebral irritation is present keep a close watch on the patient, and endeavour firmly but gently to control any irrational actions. If cerebral compression supervenes, raise the head and apply cold cloths to the face and scalp.

It must be remembered that a man may sustain a severe head injury and yet show no immediate signs of cerebral disturbance apart from a transient period of concussion. Therefore in every case of head injury it is the duty of the ambulance man to insist upon the injured person lying perfectly quiet until he has been examined by a doctor.

FRACTURES OF THE FACE.

THE LOWER JAW.—This fracture is always due to direct violence and most frequently occurs in a fight.

SYMPTOMS AND SIGNS.—Pain and loss of function cause the patient great difficulty in moving the jaw; he is unable to close the mouth, and speech is difficult owing to swelling and tenderness. There is deformity of the face and irregularity in the line of the teeth. The gums are usually torn, and blood and saliva dribble from the open mouth.

Crepitus and abnormal mobility may be elicited incidentally. The fracture is invariably compound, due to wounding inside the mouth; occasionally a wound is present on the chin externally. Shock is generally present.

TREATMENT.—1. Warn the patient not to speak.

2. Dress any external wound which may be present.

3. Steady the fragments of the lower jaw by supporting the lower teeth against the upper teeth in the following

manner. The centre of a triangular bandage folded narrow is placed under the chin, and the ends are brought up on to the top of the head, where they are tied together. The centre of a second similar bandage is placed in front of the chin, and its ends are tied together beneath the occiput. The ends of the upper bandage are then tied to the ends of the lower bandage, so as to retain them in position. In a similar manner the four-tailed bandage may be applied.   (Plate VII.)

THE UPPER JAW.—

This fracture is always due to direct violence.

SYMPTOMS AND SIGNS.—These are pain, deformity and swelling of the face ; irregularity in the line of the upper teeth and tenderness.   Tearing of the gums over the site of the fracture renders it compound and gives rise to bleeding.

TREATMENT.—Warn the patient not to try to blow his nose or to speak. In other respects the treatment is essentially similar to that for fracture of lower jaw.

FRACTURE OF THE NOSE.—

The nasal bones are always fractured by direct violence, such as a punch or a blow directly on the nose.

SYMPTOMS AND SIGNS.—Pain, swelling, deformity and bleeding are present. The fracture is nearly always compound, as the bone tears the mucous membrane lining the nose ; crepitus may be felt, and occasionally there is a wound externally.

TREATMENT.—1. Warn the patient not to try to blow his nose, since air may be driven into the tissues and cause infection.

2. Plug the nostrils very loosely with some material such as gauze soaked in antiseptic lotion ; do not attempt to stop the bleeding : it will do no harm and helps to clean the wound.

3. Dress any external wound.

FRACTURE OF THE SPINE.

A fractured spine is commonly referred to as a " broken back " or a " broken spine," and this type of fracture is especially serious on account of the damage which may be done to the spinal cord. When the spinal cord is severed or crushed as the result of such a fracture the body will be paralyzed, and sensation will be abolished below the level of the damaged vertebrae : there will also be serious interference with the functions of the urinary bladder and the rectum. It follows that the nearer the fracture is situated to the brain the more extensive will be the paralysis. If the fracture is situated high up in the neck instant death may occur ; if the cord is crushed in the mid-cervical region both arms and legs will be paralyzed, while a crush affecting the mid-thoracic or lumbar region of the spinal cord will leave the arms intact and paralyze the lower limbs. Occasionally the bones of the spinal column are fractured and the cord escapes injury : in such cases there may be few or no symptoms except some pain at the site of the fracture. There are also a few cases in which an injury to the spine is followed immediately by symptoms and signs of severe damage to the cord, although neither the spinal cord nor the bones of the spine have actually suffered any injury other than a severe shaking or sudden violent concussion. The condition of these latter cases is referred to as spinal concussion, since it would appear to be associated with jarring of the spinal cord ; recovery is the rule.

CAUSES.—These fractures are always due to violence, which may be applied directly to some particular part of the column or indirectly through a number of the vertebrae along the axis of the column. Direct violence causing such an injury may result from a severe blow on the spine, from the crush of a wheel passing over the body, or from the spine striking a beam or some other hard object in the course of a fall. Indirect violence may cause a fracture of the vertebrae when the patient falls from a height on to the feet or the head, as in diving into water, and even in jumping suddenly from a moving vehicle, when the weight is thrown violently upon the feet. When the spine is fractured by direct violence, there is usually displacement or dislocation of the fractured bones and the spinal cord is invariably damaged, whereas a fracture of the spine resulting from indirect violence is rarely complicated by injury to the spinal cord.

SYMPTOMS AND SIGNS.—There is invariably the history of an injury. Pain is complained of at or about the site of the injured vertebra. If the cord is damaged the power of movement and sensation will be partially or completely lost below the seat of injury and control over the bladder and rectum will be abolished. Tenderness is present at the site of fracture, where there may also be swelling, deformity, bruising and even wounding of the soft parts. Surgical shock is always present when the spinal cord has been damaged.

The presence of a fractured or dislocated spine should at once be assumed if there is the history of an injury to the spinal column and partial or complete loss of function in the parts below the level of the injury. When such is the case there should be no further examination.

TREATMENT.—The principal aim in the treatment of fractures of the spine is to prevent further damage to the cord incurred by unnecessary movement of the damaged vertebrae.

1. Warn the patient to lie perfectly still, and do not allow him to be moved until proper means of transport have been devised or until the arrival of the doctor.

2. Treat surgical shock by covering up the body, applying warmth in the form of hot bottles and giving hot tea or coffee to drink. Hot bottles are never to be applied directly to the skin in such cases, since the patient's skin may be insensitive and easily burned.

3. Remove the patient to hospital or to a convenient shelter in the following manner :

(*a*) Carefully place the lower limbs together and tie the feet, the legs and the thighs to each other with bandages or similar strips of cloth.

(*b*) Obtain a rigid stretcher on which to carry the patient. A wooden shutter or door might be used, or, failing this, any ordinary stretcher may be made rigid by fastening boards or similar material across the poles and covering them with a thick blanket.

(*c*) Place the patient upon the stretcher by one of the following methods :

1st Method.—Carefully pass a strong blanket or sheet under the patient, working from the head towards the feet. Lay a strong pole along each side of the sheet, and roll the sheet on each pole inwards towards the patient. First-aid assistants then arrange themselves facing each other on either side of the patient, and firmly grasp the poles together with the sheet. The rigid stretcher is then placed conveniently near to the head of the patient and in line with the body. At a word of command given by the ambulance man in charge of the case, all the helpers lift simultaneously, keeping the patient horizontal. As soon as the patient is well clear of the ground the rigid stretcher is passed under the sheet or blanket, and the patient is lowered upon the stretcher.

2nd Method.—If the injured man is wearing a coat, the garment may be opened out, and poles used as mentioned in the first method. In this case one assistant will be required to keep the lower limbs horizontal.

If a patient is found lying upon his face or upon one side, it is better not to roll him on to his back, but to remove him or keep him in this position, so as to minimise any movement required by the doctor who has later to examine him.

FRACTURE OF THE RIBS.

This is a common type of fracture, and the ribs may be broken in three different ways.

CAUSES.—1. *Direct violence.* This occurs when one or more ribs are fractured by a direct blow or kick on the chest wall. In this case the fracture occurs at the point where the blow is struck and the fragments may be driven inwards, causing damage to the pleura or lung. It will be recalled that when the lung is pierced by the broken end of a rib the fracture becomes compound, since the air within the lung has access to the site of fracture.

2. *Indirect violence.* This occurs when several ribs, usually the fourth to the eighth, are bent till they break at their most convex part just in front of the angles. This type of violence is usually the result of a severe crushing or run-over accident, as when a wheel passes over the chest. In such cases the sharp ends of the ribs are turned outwards, with the result that the internal organs of the thorax escape injury.

3. *Muscular action.* This is a relatively rare occurrence, and is most likely to happen with a sudden, violent cough or sneeze in an elderly person or in one suffering from some wasting disease. Usually only one rib is fractured in this manner.

SYMPTOMS AND SIGNS.—There is sharp pain at the site of fracture, usually severe and increased by drawing a deep breath or on coughing. It is generally described as a catching or cutting sort of pain, not unlike a stitch in the side. Occasionally the patient will feel a distinct snap as if something had cracked. The breathing becomes shallow and more rapid, while an irritating and painful cough is often present. Tenderness at the site of fracture may be elicited by pressing either over the broken rib itself or over the sternum. Occasionally crepitus can be felt by placing the hand flat on the ribs and asking the patient to take a deep breath. Deformity, swelling and discoloration are rarely ever apparent in such a fracture.

If the pleura is injured the symptoms and signs will be more severe, and if the lung is pierced there is likely to be spitting of bright red frothy blood and mucus. Some degree of surgical shock or collapse is present. More rarely, if the violence has been very severe, the liver may be damaged on the right side or the spleen on the left side : in such cases there might be evidences of internal haemorrhage. Fracture of a rib is often diagnosed by the patient.

TREATMENT.—The first essential is to discover whether the fractured rib has pierced the lung.

1. If the lung has not been damaged the principal aim will be to control the movements of the chest wall as far as possible, since it is this movement which increases so greatly the severe pain. In order to do so two triangular bandages folded broad are applied to the chest in the following manner. The centre of the first bandage is placed just below the fracture, the patient is asked to breathe out as fully as possible, and the ends of the bandage are tied on the opposite side of the chest firmly enough to limit the movement of the chest wall, but not completely to arrest it. If the correct amount of pressure has been applied, the patient will at once feel more comfortable and acknowledge the relief. The second bandage is applied in exactly the same manner with its centre just above the fracture, so as to overlap the first bandage by half its width.

A single strong towel or a broad roller bandage wound evenly round the chest and firmly pinned in position might well be substituted in the absence of triangular bandages. The forearm of the injured side should be placed in a large arm sling. (Plate VII.)

2. If the lung or any other internal organ has been damaged do not apply bandages round the chest, since this may cause further damage. Place the arm of the

injured side in a sling. Keep the patient lying down, so that the uninjured side is uppermost and has free play : support the body in this position. Cover up the patient to keep him as warm as possible and so minimize shock. If there is evidence of bleeding from the lung, apply the treatment for internal haemorrhage (*see* Chapter X.).

When ribs on both sides are fractured bandages must not be applied; the patient should be propped up and made as comfortable as possible.

In every case a patient suffering from fracture of the ribs should be removed on a stretcher, with the chest elevated and the body inclined to the injured side.

FRACTURE OF THE STERNUM (BREAST BONE).

This bone is rarely fractured.

CAUSES.—Direct violence, such as a kick or a blow directly upon the sternum, is the more common cause of fracture. Indirect violence may also cause a fracture of the sternum, when the bone is bent till it breaks. This usually occurs when the spine is fractured in the thoracic region.

SYMPTOMS AND SIGNS.—There is invariably the history of an accident. Severe pain, difficult breathing, tenderness at the site of the fracture, swelling and discoloration are present. There may also be some deformity and crepitus.

TREATMENT.—If not complicated by an injury to the organs within the thorax, treat exactly as for fractured ribs. If the fracture is complicated keep the patient warm and quiet in the most comfortable position, usually in a half-sitting posture, until the arrival of the doctor.

Treat any external wounds.

FRACTURE OF THE CLAVICLE.

This is one of the commonest fractures, especially in early life, and it happens frequently on the football field.

The fracture usually occurs near the middle of the bone, the weakest part; in young children it is generally of the green stick variety.

CAUSES.—Indirect violence is the most common cause of this fracture; it is usually the result of a fall upon the point of the shoulder, upon the elbow, or upon the hand of the outstretched arm. Rarely the clavicle is fractured by direct violence, when the bone receives a kick or a direct blow.

SYMPTOMS AND SIGNS.—Pain, increased by movement, and partial loss of power in the arm, are always present: occasionally there is experienced the sensation of something having snapped or given way. The patient usually supports the injured arm at the elbow with the opposite hand, and inclines his head towards the injured side. Since the intact clavicle acts as a prop for the shoulder, a fracture of this bone causes the shoulder to droop downwards, forwards and inwards. Tenderness at the site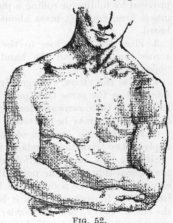

FIG. 52.

of the fracture is invariably present. Deformity is often apparent: one and sometimes both the fractured ends of the bone can be felt or, more rarely, seen, as they are apt to protrude just under the skin—especially in a slim person. Crepitus and unnatural mobility are very easily felt when the fingers are passed lightly over the bone, but these signs must not be deliberately elicited. (Fig. 52.)

TREATMENT.—The aim in the treatment of this fracture
is to prevent further overriding of the fragments. This
may be done by fixing the arm and forearm in such a
position that the downward, inward and forward displacement of the shoulder is to some extent corrected.

1. Remove the coat and, if necessary, the waistcoat, and
unfasten the brace on the injured side : commence to
undress on the uninjured side, and proceed with the
greatest possible care and gentleness. It is unnecessary to
remove any other clothing unless there is a wound.

2. Place a firm pad about as large as the patient's fist
well up into the axilla or armpit : this pad can be improvised by folding or rolling a piece of cloth or bandages
into a firm, compact mass about 2″ in diameter and 4″
broad.

3. Place the arm close to the side, and the forearm
across the chest with the hand pointing towards the
opposite shoulder.

4. Raise the elbow very gently, keeping it close to the
side, and at the same time push the shoulder well back.
In this way the downward, forward and inward deformity
of the shoulder may be corrected.

5. Maintain this position of the arm and forearm by
applying two triangular bandages in the following manner.

Slip the first bandage unfolded under the forearm of
the injured side, with the point directed over the injured
clavicle. Bring the point of the bandage down over the
front of the forearm and tuck it between the forearm and
the chest. Carry the lower border forwards and upwards,
wrapping it over the front of the forearm. The upper end
is carried over the shoulder of the uninjured side, and the
lower end is carried round behind the chest to meet the
upper end on the uninjured shoulder, where it is tied.

Finally the middle of a second triangular bandage
folded narrow is placed just above the point of the elbow
outside the sling, and its ends are carried round the body
and tied on the opposite side of the chest. By means of

this second bandage the upper end of the humerus is pulled outwards carrying the shoulder with it, since the humerus acts like a lever over a fulcrum, which is represented here by the pad. It is advisable to ascertain that the pulse can be felt satisfactorily at the wrist after application of the second bandage. (Plate XIII.)

2nd Method.—This method is especially useful when both clavicles are broken. It is easily applied and quite as efficient as the first method. Two triangular bandages are folded narrow. Each bandage is passed through one armpit, round the front of the same shoulder, and tied behind in a reef knot. The upper and lower ends of these two knots are then tied together over a pad adjusted between the shoulders. As the knots are tightened the shoulders are braced well back, in order to correct the overriding of the fragments of the clavicle on either side. Finally both forearms are supported by a narrow arm sling. (Plate XIV.)

After the treatment for a fractured clavicle has been applied, the patient may be allowed to walk if he is feeling otherwise fit : another person must always accompany the injured man in case he should become faint. If the patient shows any sign of shock, or has other injuries, he should be carried lying on his back on a stretcher. A stretcher must always be employed if both clavicles are broken.

FRACTURE OF THE SCAPULA.

This bone is rarely fractured, on account of its mobility and the muscular covering which it possesses.

CAUSE.—Direct violence, such as a severe kick or blow, is invariably the cause of fracture of the scapula.

SYMPTOMS AND SIGNS.—There is pain over the back of the shoulder, and any movement of the arm increases this pain. The power to raise the arm is partially or completely lost. Tenderness is most marked over the site of fracture. Swelling, bruising and discoloration may be present, but deformity, crepitus and unnatural mobility are rarely apparent. This fracture is very difficult to diagnose.

TREATMENT.—Remove the outer clothing and unfasten any braces or other tight bands. Apply a broad folded bandage to the chest in the following manner : the centre of the bandage is placed in the axilla of the injured side, the ends are carried round the back and front of the chest ; they are then crossed over the uninjured shoulder and tied in the axilla. The arm of the injured side is supported in a large arm sling.

The precautions advised in removing a case of fractured clavicle should be observed in dealing with a fractured scapula.

FRACTURE OF THE HUMERUS.

This fracture may be situated in any part of the bone. The commonest sites of fracture are (a) at its upper end near the shoulder joint, (b) in the shaft, and (c) at its lower end near the elbow joint. When either end of the bone is broken the adjacent joint may be dislocated.

(a) FRACTURE OF THE HUMERUS NEAR THE SHOULDER JOINT.

CAUSES.—Direct or indirect violence may cause a fracture at this site. In the latter case the fracture may result from a fall on the outstretched hand or elbow and is often impacted, the compact upper end of the shaft being driven into the softer cancellous head of the humerus.

SYMPTOMS AND SIGNS.—There is pain about the neck of the bone and partial or complete loss of power in the arm. Tenderness, swelling and deformity are usually observed : discoloration becomes evident at a later stage. Crepitus and unnatural mobility may occasionally be detected.

TREATMENT.—Remove the clothing. Place a large pad between the arm and the chest wall, and bandage the arm to the side with a broad bandage tied on the uninjured side. Support the forearm of the injured side in a narrow arm sling.

When treating a fracture of the humerus it is important to remember that so long as the patient is standing or sitting the weight of the limb below the fracture exerts a downward pull on the lower fragment of the humerus. This gravitational effect assists in the prevention of further displacement of the fragments, and should be utilized in the first-aid treatment of such fractures by supporting the upper limb from the wrist only, in a small arm sling. If a large arm sling is used in such a case the elbow is supported, and the effect of gravity is counteracted.

(b) FRACTURES OF THE SHAFT OF THE HUMERUS.— CAUSES.—Direct violence is the usual cause of a fracture in the shaft of the humerus, but a fracture in this part of the bone may also result from indirect violence, and very occasionally from muscular violence as in throwing a cricket ball.

SYMPTOMS AND SIGNS.—Pain, loss of power in the arm, tenderness, swelling, deformity, shortening, unnatural mobility and crepitus may all be well-marked features of this fracture. It is important to remember that a fracture about the middle of the humerus is particularly liable to cause damage to the large radial nerve, which winds spirally round the middle third of this bone. Injury to this nerve causes paralysis of the muscles on the back of the forearm ; these muscles are the extensors of the wrist, hand and fingers. The resulting disability is called drop wrist, since the hand droops from the wrist and cannot be raised.

TREATMENT.—1st Method.—Support the forearm at a right angle with the arm and apply two splints, one on the inner and the other on the outer surface of the arm. The splints should be at least the same width as the arm, preferably slightly wider, and they should be of sufficient length to extend from the shoulder to just below the point of the elbow. They must be carefully padded and fixed in position by means of two looped ties, the upper tie being applied before the lower tie. The forearm is then supported at the wrist in a narrow arm sling and the state of the circulation examined, either by feeling for the radial pulse at the wrist or by observing the effect of compressing the finger nails. (Plate V.)

2nd Method.—Support the forearm at a right angle as before. Make a flat pad of folded cloth or other soft material, large enough to extend from the axilla to just beyond the elbow, adjust this between the arm and the chest wall, and place the arm gently against it so that the fragments are supported on the padding. Now apply one splint of suitable size to the outer surface of the arm, and fix it in this position with two narrow folded bandages. The centre of each bandage is placed over the splint, and the ends are carried round the chest and tied on the opposite side. The forearm is then supported at the wrist by a narrow arm sling. Examine the circulation at the wrist. (Plate V.)

(c) FRACTURE OF THE HUMERUS NEAR THE ELBOW JOINT.

CAUSES.—Direct violence, such as a fall or a blow upon the elbow, is the commonest cause of fracture of the humerus near the elbow joint.

SYMPTOMS AND SIGNS.—Pain is complained of in the region of the elbow joint. This pain is increased by any movement at the joint. There is partial loss of power in the arm and forearm, and interference with the movement of the elbow joint. Tenderness, swelling and deformity are usually present; crepitus and unnatural mobility may occasionally be detected.

TREATMENT.—Support the forearm at a right angle with the injured arm, the palm of the hand facing the body.

Procure two splints, one equal in width to the thickness of the arm and of such length that it extends from the axilla to beyond the elbow ; the other equal in width to the thickness of the forearm and of sufficient length to extend from the tips of the fingers to just beyond the elbow. Cross the ends of these splints, and firmly tie them together so as to form a single right angle or " L "-shaped splint. Pad the splint carefully and apply it to the inner side of the arm and forearm, protecting the axillary vessels and nerves by placing a pad in the armpit. Fix the splint in position by three looped ties, using two for the forearm and one for the arm. Support the limb in a large arm sling. (Plate IV., A.)

In the case of a fracture near the elbow joint it is particularly important to ascertain that the circulation of the limb beyond the fracture is satisfactory. If the slightest doubt exists with regard to this important point, the ties should be undone immediately and the splint removed ; if necessary the angle of the forearm with the arm may be slightly increased until the circulation improves.

As an alternative method the forearm may be supported at the wrist in a narrow arm sling, the elbow being bent to a right angle.

FRACTURE OF THE RADIUS AND ULNA.

The radius and ulna may be fractured near the elbow joint, in the middle third of the forearm or just above the wrist joint. One or both of the bones may be broken. In adults fracture of the lower end of the radius is an extremely common accident. In children a greenstick fracture affecting the shafts of these bones is almost as frequent an occurrence.

CAUSES.—Indirect violence, almost invariably due to a fall upon the outstretched hand, is the most common cause of a fracture affecting the bones of the forearm.

E

When this happens the greater part of the force affects the lower end of the radius, which is very commonly broken just above the wrist joint; such a fracture is known as a Colles fracture. If the ulna is fractured by indirect violence, the break usually occurs at its upper end near the elbow joint.

In the case of a child a fall upon the outstretched hand usually produces a greenstick fracture of both bones about the middle of the forearm; less commonly there occurs a separation of the lower epiphysis of the radius. Occasionally the lower end of the radius is broken by the back-firing of a motor engine when starting it with a handle. The fracture caused by such an accident is called a " chauffeur's fracture "; it is another example of a fracture due to indirect violence.

Direct violence, such as a blow or a fall upon the fore-arm, is also a common cause of fracture of the radius and ulna. In this case the break usually occurs in the shafts of the bones rather than at their ends. Here again both bones or only one bone may be broken. In a fall upon the elbow direct violence may cause a fracture of the olecranon process of the ulna. This is a relatively common occurrence in the adult.

SYMPTOMS AND SIGNS.—The characteristic symptoms and signs of fracture are usually present—pain felt most acutely at the site of fracture and increased by movement of the injured part, loss of power and the sensation of something having snapped. Tenderness, swelling, deformity, unnatural mobility and crepitus may all be present when the forearm is fractured. When the lower end of the radius is fractured by a fall on the hand, as in Colles fracture, the distal fragment is displaced upwards and tilted backwards. The result is a characteristic appearance of the wrist known as the " dinner-fork deformity " (Fig. 53). As the lower end of the radius is impacted in such a fracture, there will be neither crepitus nor unnatural mobility. In a greenstick fracture there will be neither crepitus nor unnatural mobility, since the bones are merely bent and not completely broken. If only one bone is broken, the symptoms and signs are much less apparent than when both bones are fractured. Fractures about the wrist joint are often difficult to recognize, and every case in which there is the least suspicion of a fracture must be examined by a doctor. This remark applies with equal force to injuries about the elbow joint.

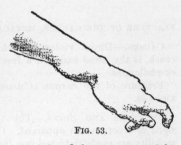

Fig. 53.

TREATMENT.—Support the injured forearm at a right angle to the arm. This should be done by grasping the injured limb above and below the site of fracture. If the right forearm is injured the assistant should grasp the patient's right hand in his own right hand and the patient's forearm near the elbow in his left hand, at the same time exerting very gentle and steady extension and counter-extension on the distal and proximal fragments respectively. When the left forearm is injured the grasp of the assistant's hands is reversed. Never apply extension and counter-extension to a Colles fracture in an old person.

Two splints of suitable size are applied to the front and back of the forearm by means of two looped ties. These ties are placed near the elbow joint proximally and the wrist joint distally. The splints should be of sufficient length to extend from the point of the elbow to the tips of the fingers, and of sufficient width to equal the thickest part of the forearm; they must be carefully and thickly padded so as to avoid pressure on the bony prominences at the joints above and below. Place the forearm in a large arm sling, and ascertain that the circulation is satisfactory by the finger-nail test. This method of treatment may be applied to any fracture of the forearm, except in the case of fracture of the olecranon process, where it is sufficient to support the forearm in a large arm sling. (Plate IV., B and C.)

FRACTURE OF THE CARPUS, METACARPUS AND PHALANGES.

CAUSES.—Direct violence, such as a severe blow or crush, is the usual cause of a fracture of the metacarpus or phalanges.

Fracture of the carpus is usually caused by indirect violence.

SYMPTOMS AND SIGNS.—The typical symptoms and signs of fracture are apparent. Crepitus and unnatural mobility are easily detected in a fracture of the phalanges. Swelling on the back of the hand is most obvious in fracture of the metacarpal bones. Fracture of a carpal bone is practically indistinguishable from a sprain of the wrist. There is frequently bruising or wounding of the soft parts.

TREATMENT.—1st Method.—Place the forearm at a right angle to the arm. Procure a splint long enough to extend from the elbow to just beyond the tips of the fingers, and broad enough to equal the width of the palm. Pad the splint evenly, and apply it to the palmar surface of the hand and front of the forearm. Secure the splint in position by means of three triangular bandages folded narrow ; one is applied in the figure of eight round the hand and wrist, the other two are applied by the looped tie method round the forearm. Support the injured limb in a large arm sling.

2nd Method.—Place a firm pad in the palm of the hand, gently flex the fingers over the pad, and apply a narrow folded triangular bandage after the manner used for the control of haemorrhage from the palm of the hand. Support the hand in a large arm sling. This method is particularly useful when there is a wound in the palm of the hand.   (Plate X.)

FRACTURE OF THE PELVIS.

This accident is always serious, as the fracture may be complicated by injury to the organs in the cavity of the pelvis.   If the sharp end of a fragment of bone pierces the urinary bladder or intestine the fracture is rendered compound ;   in this lies the extreme gravity of the injury.

CAUSES.—These fractures are caused by direct violence. They are usually produced by severe crushing, such as being squeezed between the buffers of railway waggons, run over by a heavy vehicle, or struck by a fall of rock in a mine.

SIGNS AND SYMPTOMS.—Pain, increased by movement and by coughing, is felt in the region of the pelvis.   The history of a violent crush or blow may be obtained from the patient or from a witness of the accident.   The patient is unable to stand or to move the lower limb on the affected side.   Occasionally the patient complains of a terrible feeling, as if the lower part of the body had given way.   Surgical shock and collapse are generally extremely severe.   There may be bruising and swelling over the groins and iliac crests, or in the perinaeum between the thighs.   Tenderness is marked over the site of fracture, where some irregularity of the bone may be apparent. Blood may be present in the urine if the bladder is torn. The examination of such a case should be carried out with the utmost care, and should occupy as little time as possible.   Under no circumstances is the ambulance man to examine for crepitus.

TREATMENT.—The principal aim of treatment is to prevent injudicious movement of the patient, and thus to protect the internal organs from further damage.   As soon as a fracture of the pelvis is diagnosed or even suspected, the patient must be warned not to pass water, since the urine might be forced into the soft tissues of the pelvis or into the peritoneal cavity and cause serious trouble. The patient must also be reassured and encouraged to lie quite still and flat on his back : if slight flexion of the thighs gives ease, the limbs should be supported in this position. Surgical shock is treated next by covering up the patient's body with coats or blankets, applying warmth in the form of hot-water bottles if these are available and giving hot drinks. The pelvic bones should be supported by the application of one or two triangular bandages folded broad, the one overlapping the other if two are used. These bandages must be passed round the pelvis with great care, and adjusted so that the centre of each lies over the sacrum ; the ends can then be tied securely in front, using just sufficient tension to give support and make the patient comfortable. If too much pressure is applied, the displacement of the fragments may be increased and harm done to the soft parts. A strong towel may be used as a binder round the pelvis instead of the triangular bandages. Finally, the knees and ankles are bandaged together with two triangular bandages folded narrow. The removal of the patient requires the same precautions as were indicated for the removal of a case of fractured spine.

In this fracture it is of the utmost importance to obtain medical assistance at the earliest possible moment, on account of the gravity of the complications which may rapidly develop. Whenever practicable, it is wiser to convey such a case straight to hospital rather than to the patient's home.

FRACTURE OF THE FEMUR.

This bone may be fractured in any situation, but the fracture occurs most commonly in one of three places— (a) at the upper end, (b) in the shaft, and (c) at the lower end. A fracture of the femur must always be regarded as a very serious injury.

(a) FRACTURE AT THE UPPER END.—In this situation the fracture affects the neck of the femur in the majority of cases; such a fracture is particularly common in elderly people.

CAUSES.—This fracture is usually produced by indirect violence. With advancing years the blood supply to the head and neck of the femur becomes defective and the bone is rendered brittle. Thus a relatively slight amount of violence, such as tripping over the edge of a carpet or falling out of bed, may be sufficient to break the bone.

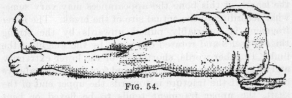

FIG. 54.

For the same reasons as render the bone brittle, repair is interfered with, and the injury may have grave consequences.

SYMPTOMS AND SIGNS.—There is usually the history of an accident, which may be quite trivial if the patient is elderly. Pain in the region of the hip joint is invariably present, and this pain is greatly increased by the slightest movement of the limb. There is loss of power in the limb, the patient not being able to raise his heel from the ground. Occasionally there is bruising and tenderness round the region of the hip joint; shortening may be noticeable, but swelling is not usually apparent. The leg is rotated outwards, and the foot lies with its outer border on the ground, giving a characteristically helpless appearance to the affected limb. The patient is usually severely shocked. (Fig. 54.)

TREATMENT.—This is essentially the same as the treatment to be applied in the case of a fracture of the shaft of the femur. The ambulance man is not expected to be able to differentiate a fracture affecting the upper end of the femur from one affecting the upper part of the shaft of this bone. Therefore the same treatment will be employed in either case.

(b) FRACTURE OF THE SHAFT.

CAUSES.—Direct or indirect violence may produce a fracture through the shaft of the femur.

SYMPTOMS AND SIGNS.—All the characteristic symptoms and signs of fracture may be present, but owing to the length of this bone the appearances may vary somewhat according to the actual site of the break. The lower fragment is invariably pulled upwards by the strong thigh muscles and rotated outwards by the weight of the limb. In other words, shortening of the lower extremity and rotation outwards of the leg and foot are nearly always obvious. If the fracture is towards the upper end of the shaft, the upper fragment tends to be flexed or bent forwards ; if the fracture occurs near the lower end of the shaft, the lower fragment is bent backwards. It is not usually difficult to diagnose a fracture of the shaft of the femur.

TREATMENT.—Place the patient flat upon his back and keep him as comfortable as possible in this position. Remove sufficient clothing to ensure that the fracture is not compound, but keep the rest of the body well covered up in order to prevent unnecessary exposure to cold. Obtain the help of one or more assistants ; whenever possible the ambulance man should have two assistants— one to hold the foot and to apply extension to the injured limb, the other to steady the splints during their application. If a third assistant is available, he may apply gentle counter-extension at the armpits of the injured man. The first assistant will take up a kneeling position at the feet of the injured man and grasp the foot of the injured limb by passing one hand under the heel and the other hand over the front of the foot. He will then apply gentle extension in the long axis of the limb, and gradually bring the foot and lower part of the limb into a natural position, so that the foot is held as nearly as possible at a right angle with the leg and with its outer border perpendicular to the ground. This position must be maintained as steadily as possible until the splints have been firmly fixed in position. Two splints are required for the treatment of this fracture. One should be of sufficient length to extend from the armpit to just beyond the heel; the other should be long enough to extend from the fork to beyond the knee. The width of these splints should as nearly as possible equal the thickness of the knee, from front to back. The splints must be adequately padded, and this is especially necessary when improvised splints are used. Before adjusting the splints to the outer and inner aspects of the thigh, a soft pad should be placed in the armpit and in the fork. The second assistant will now steady the splints in position while the ambulance man fixes them by means of seven triangular bandages. The long outer splint is fixed to the trunk by two triangular bandages folded broad; one is applied round the hips and pelvis, and the other round the chest just under the armpits. The shorter inner splint is fixed to the thigh and leg and to the outer splint by three triangular bandages folded narrow and using the looped tie method, one being placed just above and a second just below the supposed site of fracture; the third bandage is placed just below the knee. Two more triangular bandages folded narrow are now applied—one tying the two limbs together just above the knees, and the other tying both feet together above the ankles. The last bandage is applied in a figure of eight fashion by placing its centre behind and between the ankles, crossing the ends over the insteps in front of the feet and tying off on the outer splint. (Plate XV.)

If the injured person is a woman.—The inner splint may be dispensed with, and the skirt used as padding between the limbs. Each of the lower five bandages is passed round both limbs, the ends being tied off on the splint as described above.

(c) FRACTURE OF THE LOWER END.

CAUSES.—Direct or indirect violence may produce fracture in this region.

SYMPTOMS AND SIGNS.—The usual symptoms and signs of a fracture are present. The short lower fragment is apt to be drawn forcibly backwards, and may injure or press upon the popliteal artery and endanger the circulation of the limb. Should the fracture involve the knee joint, there will be excessive swelling in this region.

TREATMENT.—This is the same as that for a fracture of the shaft. Special care must be taken to ascertain that the circulation is satisfactory. If there is evidence of grave interference with the circulation after such a fracture, the leg should be slightly flexed at the knee, and if the circulation improves with this alteration in position splints should not be applied, but the patient made as comfortable as possible until the arrival of a doctor. Under these circumstances it would be advisable and justifiable to remove the patient on a rigid stretcher without the application of splints.

In all cases of fracture of the bones of the lower extremity, with the exception of the patella and the bones of the foot, the limbs should be tied together and the patient removed lying upon his back on a stretcher.

FRACTURE OF THE PATELLA.

CAUSES.—This fracture may be produced either by direct violence or by excessive muscular action. When the strong quadriceps muscle in front of the thigh is suddenly thrown into contraction in order to save oneself from falling backwards, the full force of the muscle is suddenly thrust upon the patella, which may be split transversely across about its middle, wide separation of the fragments resulting.

SYMPTOMS AND SIGNS.—There is great pain over the knee-cap, and partial or complete loss of power to extend or straighten the leg. The patient falls to the ground, and is unable to rise or to walk if the fragments are separated at the instant of fracture. In some cases, when the fracture is due to direct violence, the bone may be cracked into several pieces, but there is no separation of the fragments : in such a case there may be sufficient power to move the limb. The knee joint is greatly swollen, and the skin may be bruised if the fracture has been caused by direct violence. Tenderness is invariably present over the fractured bone : a space may be felt in the interval between the fragments ; crepitus and unnatural mobility are occasionally elicited.

TREATMENT.—Place the patient in a semi-sitting position, with the head and shoulders supported in order to relax the muscles in front of the thigh. Procure a splint of sufficient length to extend from the fold of the buttock to just beyond the heel and as wide as the patient's knee. Pad the splint and place it along the back of the thigh and leg, support the lower end of the leg on a pillow, stool, or rolled-up coat, so as further to relax the muscles in front of the thigh. Fix the splint to the lower limb by applying three triangular bandages folded narrow. The first and second bandages are passed round the upper end of the thigh and the lower part of the leg respectively ; in each case the looped tie method is employed, and the knots are tied towards the outer side instead of over the splint. The third bandage is applied with its centre immediately above the knee-cap, the ends are crossed over the splint behind, and then brought forward and tied off in front immediately below the knee-cap. By applying the third bandage in this manner the fragments of the patella are approximated to some extent and held steady.

When treating this fracture the help of one assistant is preferable, but the ambulance man may apply the necessary treatment without the aid of a second person. The legs need not be tied together in the case of a fractured patella; the affected limb should be kept elevated. (Plate XVI., A.)

FRACTURE OF THE TIBIA AND FIBULA.

These bones are frequently broken; one or both may be fractured. It is uncommon to find the tibia fractured alone, whereas fracture of the fibula alone is a very common accident. When the tibia is fractured there is great danger of the fracture becoming compound, since the sharp end of a fragment may easily pierce the skin, practically the only soft tissue covering the shin bone along the greater part of its length.

CAUSES.—The bones of the leg may be fractured by direct or by indirect violence. An example of the former type of violence is seen when a wheel passes over the leg. Both bones are likely to be broken ; more rarely the tibia alone is fractured. Indirect violence is often the cause of a spiral fracture of the lower third of the tibia and, concurrently, of the upper third of the fibula : it is especially common in children when the leg or foot is twisted in falling. Fracture of the fibula alone occurs most commonly near the lower end of the bone. It is almost invariably caused by indirect violence—for example, in stepping off the kerb and forcibly everting the foot. Such a fracture is referred to as a Pott's fracture when associated with tearing of the ligaments on the inner side of the ankle joint.   (Fig 55.)

SYMPTOMS AND SIGNS.—The usual evidences of fracture are present, but the symptoms and signs vary somewhat according to the site of the fracture. If only one bone is broken the other bone acts as a natural splint, and the signs of fracture will be less evident. There is localized pain and partial loss of power in the limb; occasionally there is the sensation of something having snapped or given way. Tenderness, bruising, swelling and deformity are usually present. Unnatural mobility and crepitus may be detected, but the ambulance man must never make the slightest attempt to discover these signs when a fracture of the tibia is suspected, because he may so easily render such a fracture compound. A fracture of the fibula near its lower end is generally associated with tearing of the ligaments on the inner aspect of the ankle joint, and the foot is usually somewhat everted. There is often, however, so much swelling around the ankle joint that the fracture may easily be overlooked.

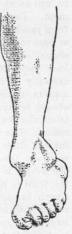

FIG. 55.

The warning which was given regarding fractures in the region of the wrist joint applies with equal force to the region of the ankle joint : every case in which there is the slightest suspicion of a fracture must be treated as such.

TREATMENT.—Lay the patient upon his back and endeavour to keep him quiet and comfortable. When the tibia is fractured the greatest care must be taken in handling the limb, since even the weight of the foot, if suddenly allowed to fall backwards, may cause the bone to pierce the skin. Whenever possible, obtain the help of two assistants : one to hold the foot and steady the lower portion of the limb, the other to steady the splints during their application by the ambulance man. The assistant will grasp the foot in the same manner as was described in the case of fracture of the femur, and he will endeavour to keep it steady at right angles to the leg and with its outer border vertical to the ground. At the same time he will exert very gentle extension upon the lower fragment. Two splints are required. Each should extend from just beyond the heel to the upper end of the thigh, or at least to beyond the knee joint. The width of each splint should equal as nearly as possible the thickness of the knee joint from front to back. These splints must be carefully padded, and applied to the outer and inner aspects of the limb : if only one splint is available, it should be applied to the outer side of the limb. Five triangular bandages folded narrow are used to fix the splints. The first three bandages secure the splints to the injured limb and are applied by the double loop-tie method ; the first is placed just above the site of fracture, the second is placed just below the site of fracture, and the third is placed near the upper end of the thigh ; the fourth bandage is applied just above the knees, passes round both legs, and includes the outer splint ; the fifth bandage is applied in a figure of eight fashion, in order to keep the feet together, in the same manner as was described under the treatment of fractured femur. With the exception of the last bandage, all the knots are tied off over the outer splint. (Plate XVI., B.)

FRACTURE OF THE TARSUS, METATARSUS AND PHALANGES.

CAUSES.—Direct violence, such as the crushing force of a heavy wheel, is commonly the cause of a fracture involving the bones of the foot. When the foot is injured by a wheel passing over it or by some heavy object falling upon it, the soft tissues are often so severely damaged that a compound fracture results. Less commonly, one of the bones of the foot is fractured by indirect violence as the result of jumping from a height on to the foot. The calcaneus or bone of the heel is especially liable to fracture in this way.

SYMPTOMS AND SIGNS.—There is usually pain and partial loss of power in the affected foot. Tenderness, swelling, deformity, discoloration, bruising or wounding may all be present ; crepitus and unnatural mobility are easily detected in fracture of the phalanges.

TREATMENT.—Place the patient in a comfortable position, preferably lying upon his back. Carefully remove the boot and stocking, if necessary cutting the seams or lacing of the boot. Apply a dressing to any wound or abrasion which may be present. Procure a splint of the same width as the foot, and long enough to extend from the heel to the toes. Pad the splint, and fix it to the sole of the foot by means of a triangular bandage folded narrow. The centre of the bandage is placed over the instep, and the ends are passed round the splint under the foot, where they are crossed and then carried backwards behind the heel, and finally passed over the instep again in a figure of eight fashion. The ends are tied off under the foot on the splint. The limb should be elevated, but the feet should not be tied together.

CHAPTER VIII.

DISLOCATIONS, SPRAINS AND STRAINS.

A DISLOCATION is the displacement of the articular surface of one or more of the bones which take part in the formation of a joint. In a dislocation the fibrous

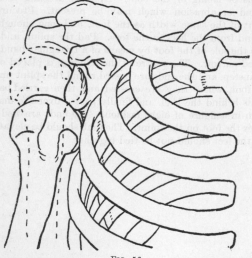

FIG. 56.

capsule of the joint is torn, the ends of the bones are partially or completely separated, and the surrounding ligaments, tendons and blood vessels may also be ruptured. Owing to the tearing of small blood vessels, bleeding occurs into the soft tissues under the skin, and is evidenced by the great swelling which soon develops around the joint ; for the same reason considerable discoloration of the surrounding skin appears at a later stage. Less commonly a large nerve or vessel is pressed upon : this happens not infrequently when the humerus is dislocated at the shoulder joint. Dislocations are most commonly seen affecting the shoulder, the elbow, the jaw, the hip and the finger joints. (Fig. 56.)

CAUSES OF DISLOCATIONS.—For the purposes of first-aid we are only concerned with dislocations which are produced by violence, either external or muscular, but it is important to remember that certain dislocations are present at birth, notably of the hip joint, while others are caused by disease. The great majority of dislocations result from external violence, as in severe twisting injuries and falls when a limb is doubled up under the body in an awkward manner. Dislocations resulting from excessive muscular violence are seen occasionally when an unusual degree of movement is suddenly performed by an individual ; thus in yawning the lower jaw may be dislocated.

VARIETIES OF DISLOCATION.

1. COMPLETE.—A complete dislocation is one in which the articular surfaces of the bones are completely separated.

2. INCOMPLETE.—An incomplete dislocation is one in which the articular surfaces of the bones are displaced, but not completely separated from one another.

3. COMPLICATED.—A complicated dislocation is one which is associated with injury to some important adjacent structure, such as a large nerve or a blood vessel.

4. COMPOUND.—A compound dislocation is one attended by a wound of the overlying soft parts, the wound being f such a nature as to place the outer air in communication '' the cavity of the joint.

5. A FRACTURE-DISLOCATION.—A fracture-dislocation is one in which the articular end of the bone is fractured as well as dislocated.

SYMPTOMS AND SIGNS OF A DISLOCATION.—There is usually the history of an injury or of some excessive and unusual muscular action. Pain is felt about the affected joint, and is greatly increased by any attempt at movement. Occasionally numbness is complained of in the limb below the injured joint. There is complete loss of power, and the patient is unable to move the limb at the affected joint. Swelling, tenderness and deformity are invariably present. The joint is more or less fixed in a characteristically abnormal position, and its mobility is greatly restricted : shortening of the limb may be apparent. Crepitus is only elicited when a fracture is present at the site of the dislocation. The patient may suffer from some degree of surgical shock.

When a joint is injured there is often great difficulty in deciding whether a dislocation or a fracture has occurred. While it is entirely outwith the scope of an ambulance man to carry out any elaborate examination or to make a diagnosis, it is important for him to remember certain rules.

(a) If, for any reason, a fracture is suspected, the case must be treated as one of fracture without further examination or delay.

(b) A dislocation and a fracture quite often co-exist.

(c) In a dislocation there is absence or limitation of mobility at a place where mobility should exist, whereas in a fracture unnatural mobility is present when there should be rigidity.

TREATMENT OF DISLOCATIONS.—Place the patient in the position which he finds most comfortable. Support the affected joint or limb in whatever position gives most relief. For this purpose a triangular bandage, a sling or even a splint may be required, and cold water cloths be applied if pain is severe. Every case of dislocation should be seen by a doctor at the earliest possible moment, since the longer a dislocation is left untended the more difficult does its reduction become. The ambulance man must never attempt to reduce a dislocation except in the case of the lower jaw when external violence can be excluded as a cause of the condition. If there is any evidence whatever that a fracture is present, the case must be appropriately treated as one of fracture.

DISLOCATION OF THE LOWER JAW.

This accident is a relatively common form of dislocation, and in most cases it is the result of some unusually sudden or severe muscular action, such as yawning or excessive laughter. The condyle of the mandible on one or on both sides is forced forwards and slips out of the glenoid fossa, the depression on the base of the skull which normally retains it ; the mouth remains open, and cannot be closed ; speech is almost impossible, and saliva dribbles from the open mouth. If only one side is dislocated there is particularly marked deformity of the face. Pain is felt over the temporo-mandibular joint on the affected side or sides.

TREATMENT.—In the case of a dislocated jaw the ambulance man, so long as he is satisfied that the condition did not result from external violence, is permitted to depart from the general rule that " no attempt is to be made to reduce a dislocation." He may attempt to replace the dislocated bone in the following manner. Place the patient sitting in a strong chair with his back upright, and stand in front of him. Protect the thumbs with a thick piece of towelling or other similar cloth, and place a thumb thus protected along the alveolar or upper margin of the mandible on each side ; with the thumbs in this position exert firm pressure in a downward direction, and at the same time endeavour to direct the lower jaw backwards into its proper place. If the condyle does not slip back quite easily after applying steady pressure for several minutes, no further attempt should be made to reduce the dislocation.

It is important to remember that any case of dislocated jaw must be seen by a doctor as early as possible, whether it has been reduced or not. If the ambulance man is successful in the use of the method described above, he should apply two triangular bandages folded narrow so as to keep the jaw in position. The centre of one bandage is placed under the chin and the ends tied over the top of the head : the centre of the other bandage is placed in front of the chin and its ends are tied behind the neck. Finally, it should be clearly understood that a dislocated jaw may be left entirely alone for several hours, and little harm will occur while awaiting medical assistance. It is only because of the alarm which this dislocation causes, and the ease and safety with which it can usually be replaced, that an ambulance man is allowed to attempt reduction.

SPRAINS.

A sprain is the result of a sudden violent stretching of the soft tissues surrounding a joint. The articular surfaces of the bones are moved beyond their normal limit in one or other direction, but the force is not sufficient to separate or dislocate the bones. The ligaments of the joint and the surrounding muscles, tendons and vessels are overstretched or even torn ; the part soon becomes greatly swollen and discoloured on account of the bleeding which occurs into the soft tissues under the skin ; swelling of the joint may also be caused by bleeding within its capsule.

CAUSES.—A sprain is usually produced by a sudden severe twisting injury. It may also be caused by a fall or by any accident which results in a sudden violent movement of the joint. Sprains are most commonly seen affecting the ankle, the wrist, the shoulder and the knee joints.

SYMPTOMS AND SIGNS.—There is usually the history of an accident involving some sudden violent movement of a joint. Pain, increased by almost any movement, is complained of around the injured joint. Loss of power may be partial or complete. Swelling is invariably present, and may be slight if the joint is examined immediately after the accident, but the swelling increases very rapidly. Tenderness is present over the torn ligaments, and, at a later stage, discoloration of the skin may occur; this latter sign may extend to a considerable distance from the actual site of injury. Apart from the swelling, there is no deformity of the affected part.

TREATMENT.—The treatment of a sprain is principally directed towards the protection of the damaged ligaments or tendons from further stretching and the limitation of bleeding and effusion into and around the joint. This is done by supporting the part in the most comfortable position. The affected region should be firmly bandaged as soon as possible, and cold water cloths should be applied. Absolute rest is essential, and in order to secure this rest it may be necessary to apply a splint and to elevate the injured part. In the case of the upper limb, it is usually sufficient to place the forearm in a large sling after a firm bandage has been applied.

SPRAINED ANKLE.—This is an extremely common accident, and it is frequently associated with fracture of the lower end of the tibia on its inner side or of the lower end of the fibula. Whenever a fracture is suspected the patient should be treated for the more serious condition.

TREATMENT.—(a) If the accident happens out of doors —at some distance from home or where assistance is unavailable—keep the shoe or the boot on the foot, lace it firmly, and bandage the foot as tightly as possible with a triangular bandage folded narrow in the figure of eight fashion. The swelling will thus be limited, and greater comfort secured. The patient may thus be enabled to walk with support for some distance to a conveyance.

(b) If the accident occurs at home, the first thing to do is to remove the boot or shoe and elevate the part. At the same time the joint should be bandaged firmly and cold water cloths applied.

STRAINS.

The word strain usually refers to the result of excessive action on the part of a muscle or tendon. After very severe muscular exertion we may speak of a strained muscle or a strained tendon; similarly when a joint has been used to excess the joint may be strained, or some particular ligament of that joint may be strained. If a muscle or a tendon is completely torn across, the condition may be referred to as a ruptured muscle or a ruptured tendon. The large tendon at the back of the heel, known as the tendo Achillis, is quite frequently strained or ruptured while playing such games as badminton or tennis. When this accident occurs the patient experiences a sudden sharp pain in the region of the tendon, he is conscious of something having snapped in the leg, and he either falls to the ground or finds that he is quite unable to walk.

TREATMENT.—When a muscle is strained, the limb should immediately be placed at rest in the most comfortable position; no further treatment is required, apart from supporting the injured part. If a muscle or a tendon is ruptured, it should be placed in such a position as will relax the muscle and allow its ends to come together. Cloths soaked in cold water may be applied if the pain is severe.

CHAPTER IX.

THE CIRCULATORY SYSTEM.

THE circulatory system may be defined as that system whereby blood is conveyed to the tissues of the body and whereby it is re-collected for oxygenation and redistribution. The mechanism of the circulation of the blood has been understood only since the middle of the seventeenth century. Although many attempts were made to explain how blood circulated through the body, attempts by Greek, Roman, Arabic and mediæval physicians including the celebrated Leonardo da Vinci, the actual discovery falls to the credit of William Harvey, a distinguished English physician who flourished during the reign of Charles I.

The main organ of the circulation is the heart. It is a hollow, muscular organ which is placed in the thorax. To gain an appreciation of the situation and size of the heart, the reader might close his left fist, hold his left arm close to his side, bend his forearm and place the fist so that the middle bones of his fingers are just directly over the breast bone and the lower margin of the hand is just at the lower end of the breast bone. The closed fist over the chest represents roughly the situation and size of the heart. The fist will cover an area bounded above by the third rib; on the right by the right border of the sternum; and on the left by a curved line drawn, with its convexity upwards, from the junction of the third rib with the sternum to a point in the space between the fifth and sixth ribs 3½ inches from the mid-line of the body. The boundaries described above are the surface markings of the heart. The apex beat may be felt in adults in the fifth interspace; in children, however, the apex beat is usually in the fourth interspace.

The heart is divided into four chambers, two auricles or atria and two ventricles. There is a right and a left auricle and a right and a left ventricle. The auricles are the upper chambers and the ventricles are the lower. It is to be remembered that there is direct communication between the auricle and ventricle of the same side but blood never flows directly from the one side of the heart to the other. To make the position clear, blood flows from auricles to ventricles through orifices guarded by one-way valves, which prevent a flow in the reverse direction; owing to an impenetrable septum or wall between the right and left sides of the heart, blood never flows directly from auricle to auricle or from ventricle to ventricle.

The walls of the heart chambers are made up of muscle which has the characteristic power of contraction and relaxation, thus rendering the various chambers of the heart large or small. Contraction and relaxation takes place in a regular way so that a pump-like action—referred to as pulsation—occurs. Simultaneous contraction of both auricles, immediately before simultaneous contraction of both ventricles, causes blood to pass from auricles to ventricles. When the ventricles are filled they immediately contract, and, were it not for the presence of valves, the blood would be driven back again into the auricles. These valves are flap-like structures which, projecting downwards into the ventricles, are attached at their broad upper ends to the orifices between the auricles and ventricles, and at their lower free ends by strong cord-like strands to finger-like processes of muscle which project up from the lower parts of the ventricles. The action, therefore, of the contracting ventricles is to force blood against these flaps and to pull their free ends together by the contraction of the finger-like muscular processes acting on the cords. This mechanism completely closes the orifices between auricles and ventricles. Between the right auricle and the right ventricle there are three flaps or cusps which form the tricuspid valve, and similarly between the left auricle and ventricle there are two cusps which make up the mitral valve. When the ventricles contract, the blood which they contain is forced through orifices into great blood vessels. Here again a valvular arrangement exists to prevent blood from flowing back into the ventricles when they relax. These valves each have three cusps which are pocket-like. In the great vessels leaving the heart the blood under pressure forces back the cusps, so that their free edges meet and prevent a flowing back of blood from these great vessels into the ventricles when the latter relax. It will be apparent that the ventricles have to work against the pressure existing in the vessels ; they are therefore provided with very thick muscular walls. On the other hand, the thin auricular walls have merely to drive blood into fully relaxed ventricles.

The left ventricle empties its contents into the main artery, the aorta, which, through its various branches, distributes blood to all parts of the body with the exception of the essential tissue of the lungs. The orifice of the aorta is guarded by the aortic valve, the function of which has been described. In a similar way the right ventricle empties its contents into the pulmonary artery, the valve of which is termed the pulmonic valve. The pulmonary artery conveys blood to the lungs. The heart wall itself has a rich blood supply of its own in spite of the fact that its cavities are filled with blood. This blood supply comes through the coronary arteries, which are the first branches of the aorta, and returns by the coronary veins, which empty into the right auricle. To complete the anatomical survey of the heart the pericardium and the endocardium require consideration. The pericardium is a sac-like membrane which envelops the heart, while the endocardium is the lining membrane of the heart cavities. Further, the cusps of the valves are merely fibrous tissue covered by endocardium. The vessels of the body are lined by endothelium which is continuous with the endocardium.

THE CIRCULATION OF THE BLOOD.—Let us follow the course of blood through the complete cycle of the circulation. Pure blood is constantly being pumped from the left ventricle into the aorta through the aortic valve. With each contraction of the left ventricle some two to three ounces of blood pass into the aorta. Normally this occurs 72 times per minute, and corresponds to the pulse rate as felt at the wrist. The blood, driven into the aorta at pressure, closes the aortic valve and flows out through the aorta to its branches, the arteries, which divide and subdivide until the capillaries are reached. These latter are the finest vessels in the body and are present everywhere. They join up to form veins which convey the blood back to the main veins of the body, the superior vena cava and the inferior vena cava. The superior vena cava collects blood from the upper parts of the body and the inferior from the trunk and lower extremities ; both enter the right auricle. This blood entering the right auricle, after its journey through the body, is deficient in oxygen, overladen with carbon dioxide and is called impure blood. The contracting right auricle passes blood on through the open tricuspid valve into the right ventricle. The right ventricle, when full, contracts, the tricuspid valve closes, and blood is forced through the pulmonic valve into the pulmonary artery. The action of the pulmonic valve is exactly similar to that of the aortic and closes when the ventricle relaxes. The pulmonary artery divides into two to convey blood to the lungs. The artery to each lung branches and rebranches to form a capillary system through which blood passes on to the pulmonary veins. These are four in number and two from each lung convey blood to the left auricle. While circulating through the lung capillaries, blood becomes pure by giving up its excess of carbon dioxide and replenishing its store of oxygen. We have now only to follow blood through the mitral valve, from the left auricle to the left ventricle, to complete the entire circulation.

The reader may be puzzled by the complexity of the mechanism which keeps blood circulating through the body. It may seem to him to be an aimless, complicated system. Let him remember that, for the human being to exist, there are two essential functions necessary: first, the distribution of oxygen to all the tissues of the body, and, second, the elimination of waste products. Nature has devised a means whereby there are two primary circulatory systems. They are the systemic circulation and the pulmonary circulation. The systemic circulation refers to the course of blood from the left side of the heart through the body as a whole to the right side of the heart; the pulmonary circulation refers to the course of blood from the right side of the heart through the lungs to the left side of the heart. The systemic circulation exists for the distribution of pure blood, which has just been replenished with oxygen, to the tissues of the body and the re-collection of that blood now deficient in oxygen. The pulmonary circulation exists for the conveyance of impure blood to the lungs in order that it may become rich in oxygen once more and in order that it may part with its excess of carbon dioxide. Not only does the pulmonary circulation distribute blood to the lungs for purification, but it also conveys pure blood from the lungs back to the heart. (Fig. 57.)

THE BLOOD VESSELS.—Some description of the blood vessels of the body is now demanded. With the exception of the capillaries all blood vessels which carry blood away from the heart are termed arteries and all blood vessels which carry blood towards the heart are termed veins. Capillaries are very fine vessels which connect the arteries to the veins. The direction in which the blood is flowing in a blood vessel at once determines its nature. The aorta

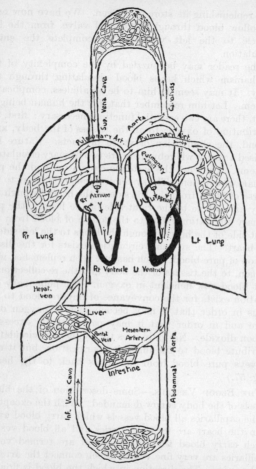

FIG. 57. DIAGRAMMATIC SCHEME OF THE CIRCULATION OF THE BLOOD.

is an artery because it conveys blood away from the heart ; the vessel between the right ventricle and the lungs is an artery for the same reason. The aorta carries pure blood, the pulmonary artery carries impure blood. We can now make a further generalization by saying that all the arteries of the systemic circulation carry pure blood while the pulmonary arteries contain impure blood. The inferior vena cava is a vein because it carries blood towards the heart ; so are the vessels between the lungs and the left side of the heart, veins, for the same reason. The inferior vena cava carries impure blood while the pulmonary veins carry pure blood. We may again make another general statement. All the veins of the systemic circulation carry impure blood while the veins of the pulmonary circulation carry pure blood.

THE ARTERIES.—Ancient anatomists, on dissecting the body, found that these vessels were empty ; they believed, erroneously, that the arteries contained air and accordingly the name artery was applied. The misconception was completely dispelled when William Harvey, in making his momentous discovery, described their true function. It has been stated that the arteries carry blood away from the heart ; as a consequence of this function it will be seen that these blood vessels have to withstand great and sudden alterations in the pressure of blood. Every time the ventricles contract they drive blood into the arteries of the systemic and pulmonary circulations. Each beat of the ventricles means a sudden increase in the pressure of blood in the arteries. The arteries are therefore thick and have a considerable amount of elastic tissue in their walls. This amount of elastic tissue, which is the most admirable tissue for taking sudden alterations in pressure, diminishes in amount as the arteries become smaller. In addition to elastic tissue there is also visceral muscle in the arterial wall. By the contraction of the visceral muscle the bore of the tube diminishes and consequently less blood flows through the vessel. Relaxation of the muscle means that the calibre of the vessel is increased and that more blood can find its way through the channel. Visceral muscle is the prominent constituent of the walls of the small arteries or arterioles. A blanching of the skin occurring suddenly, as when a person gets a severe fright, is accounted for by the contraction of the muscle tissue in the arterioles of the skin. A blush is accounted for by a relaxation of visceral muscle in the same vessels and consequently allowing a greater flow of blood in these vessels.

Another consequence of the regularly contracting ventricles pumping blood into the arteries is that these sudden alterations in pressure give rise to waves of pressure which pass through the arteries. The regular succession of waves of pressure may be felt not only at the wrist in the radial artery, but also in the superficial arteries of the body, and is known as the arterial pulse. It is a direct indication of the functioning of the heart muscle, and consequently the facts relating to the production of the arterial pulse must be borne in mind. It is enough here simply to indicate that the normal arterial pulse rate is 72 per minute and that it corresponds in the normal individual to the frequency of the heart beat; references will be made to its importance in various emergencies when they are being considered in detail.

THE VEINS.—As has been indicated before, the veins are those vessels which carry blood back to the heart. These particular vessels are not called upon to withstand the great changes in pressure to which the arteries of the body are subject. It is therefore unnecessary that the veins should have the same amount of elastic tissue and visceral muscle composing their walls. We find accordingly that the wall of a vein is comparatively thin, is poor in elastic and muscular tissue, but is rich in fibrous tissue. In the circulatory system the propulsive force, initiated at the heart, driving blood through the vessels diminishes in passing from the large arteries through the capillaries into the veins. This attenuated force necessitates the presence of one-way valves in the veins, in order that any tendency for blood to flow in the reverse direction to its normal course may be overcome. This tendency is all the more marked in the veins of the legs; since, when the individual rises to the erect posture, there is the addition of the weight of a column of blood stretching from the foot to the level of the right auricle. When there is a liability for back pressure on the veins to occur, the valves which are pocket-like structures may become incompetent, and, as a consequence, varicose veins result.

THE PULSE.—The arterial pulse may be felt in any of the superficial arteries of the body. It is usual to feel this pulse at the wrist, where the radial artery is comparatively superficial and lies upon the radius. We are able to feel the actual pulsation in the vessel because the arterial wall is elastic. The pulse is the transmission of a wave of pressure initiated at the heart. It may be felt in situations other than at the wrist; for example, pulsation may be felt in the neck over the carotid arteries, in the temple and at the ankle just behind the internal malleolus. In severe injuries to the leg or thigh, an attempt should be made to feel the pulse on the inner side of the ankle in order to determine the state of the circulation below the site of the injury. Here it is necessary to compare the pulse at the ankle of the injured side with the pulse at the other ankle. There is one correct and many wrong ways of feeling the radial pulse. The thumb should be placed behind the wrist on the radial side and the index, middle and ring fingers should be placed over the line of the radial artery. The pulse must not be felt by the observer's thumb because confusion may arise owing to the fact that his own pulse may be felt in the thumb.

The following observations in feeling the pulse may prove useful under certain conditions: the rate, the rhythm, and the quality of the pulse.

THE PULSE RATE in the normal individual while sitting

is 72 beats per minute. When a man rises to his feet his pulse may become slightly faster, and when he is at rest in bed or asleep his pulse may be slower. Athletes have often very slow pulses. It is not to be imagined that, because a strong man has a pulse rate of 60 beats per minute, he is necessarily ill : nor is it to be thought that, because a young girl, in a state of emotional excitement, has a pulse rate of 100, she is in danger. The main factors to be considered in assessing the value of the pulse rate are the age—in children the pulse is normally faster than in the adult—and the state of the individual at the moment ; the pulse rate may be elevated during emotional strain from whatever cause, and after exercise the pulse rate may be doubled in the normal person.

THE RHYTHM OF THE PULSE in the normal person is regular and the length of each beat, as well as the interval between consecutive beats, is constant. The heart beats are directly reflected in the arterial pulse, and therefore if the heart be beating irregularly from some cause this irregularity will be felt in the pulse and may suggest heart disease.

THE QUALITY OF THE PULSE normally is constant with reference to each individual beat. Notice should be taken as to whether the pulse is strong or feeble. The quality may be ascertained by the pressure necessary to obliterate the pulse and this pressure may be taken roughly as an indication of the efficiency of the heart muscle.

THE BLOOD.

The blood is a tissue apparently fluid but having a proportion of solid material in it. The solid material is in the form of cells, the blood corpuscles, while the fluid is of a very special nature and is termed the blood plasma. The plasma consists of serum, together with fibrinogen, a fluid substance, which when subjected to any influence causing clotting of the blood is converted into a solid material called fibrin. When a quantity of blood is exposed in a glass vessel for a period of time, the solid material, forming a clot, will separate out, leaving behind straw-coloured serum. The clot is formed of two things, the fibrinous network which comes from the plasma, and the cellular elements of the blood which are found in the meshes of the network of fibrin.

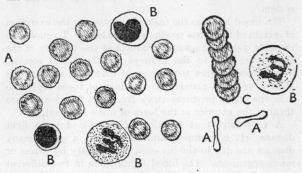

FIG. 58.

A. Red blood corpuscles.
B. White blood corpuscles.
C. Red blood corpuscles in rouleaux.

The cells of the blood are of two very distinct types. The red cells are small discs without a nucleus which gain their colour from their principal content, hæmoglobin. The white cells are of various sizes and shapes and have each a nucleus. (Fig. 58.)

The principal function of the blood is to carry oxygen by the arteries to the tissues and to transport carbon dioxide by the veins to the lungs. The red blood corpuscles are responsible for the carriage of oxygen to the tissues. The hæmoglobin which they contain fastens on to the available oxygen as blood passes through the lungs. This oxygen is readily given up to the tissues in the transport of the

F

blood through the systemic circulation. The carbon dioxide which comes from the tissues is carried to the lungs for liberation by the blood plasma.

Possibly the next most important function of the blood is to transport nourishment to the various organs and tissues of the body. Here the blood plasma is mainly responsible. It carries in solution the simplest of food stuffs which have been carefully prepared by the digestive system.

The blood has also the task of assisting in the excretion of certain of the waste products of the body. To quote one example, part of the waste products of the activity of the liver is carried to the kidneys by the blood stream. When blood reaches the organs of excretion such as the kidneys or sweat glands it is the duty of these organs to take the waste products away from the blood and pass them to the exterior in the form of urine or sweat.

A very important function of the blood is to fight disease. It is common knowledge that a great many diseases are due to the invasion of the body by germs or micro-organisms. The blood fights these in two different ways ; firstly by the white cells swallowing up whatever germs they can, and secondly by the development of certain substances in the blood plasma. Some of these substances make the germs palatable to the white cell, while others tend to counteract the poisons which are elaborated by germs. This last kind of substance is familiar to many in the form of diphtheria antitoxin.

The last function of the blood which we will notice particularly is that which prevents its own loss to the body. This function is that of clotting. When a wound is inflicted to the effusion of blood there is the simultaneous liberation of a special substance which is the product of injured tissue. This substance activates fibrinogen and there is formed a fine network of fibrin, in the interstices of which blood corpuscles become enclosed. The effect of the formation of such a clot is to seal up the wound, to

prevent further bleeding and the entrance of foreign
material which might be of a harmful nature.

ANATOMY OF THE CIRCULATION.

THE HEART.—This organ has already been referred to as
the main organ of the circulation and described as a hollow
muscular structure enclosed in the pericardium. It is
somewhat conical in shape, lies in the thorax between the
lungs and is disposed in such a manner that about one-
third of it lies on the right side and two-thirds on the left
side of the median plane. It is situated obliquely behind
the sternum and the adjoining rib cartilages, and is partly
covered by the lungs. Its base, formed mainly by the
left auricle and partly by the right auricle, is directed
upwards, backwards and to the right. From this aspect
of the heart spring the great vessels which help to support
it. The apex, formed by the left ventricle, is directed
downwards, forwards and to the left, so that it comes to
lie behind the fifth left intercostal space about $3\frac{1}{2}$ inches
from the middle line. During life each contraction of the
heart causes its apex to beat or pulsate against the inside
of the chest wall at this point. This accounts for the
visible apex beat or the cardiac impulse. The inferior
surface of the heart, formed mainly by the ventricles, rests
upon the diaphragm : the anterior surface is formed principally by the right ventricle and the right auricle : the
right margin is formed by the right auricle : the left
margin is formed by the left ventricle and to a slight
extent by the left auricle.

THE CHAMBERS OF THE HEART.—The right auricle is
situated on the right side of the heart and forms the
anterior portion of its base. It has two large openings at
its upper and lower posterior angles for the superior and
inferior venae cavae respectively. The right ventricle
occupies the greater part of the anterior surface of the

heart and forms its lower border resting upon the diaphragm. Towards the right side of the base of this ventricle lies the auriculo-ventricular orifice guarded by the tricuspid valve with its three large flaps. Through it blood passes from the right auricle to the right ventricle. Above and to the left it becomes continuous with the pulmonary artery by an opening which is guarded by three semi-lunar cusps—the pulmonary valve, through which the blood passes from the right ventricle into the pulmonary artery. (Plate XVII.)

The left auricle lies posteriorly at the base of the heart and is inclined towards its left side, being obscured from the front by the commencement of the aorta and the pulmonary artery. On each side there are two openings through which blood from the pulmonary veins enters this chamber. These four orifices have no valves. The left auricle is smaller than the right auricle and its walls are thicker. The left ventricle forms the left border of the heart, its apex and the greater part of its under surface. At its base there are two orifices. The mitral or bicuspid valve is situated behind and towards the left: it has two large valvular flaps. Through it blood passes from the left auricle to the left ventricle. The aortic opening lies in front and towards the right: it is guarded by three semi-lunar cusps which form the aortic valve. Through it blood passes from the left ventricle into the aorta.

THE BLOOD VESSELS.—In the performance of first-aid work it is essential that the ambulance pupil should be acquainted with the position and general arrangement of the main blood vessels of the body. Life may be lost in a very few minutes if an individual. lacking this anatomical knowledge, fails to do immediately what is required of him when he is confronted with a case of haemorrhage from a large vessel.

THE ARTERIES.—The aorta is the main artery of the systemic circulation and gives off branches to the head and neck, a branch to each upper limb, branches to the organs of the trunk and ultimately divides into two branches for the supply of the pelvis and the lower extremities. It arises from the left ventricle, passes upwards for a short distance along the right side of the vertebral column, curves horizontally across the column and continues backwards and downwards along the left side of the column to the level of the fourth lumbar vertebra which corresponds on the surface of the abdomen to a point just below and to the left of the umbilicus or navel.

The aorta is divisible into the following portions : the ascending aorta, the aortic arch and the descending aorta with its thoracic and abdominal portions above and below the diaphragm.

The ascending aorta gives off only the coronary arteries which supply the heart muscle. The aortic arch gives off the innominate artery (the common trunk of origin of the right subclavian and the right common carotid arteries), the left common carotid artery and the left subclavian artery. The thoracic portion of the descending aorta gives off intercostal branches which supply the chest wall. It also supplies branches to the pericardium, the air passages of the lungs (bronchi), the gullet and the diaphragm.

The abdominal aorta gives off branches which supply the alimentary tract and its associated digestive organs in addition to the kidneys, the liver and the spleen. There are also lumbar branches from this part of the aorta which supply the lower trunk walls. The terminal portion of the aorta divides into two large trunks—the right and left common iliac arteries which are of equal size and diverge in a downward and outward direction. At the junction of the last lumbar vertebra with the sacrum each common iliac artery divides into an external and an internal iliac artery : the former supplying the greater part of the lower extremity, the latter the walls of the pelvis and the organs contained in that cavity.

The principal branches of the aorta may be conveniently

classed as those of the head and neck, those of the upper extremity and those of the lower extremity. The branches of the aorta which supply the various organs of the thorax, the abdomen and the pelvis are of very little practical importance in first-aid work and therefore require no further description.

THE ARTERIES OF THE HEAD AND NECK.

These are the common carotid arteries and their branches; the right common carotid arises from the innominate artery whereas the left comes directly off the aortic arch. (Plate XVIII.)

THE COMMON CAROTID on each side ascends in the neck in a line from the sterno-clavicular joint towards a point just behind the angle of the jaw. At the level of the thyroid cartilage (Adam's Apple) each divides into an internal and an external carotid artery.

THE INTERNAL CAROTID courses deeply and enters the base of the skull to supply the brain.

THE EXTERNAL CAROTID continues in the line of the common carotid as far as the condyle of the lower jaw. It lies nearer the surface and gives off three important branches, the facial, the temporal and the occipital.

THE FACIAL passes upwards and forwards over the side of the lower jaw about one inch in front of the angle. It supplies the front and lower portion of the face.

THE TEMPORAL passes upwards over the region of the temple to supply the side of the face and scalp. It lies about one finger's breadth in front of the opening of the ear as it ascends across the zygomatic process of the temporal bone.

THE OCCIPITAL runs upwards and backwards about two fingers' breadth behind the back of the ear. It supplies blood to the occipital region or the back of the head.

THE ARTERIES OF THE UPPER EXTREMITIES (Plates I. and II.).—These are the right and left subclavian arteries which are continued through the armpit and arm as the axillary and brachial arteries respectively. In the forearm we find the radial and ulnar arteries the terminal branches of the brachial. The right subclavian arises from the innominate artery whereas the left subclavian comes directly off the aortic arch.

THE SUBCLAVIAN on each side runs laterally from the sterno-clavicular joint, arches slightly upwards and crosses over the upper surface of the first rib at a point just behind the middle of the clavicle. From this point the subclavian artery continues into the axilla or armpit as the axillary artery.

THE AXILLARY passes over the apex of the axilla and along its outer wall into the arm where it becomes the brachial. When the arm is held at right angles to the body the axillary artery follows the first part of a line drawn from the middle of the clavicle to the centre of the bend of the elbow.

THE BRACHIAL extends downwards along the inner side of the arm, then inclines forwards following the inner border of the biceps muscle to a point about one inch below the centre of the bend of the elbow. There it divides into the radial and ulnar arteries. When the arm is raised horizontally from the side the brachial follows the lower part of the line given for the axillary. In the middle of the arm it can easily be compressed against the humerus by applying pressure from the medial side.

THE RADIAL runs along the outer side of the forearm towards the thumb. Immediately above the wrist it lies superficially and it has already been mentioned that the pulse can be felt most conveniently at this point. The radial artery then curves round the outer side of the lower end of the radius, crosses the side of the carpus and reappears in front to traverse the palm and join with the deep branch of the ulnar artery. Just before the radial turns towards the back of the carpus it gives off a superficial volar or palmar branch which anastomoses or joins with the lower end of the ulnar artery.

THE ULNAR passes down the inner side of the forearm to the wrist where it lies superficially. It is continued into the palm of the hand where it ends by joining the superficial volar branch of the radial. In the palm of the hand the ulnar gives off its deep branch which joins the terminal portion of the radial artery.

THE PALMAR ARCHES are two in number and are formed by the anastomoses of the radial and ulnar arteries in the palm of the hand. These arches give off branches to supply the fingers.

THE DEEP PALMAR ARCH is mainly formed by the terminal portion of the radial which unites with the deep branch of the ulnar to form an arterial arch. It lies deeply under tendons and upon the bases of the metacarpal bones.

THE SUPERFICIAL PALMAR ARCH is formed mainly by the terminal portion of the ulnar which joins with the superficial volar branch of the radial to form a second arterial arch lying superficial to the tendons. It crosses the palm about one finger's breadth distal to the deep palmar arch. It may be marked upon the surface by drawing a line across the palm at the level of the outstretched thumb.

THE ARTERIES OF THE LOWER EXTREMITIES (Plate I.).

These are the external iliac arteries and their branches.

THE EXTERNAL ILIAC arises on each side from the common iliac artery of the same side and is the larger of

THE VEINS (Plates I. and II.).

In the practice of first-aid, anatomical knowledge of the veins is of less importance than it is in the case of the arteries. Therefore only a brief account of the more important veins will be given. The veins convey the blood back to the heart from the capillaries of every part of the body. As the blood commences on its return journey it flows through a continuous series of veins which become successively larger as the heart is approached.

The veins of the systemic circulation are distributed in such a manner that a superficial and a deep set of veins may be distinguished: the superficial veins lie immediately beneath the skin in the fatty layer superficial to the muscles; the deep veins accompany the arteries under cover of muscles and other structures. The superficial veins branch more frequently than the arteries, but they pursue a course which is less constant. They communicate with the deep veins by side branches, and the large venous trunks, which the superficial veins eventually form, also join the deep veins: in the case of the extremities this union occurs towards the proximal end of the limb. Thus it will be seen that blocking of a deep vein will lead to rapid engorgement of superficial veins. The deep veins run alongside of the arteries, and in the case of the largest vessels similar names are usually applied to both the artery and its accompanying vein; for example we have the femoral artery and vein.

All the blood from the head, the neck, the upper extremities and the thorax, with the exception of the lungs, is collected into one great venous trunk, the superior vena cava, which enters the right auricle at its posterior superior angle. Similarly, all the blood from the lower extremities, the pelvis and the abdomen, is collected into the inferior vena cava which joins the right auricle at its posterior inferior angle.

In the neck, on either side, there is a large deep vein,

PLATE XVII.

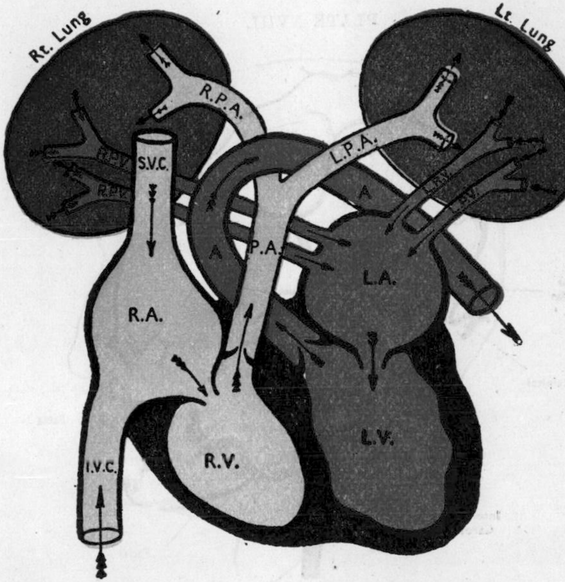

R.A.	=Right Auricle.	P.A.	=Pulmonary Artery.
R.V.	=Right Ventricle.	R.P.A.	=Right Pulmonary Artery.
L.A.	=Left Auricle.	L.P.A.	=Left Pulmonary Artery.
L.V.	=Left Ventricle.	A.	=Aorta.
I.V.C.	=Inferior Vena Cava.	R.P.V.	=Right Pulmonary Veins.
S.V.C.	=Superior Vena Cava.	L.P.V.	=Left Pulmonary Veins.

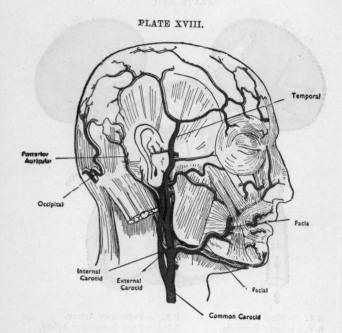

PLATE XVIII.

Temporal

Posterior
Auricular

Occipital

Facia

Internal
Carotid

External
Carotid

Facial

Common Carotid

the two branches into which the common iliac divi Each external iliac curves round inside the back wall the pelvis to the middle of the fold of the groin where passes over the middle of the pubic bone and enters t thigh to become the femoral artery.

THE FEMORAL passes down the front of the thigh, in clines to the inner side of the knee and enters the ham o back of the thigh where it is continued as the poplitea artery. The femoral extends from the middle of the fold of the groin to a point immediately behind the internal condyle of the femur.

THE POPLITEAL runs along the middle of the ham and behind the knee joint. Just below the bend of the knee it divides into two branches, the anterior and posterior tibial arteries.

THE ANTERIOR TIBIAL turns forwards between the two bones of the leg immediately below the point where the head of the fibula articulates with the tibia. It passes down the front of the leg but lies deeply until it reaches a point midway between the malleoli of the ankle : here it becomes more superficial and is continued over the upper surface of the foot as the dorsalis pedis artery.

THE POSTERIOR TIBIAL passes downwards and medial-wards in the back of the leg towards the inner side of the ankle. It then runs midway between the medial malleolus of the ankle and the inner border of the tendo Achillis and turns forwards into the sole of the foot where it divides into the medial and lateral plantar arteries which supply the toes and the sole of the foot.

THE PLANTAR ARCH.—It is of interest to note that an arterial arch is formed in the sole of the foot by the union of the terminal branch of the posterior tibial artery with the deep plantar branch of the dorsalis pedis. This arch is known as the plantar arch.

the internal jugular, which runs along the outer side of the common carotid artery and is represented on the surface by the same line which has already been given for that artery. It is not visible on the surface. There is also, on each side of the neck, a large superficial vein, the external jugular, which is frequently visible on the surface running along a line from the angle of the jaw to the middle of the clavicle.

In the upper extremity the basilic vein runs superficially along the medial side of the forearm to the arm, near the middle of which it passes deeply to run alongside of the brachial artery. In the arm this vein is called the basilic : in the armpit and below the clavicle it is continued as the axillary and the subclavian veins which follow the corresponding arteries. The cephalic vein is a large superficial vein which runs up the outer side of the forearm and arm to cross the front of the shoulder where it passes deeply to join the axillary vein. At the bend of the elbow the median cubital vein runs upwards and medially from the cephalic on the outer side to join the basilic on the medial side. It is usually visible upon the surface.

In the lower extremity there are two large superficial veins which are important mainly because of the frequency with which they become varicose. The great saphenous vein passes up the inner side of the leg and knee towards the front and inner aspect of the thigh to just below the fold of the groin where it unites with the deep femoral vein. On the outer side of the leg there is the small saphenous vein which, behind the knee, joins the deep vein accompanying the popliteal artery.

THE LYMPHATIC SYSTEM.

There is in addition to the circulation of blood through the body a circulation of clear fluid termed lymph. The fluid lymph is the product of the filtration of blood through the walls of the blood capillaries. This fluid bathes the tissues of the body generally and is collected by very fine hair-like tubes, the lymphatic vessels or lymph capillaries. These tubes drain into small bean-shaped glands, the lymph glands, the function of which will be described later. From the lymph glands fresh tubes arise which ultimately open into the veins at the root of the neck where the blood pressure is at its lowest. This system of lymphatics is general throughout the body and the lymphatic vessels largely follow the course taken by the veins. Germs which find their way into the body through a wound travel in many instances by the lymphatics. When the resistance of the lymphatic system is at its lowest the infection becomes general and a fatal issue terminates the condition. The lymphatic system resists by the multiplication of lymph cells in the lymph glands, these lymph cells having the faculty of fighting germs of disease by swallowing up the germs and digesting them. When an individual has a whitlow or a festering finger, the lymph glands swell, first inside the elbow and later in the armpit. Should the infection continue, the lymph glands above the clavicle may swell, and as a result of the poor resistance the germs find their way into the general circulation and very grave blood poisoning results. The lymph glands are the sentinels of the body to guard it against infection by germs.

There is another function of the lymphatic system. The lymphatics of the intestine drain into a special lymph bag, the receptaculum chyli. From this a duct or tube arises which passes through the diaphragm to become the thoracic duct. The thoracic duct ultimately opens into the left subclavian vein. This system is concerned with the absorption of fat from the intestine and it will be more adequately considered in the chapter on the alimentary or digestive system.

CHAPTER X.

HAEMORRHAGE AND ITS ARREST.

HAEMORRHAGE or bleeding is an emergency of frequent occurrence and one which demands the most urgent and decisive first-aid treatment. Before attempting to study the different varieties of haemorrhage and the appropriate methods of treatment to be applied, it is essential that the ambulance man should be thoroughly acquainted with the anatomy and physiology of the circulatory system.

Haemorrhage may be defined as the escape of blood from its normal confines in the blood vessels. Haemorrhage may occur on the surface of the body externally or on any mucous surface of any internal hollow organ ; blood may also escape into any of the serous cavities or into the body tissues.

There are three principal varieties of haemorrhage :

> (a) Arterial.
> (b) Venous.
> (c) Capillary.

(a) ARTERIAL HAEMORRHAGE occurs when an artery is injured so that blood escapes from it. In arterial haemorrhage the blood is of a bright red or scarlet colour and escapes in spurts or jets which correspond in their frequency with the arterial pulse. The blood from an artery is shed at higher pressure than in the other two varieties. Arterial bleeding is more serious than venous bleeding owing to the rapid escape of blood.

(b) VENOUS HAEMORRHAGE occurs when a vein is injured so that blood escapes. The colour of the blood is dark red or purple and the blood escapes in a steady flow.

In contrast with the intermittent spurting of arterial blood at high pressure, the blood from a vein wells out of the wound at low pressure. Venous bleeding is more easily controlled and therefore is a less serious condition.

(c) CAPILLARY HAEMORRHAGE occurs when a network of capillary blood vessels is injured. The colour of the blood is usually bright red. In capillary haemorrhage the escape of blood may be described as an oozing ; it is at comparatively low pressure and is seldom of a serious nature.

Any one of these types of haemorrhage may be either external or internal. *External Haemorrhage* occurs when the skin is wounded ; the source of the bleeding is easily detected and the discharge of blood is always evident. Since external haemorrhage is obvious, the condition is more amenable to treatment.

Internal Haemorrhage signifies the escape of blood from a source inside the body. The blood may escape on to the surface of the body through any of the natural orifices according to the site of the bleeding point ; on the other hand, when bleeding has occurred into the tissues or into a closed serous cavity, only the constitutional symptoms and signs of haemorrhage are present, there being no external evidence of bleeding. The term " Concealed Haemorrhage " might well be applied to this latter variety of bleeding, since the blood is concealed as well as the source from which the blood is escaping.

CAUSES OF HAEMORRHAGE.

There are two causes of haemorrhage : (a) injury or violence, (b) disease or constitutional disturbances.

(a) HAEMORRHAGE DUE TO INJURY occurs as the result of violence, usually of a mechanical nature. Bleeding occurs in all types of wounds. The relative amount of haemorrhage in the various kinds of wounds is considered in the chapter on wounds, where it will be also learned that cut vessels bleed much more freely than vessels which have been torn or crushed.

(b) HAEMORRHAGE DUE TO DISEASE occurs when the wall of a blood vessel is perforated by the process of some disease. The onset of such haemorrhage is frequently sudden and occurs without warning. This type of haemorrhage may equal in severity haemorrhage due to the wounding of a large vessel and varies according to the calibre and site of the affected vessel.

Haemorrhage may be further classified according to its cause and time of onset. The following terms are applied :

<blockquote>
(a) Primary Haemorrhage.
(b) Reactionary Haemorrhage.
(c) Secondary Haemorrhage.
</blockquote>

(a) PRIMARY HAEMORRHAGE occurs at the time of the injury. This type of bleeding tends to diminish or even to cease naturally except when a large artery is severed.

(b) REACTIONARY HAEMORRHAGE occurs some time after the primary haemorrhage has stopped. It is a recurrence of the bleeding which generally takes place within the first twelve or twenty-four hours, and is usually due to the rise in blood pressure which accompanies recovery from surgical shock. The condition is specially apt to occur if the initial treatment has been inadequate ; under such conditions any sudden movement or effort on the part of the patient may cause the dislodgment of a clot of blood from an open vessel with resulting reactionary bleeding.

(c) SECONDARY HAEMORRHAGE occurs rarely and is seen at a later stage—some days after the bleeding has ceased. In most cases this is a very urgent and grave condition which results from sepsis or suppuration in the wound : either the clot which normally plugs the wounded vessel is dissolved or the vessel wall becomes eroded and ruptures spontaneously.

SYMPTOMS AND SIGNS OF HAEMORRHAGE.

During the active stage of external haemorrhage the signs of bleeding are obvious and may be either those of the arterial, the venous or the capillary variety. Apart from these obvious local manifestations of external haemorrhage certain general symptoms and signs are produced by loss of blood. These general symptoms and signs are the same, irrespective of the variety of bleeding, but they vary in their intensity with the volume of blood which is lost from the circulatory system and with the rate at which the loss of blood occurs. The recognition of the group of symptoms and signs which are presently to be described is most valuable when the bleeding is of the internal variety and, more particularly, when the blood remains concealed within one of the body cavities.

SYMPTOMS :

(a) Thirst.
(b) Dimness of vision or black spots floating in front of the eyes.
(c) Nausea and faintness.
(d) Coldness.
(e) Noises in the ears.
(f) Tightness across the chest or a sense of suffocation.

SIGNS :

(a) Pallor of the face and body.
(b) Increasing rapidity of the pulse rate ; it may disappear altogether at the wrist.
(c) Difficult and rapid gasping or sighing respiration.
(d) Cold, clammy, sweating skin—subnormal temperature.
(e) Dilated pupils.
(f) Restlessness.
(g) Faintness and syncope.
(h) Collapse and surgical shock.
(i) Complete unconsciousness.

THE NATURAL ARREST OF HAEMORRHAGE.

It is all important to realise that nature has endowed the human body with certain vital reactions which play an essential part in the arrest of haemorrhage. The process by which haemorrhage is arrested is referred to as haemostasis, and any substance which assists in this process is called a haemostatic. In every case of haemorrhage there is a natural tendency for the bleeding to diminish or to cease altogether, but, in any case of severe bleeding, the loss of an amount of blood sufficient to endanger the patient's life might occur before the bleeding could be arrested in this manner. None the less it should be remembered that, without this natural tendency towards haemostasis, every case of haemorrhage would end fatally, since first aid merely assists nature in her efforts to stop bleeding. Some conditions are favourable to the natural arrest of haemorrhage while others act in an adverse manner. It is, therefore, necessary for the ambulance man to become thoroughly acquainted with the factors which take part in the process of natural haemostasis, and with the various conditions which help or hinder this process. He will then be in a better position to understand the methods to be employed for the artificial arrest of haemorrhage. When a blood vessel is completely severed, as frequently happens in an incised wound, the involuntary muscle fibres encircling the vessel contract locally and reduce the size of the opening ; at the same time, owing to the release of natural tension, there is a retraction of the ends of the vessel due to recoil of the elastic tissue fibres. This process further diminishes the calibre of the vessel at the site of injury. Simultaneously, blood clots in the wound and surrounds the cut ends of the vessel ; inside the severed vessel itself blood clot forms to plug the lumen for a variable distance from the site of severance. Ultimately, the clot is transformed into living fibrous tissue which permanently occludes the opening in the wounded vessel.

Syncope or collapse of the patient, accompanied by a marked fall in blood pressure, is a very important contributory factor in diminishing haemorrhage and in promoting clotting, this process occurring most readily when the circulation of the blood has been slowed down.

The conditions which interfere with natural haemostasis are :

(a) Incomplete division of a vessel so that the contraction of involuntary muscle is prevented.

(b) Deficiency in the clotting power of the blood as in certain diseases, such as haemophilia and haemorrhagic anaemia.

(c) Excessively high blood pressure as occurs permanently in certain diseases and temporarily and suddenly during coughing or vomiting.

(d) Stimulation of the heart's action by drugs such as alcohol.

(e) Sudden violent movement of the part which prevents the formation of a clot or loosens the clot once it has formed.

The conditions which assist natural haemostasis are :

(a) Contusion or crushing of the walls of the blood vessel.

(b) Increased clotting capacity of the blood.

(c) Abnormally low blood pressure as occurs when an injured person faints and falls to the ground.

HAEMORRHAGE FROM DISEASE.

Haemorrhage may arise from causes which are not the result of injury. These causes may be divided into two great classes according to whether blood appears externally or not. Where blood is in evidence, the diagnosis is comparatively easy, but where grave internal bleeding has occurred, there may be considerable doubt as to its source.

I. Haemorrhage with evidences of blood externally.

    (a) Epistaxis (bleeding from the nose).

    (b) Haematemesis (bleeding from the stomach).

    (c) Haemoptysis (bleeding from the lungs).

II. Haemorrhage with no evidences of blood externally (concealed haemorrhage).

    (a) Bleeding into the chest cavity.

    (b) Bleeding into the abdomen.

I. Haemorrhage with evidences of Blood externally.—(a) Epistaxis.—This condition means bleeding from the nose. Occasional bleeding from the nose is not an uncommon phenomenon in normal people, and it must not be imagined that such bleeding is harmful or is to be regarded as evidence of grave internal disease. Bleeding from the nose, however, may be due to a variety of causes apart from actual injury. Gross local disease in the nose may be accompanied by great haemorrhage, but, in addition to these cases where local factors are at play, there are certain constitutional disorders which are liable to be complicated and in certain instances relieved by epistaxis. In some cases of anaemia the blood is vitiated to the extent that bleeding often occurs from an unbroken mucous surface, and the mucous surface through which blood is most likely to ooze is that of the nose. This must be regarded as a complication of these forms of anaemia, since no haemorrhage can possibly do anaemia good. Epistaxis may come as a relief to the condition of high blood pressure, and it is generally believed that a profuse epistaxis has often saved a man from some much more serious catastrophe. Epistaxis is not serious in the great majority of cases, and it is only when long-continued haemorrhage from the nose causes evidence of weakness from loss of blood that the condition has to be regarded as endangering life.

    All cases of epistaxis should be treated by first-aid measures. Those cases which will do harm are alleviated and those cases in which haemorrhage is likely to do good are not amenable to the treatment.

TREATMENT.—The patient should be kept at rest and reassured that the condition is not serious. Unless obviously faint he should be kept sitting up with the head in a comfortable forward position and not thrown backwards. If he is faint he should be laid flat on his back with his head turned to one or other side and supported on a pillow. Any tight clothing, especially around the neck, should be loosened. In some cases the bleeding may be controlled by compression of the nostrils between the forefinger and thumb. Cold compresses or cloths wrung out of cold water may be placed over the bridge of the nose and over the forehead. The application of cold to the back of the neck is also useful. Should severe bleeding continue in spite of these measures narrow strips of lint or clean rag wrung out of cold water may be packed into the nostrils by a blunt instrument such as a pencil. The packing should be directed backwards and slightly upwards. If the loss of blood is severe the patient must be kept warm and warned not to blow his nose even after the bleeding has ceased.

(b) HAEMATEMESIS.—This word literally means vomiting of blood. Only when large quantities of fresh blood have escaped into the stomach and are vomited up immediately can anything suggestive of blood be seen in the vomit. Blood leaking into the stomach soon becomes altered to a dark material, and hence the typical appearance of the vomit in haematemesis is dark brown and is often spoken of as " coffee-grounds " vomit. Blood in the stomach may come from a variety of sources ; *first*, disease of the stomach may cause erosion of a blood vessel in the stomach wall and give rise to considerable haemorrhage ; *second*, blood from epistaxis may trickle from the back of the nose into the stomach and ultimately manifest itself in a dark vomit ; *third*, bleeding from the lungs may be coughed up and swallowed, later to manifest itself also in a dark vomit.

This last condition is more liable to occur in young children who have not yet learned to spit. In haematemesis the source of blood is usually an ulcer or erosion of the mucous membrane lining the stomach. In the process of disease the ulcer erodes the wall of a blood vessel. According to the calibre of the vessel so is the seriousness of the condition. There is usually a long history of indigestion in these cases, but it may happen occasionally that an individual may have a haematemesis without having had any previous indigestion. The patient with haematemesis is cold and collapsed ; the pulse is feeble and rapid ; the skin is moist and cold ; the face is white and pinched ; the mental state is one of anxiety and alarm.

TREATMENT.—The most important thing in dealing with a case of haematemesis is to disturb the patient as little as possible. Movement or disturbance has a tendency to increase the liability to further haemorrhage. The patient must be reassured without any ostentation or flurry on the part of the ambulance man. Transport of the patient must be carried out with the care and gentleness which is demanded by a case of fractured spine. The patient must be covered with warm blankets or coats, as the condition is attended by the most profound collapse ; hot-water bottles may be applied with advantage to the soles of the feet. Haematemesis is seldom if ever immediately fatal; hence the treatment, further than the measures already indicated, is a matter for a doctor. On no account should the first-aid man give the patient any stimulant; nothing, not even water, should be given by the mouth.

(c) HAEMOPTYSIS.—This word means spitting of blood, but its significance has become somewhat more confined to the spitting of blood from a source of haermorrhage in the lungs. It is true that a wound of the pharynx or of the mouth may give rise to spitting of blood, but such a condition is not described as haemoptysis. True haemoptysis is always the result of disease and is never regarded by the medical profession with equanimity. It usually indicates well-established lung disease the treatment of which is prolonged and demands much patience. Haemoptysis may occur in an individual who appears to be in normal health ; he may be going about his ordinary work when, suddenly, without any warning, he coughs slightly and large amounts of blood are expectorated. The rapid onset of the condition and the large amount of blood which may be lost in a short period of time render it a first-aid emergency of grave portent. As in haematemesis the patient becomes alarmed and extremely apprehensive. The blood brought up from the lungs is bright red in colour, is mixed intimately with mucus and presents a frothy appearance. The general symptoms are those of haemorrhage : the patient is pale and anxious ; he is restless ; the skin is cold, the pulse rapid and the breathing frequent. In certain circumstances it is difficult to distinguish haemoptysis from haematemesis, but, as the first-aid treatment in either condition is largely similar, time should not be spent in endeavouring to differentiate between them.

TREATMENT.—Again the main duty of the ambulance man is to reassure the patient and to keep him quiet mentally and physically. Muscular movement stimulates the circulation and increases the liability to further haemorrhage. The patient must be kept warm by blankets and hot-water bottles ; no stimulant drinks should be administered. To alleviate thirst it may be grateful to give the patient ice to suck. Lastly, that amount of care which is exercised in transporting a patient with grave surgical injuries has to be exercised in an equal degree when conveying the patient to a hospital.

II. HAEMORRHAGE WITH NO EVIDENCES OF BLOOD EXTERNALLY (CONCEALED HAEMORRHAGE).—There is no point in giving a detailed description of the causes of haemorrhage into the chest and abdomen ; suffice it merely to remark that haemorrhage into the chest cavities occurs with lung disease, disease of the great vessels, particularly from syphilis, and, very occasionally, with heart disease, while haemorrhage into the abdomen occurs most frequently during the early months of abnormal pregnancy. Towards the end of pregnancy severe haemorrhage into the womb may occur without evidence of blood externally.

(a) HAEMORRHAGE INTO THE CHEST.—The condition is sudden in its onset, is accompanied by a feeling of constriction in the chest, and frequently is almost immediately fatal. There is considerable interference with respiration; the patient finds it difficult to breathe. There is great pallor and the skin presents a greyish tint. The pulse is feeble and rapid. The skin is cold and moist. Mentally the patient is anxious; there is great restlessness.

TREATMENT.—The patient must be placed comfortably. The head and shoulders should be slightly raised on cushions or folded clothes in order to facilitate breathing. The patient must be kept warm by covering him well with blankets and the use of hot-water bottles. The mental condition calls for reassurance. No stimulants should be given. Transport demands excessive care, since any movement necessarily aggravates the condition.

(b) HAEMORRHAGE INTO THE ABDOMEN.—This condition may come on with great suddenness; collapse soon follows with the usual signs of grave bleeding. It is noteworthy that the greyish appearance of the pallid skin is not found in this condition in contrast to the appearance of the patient with haemorrhage into the chest. There is frequently much pain and sickness at the commencement of the condition. Often the patient with abdominal haemorrhage lies curled up; usually there is great restlessness.

TREATMENT.—While it is impossible to relieve the patient of the condition, much can be done to allay fear. The patient should be kept warm by ordinary means; the knees may be supported on a pillow, so that the thighs are slightly flexed, and, without any disturbance to the patient, immediate transport to a hospital should be carried out.

This procedure involves the use of some mechanical means calculated to assist the natural process of haemostasis. There are three ways in which one may aid nature in this respect.

1. DIRECT OCCLUSION BY LOCAL PRESSURE.

(a) DIRECT DIGITAL PRESSURE.—This is the first method to use in a dangerous emergency. When serious arterial haemorrhage occurs the natural and most obvious action is to clap the fingers over the source of the bleeding. The thumb or fingers are instantly applied to the spouting wound and steady pressure is maintained until a more permanent means of controlling the haemorrhage can be accomplished. This method is known as the method of direct digital pressure. When the control of haemorrhage by this means is particularly difficult and requires considerable and prolonged pressure it is advisable to reinforce the pressure of the fingers or thumb controlling the bleeding by pressing on them with the thumb or fingers of the other hand. Furthermore, it is advisable when pressure has to be maintained for any length of time that the ambulance man should place himself in a position which will enable him to hold his arms fully extended ; should he attempt to maintain pressure by transmitting his weight through flexed arms he will find that he quickly tires. Direct digital pressure has certain disadvantages in that it may introduce germs of disease into the wound. This consideration is purely a secondary one in critical cases of arterial haemorrhage. In very large wounds direct digital pressure may be inapplicable, and in such cases one of the other methods to be described must be resorted to. Direct digital pressure should always be used in cases of arterial haemorrhage threatening life without regard to any disadvantage ; in minor degrees of haemorrhage it is not indicated.

(b) PRESSURE BY PAD AND BANDAGE.—The same principle of direct application of pressure should be observed in the use of any first dressing or pad over a wound, the pressure being maintained by a tight bandage. This method is admirable for the control of lesser degrees of haemorrhage, whether arterial, venous or capillary. In cases of very severe haemorrhage there is no time to search for a dressing, and consequently direct digital pressure is essential.

(c) FORCIBLE FLEXION.—This is a method of applying local occlusion pressure to a site of haemorrhage where bleeding proceeds from a large vessel situated over the flexor aspect of certain large joints. The principle consists of compressing the artery by bending it acutely over a pad. Forcible flexion is applicable to groin, axilla, knee and elbow wounds, though in the case of the axilla the term is a misnomer as forcible adduction is what is really performed. The use of forcible flexion for the control of haemorrhage is not recommended when other methods are applicable.

In order to apply forcible flexion a pad of lint or any available dressing material is placed in the bend of the joint, which is then forcibly flexed and bandaged in this position.

In the axilla a pad, about the size of the fist, should be used. The pad is kept in position by placing over it a narrow fold triangular bandage, the ends of which are brought up and crossed over the shoulder of the same side, then carried across the chest and back under and tied in front of the armpit of the opposite side. The arm is then brought firmly against the side of the chest and held in this position by means of a triangular bandage folded broad ; the forearm is flexed to a convenient angle at the elbow. In other situations the ambulance man may use his own ingenuity in the use of the triangular bandage so as to maintain forcible flexion. (Fig. 59.)

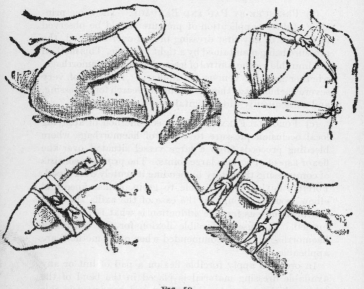

FIG. 59.

It is most important to remember that this is a method which should only be used over a relatively short period of time ; to be efficient it requires very forcible flexion which is necessarily uncomfortable and even painful. During the period of application the circulation of the limb is entirely strangled beyond the flexed joint, and if this is not relieved at least every thirty minutes serious harm may be done.

2. Indirect Occlusion by Pressure over a Main Vessel at some Distance from the Site of Haemorrhage.

This method may be employed in two forms :

(*a*) Indirect Digital Pressure.—There are certain well-recognised anatomical points at which this form of pressure may be applied in order to stop the flow of blood through a main artery. These points are situated where the larger arteries cross some bony structure against which they may be compressed. Obviously, when arterial haemorrhage has to be controlled by this method the point of application of pressure is necessarily situated between the heart and the wound. The most important pressure points will be described later ; at present it is sufficient to state that no useful purpose is served by describing pressure points distal to the elbow and knee, since compression of the main arteries of the forearm and leg is insufficient owing to their position relative to the bones and to the freedom of the anastomosis.

One or both thumbs may be used to maintain compression, except in the case of the brachial artery, where the fingers are employed. Compression of the artery alone against the underlying bone can be effected, and the same mechanical principles with regard to the position of the arms and fingers as in direct digital pressure should be observed. The efficacy of the method is readily tested by observing to what extent haemorrhage is controlled. Should haemorrhage continue, the pressure is probably being applied over the wrong place or is insufficient. The advantages of this method are that the risk of infection of the wound by germs is not increased and that it can be applied in the case of large wounds. In cases of great emergency indirect digital pressure can be applied by a second person after the haemorrhage has been controlled by the initial measure of direct digital pressure.

The disadvantages of this method are that it can only

be applied in certain situations to be described and that it can be efficiently maintained by one person only for about a quarter of an hour. If indirect digital pressure has to be maintained for any considerable period of time it should be momentarily relaxed at least every thirty minutes.

(*b*) TOURNIQUET PRESSURE.—A tourniquet is an instrument or appliance which can be employed to compress the main artery of a limb. When a tourniquet is used, haemorrhage beyond it is arrested by strangulation or compression of the vessels at the point where the tourniquet is applied. This method of arresting haemorrhage is only to be used as a last resort in cases of extremely severe bleeding. Many forms of tourniquet have been devised, but for first-aid work two types are recommended ; one is the improvised tourniquet involving the use of a triangular bandage and pad, and the other is the Esmarch elastic web bandage.

THE IMPROVISED TOURNIQUET.—This consists of three essential parts :

(*a*) a narrow folded triangular bandage, strip of strong cloth or any other available strap-like piece of material with which to encircle the limb ;

(*b*) a small pad of suitable size such as a piece of rolled-up cloth, a block of india-rubber or even a flat oval stone or pebble rolled in cloth to place over the line of the artery ;

(*c*) a strong piece of stick, such as a large pencil, a ruler, or other similar object, with which to tighten the band round the limb.

To apply this form of tourniquet place the pad over the line of the main artery above the site of haemorrhage, adjust the narrow bandage so that its centre lies over the pad and tie its ends in a knot on the opposite side of the limb ; place the stick over the knot and over the stick tie a reef knot. Now twist the stick so as to tighten the pad on the artery and lock the stick in position by another bandage passed round both the limb and the stick. (Plate XIX.)

THE ESMARCH ELASTIC WEB BANDAGE.—This appliance consists of a length of elastic webbing of good quality about two and a half inches broad and four feet long. At one end there are two tapes sewn on to the bandage for fixing after application of the tourniquet. In order to apply this form of tourniquet the elastic webbing is wound firmly round the limb, each turn of the bandage being placed directly over the preceding one. While encircling the limb with the bandage the rubber is stretched to the limit of its elasticity as each turn is applied; in this way strong compression is brought to bear on the limb and the circulation is completely arrested. To secure the bandage in position and to prevent it from slackening the tapes of the bandage are tied securely round the limb over the coils of the tourniquet, care being taken not to allow the bandage to slip while this knot is being tied.

GENERAL PRINCIPLES TO BE OBSERVED IN THE USE AND APPLICATION OF A TOURNIQUET.

1. The method is only to be used in cases of severe haemorrhage when it is impossible to control the bleeding by other means, or where severe haemorrhage is likely to occur.

2. A tourniquet of the improvised type should be placed in position without actually tightening it in all cases of compound fracture, in order to be ready for possible reactionary haemorrhage.

3. The Esmarch elastic web tourniquet should not be used in any case where a fracture is present or is suspected.

4. In certain cases of poisonous bites a tourniquet may be applied with advantage, not, however, with the idea of arresting haemorrhage, but with a view to preventing the return of blood from the poisoned wound to the general

circulation ; in such cases either type of tourniquet may be used.

5. A tourniquet is applied only to the arm or the thigh, never to the fore-arm or the leg.

6. When a wound is situated proximally in a limb, for example in the axilla or groin, the efficient application of a tourniquet is impossible and the haemorrhage must be controlled by forced flexion or by some other means.

7. It is always to be borne in mind that a tourniquet is to be placed between the heart and the wound.

8. Whenever possible the limb should be elevated almost to a vertical position before applying a tourniquet, in order to reduce the amount of blood in the limb.

9. An improvised tourniquet should be tightened just sufficiently to control the haemorrhage.

10. In no case should a tourniquet be allowed to remain taut in position for longer than thirty minutes at a stretch, since devitalisation of the limb below the site of the tourniquet may lead to permanent damage and ultimately cause loss of the limb. At intervals of not longer than thirty minutes the tourniquet should be slackened so as to flush the limb with fresh blood.

(3) POSTURAL TREATMENT.—

The systemic blood pressure may be lowered by causing the patient to lie flat on the ground. This is the first essential in the treatment of all cases of haemorrhage except in head wounds. It has to be remembered that the heart's action becomes more forcible when the patient is standing, owing to the general expenditure of muscular energy required to maintain the upright posture. When the patient is in the recumbent position this expenditure of energy is abolished because the general musculature of the body is relaxed ; the blood pressure under these conditions is correspondingly low. The local blood pressure may be diminished in a limb by elevating it ; in this case the result is produced by the effect of gravitation on the blood flow. It follows, as a principle of treatment, that a bleeding limb should be raised and supported. This, however, should never be done in the case of a suspected fracture. In the case of head wounds the patient should have the head and shoulders raised on pillows, since elevation of the bleeding part diminishes the flow of blood to it.

PRESSURE POINTS FOR THE DIGITAL COMPRESSION OF ARTERIES.

1. ARTERIES OF THE HEAD AND NECK—(*a*) TEMPORAL.—The temporal artery passes almost vertically upwards over the region of the temple. It should be compressed where the vessel crosses the zygomatic process of the temporal bone at a point one finger's breadth in front of the external opening of the ear. (Plate XX.)

(*b*) FACIAL.—The facial artery passes upwards over the outer aspect of the lower jaw in a small groove which may be felt as the finger is passed along the lower edge of the bone. The vessel should be compressed against the bone at this point about two fingers' breadth in front of the angle of the mandible. In some wounds about the lower part of the face it is advisable to compress both facial arteries simultaneously owing to the free anastomosis or inter-communication between these vessels. (Plate XXI.)

(*c*) OCCIPITAL.—The occipital artery passes upwards and backwards behind the ear. It should be compressed against the occipital bone at a point about two fingers' breadth behind the opening of the ear. (Plate XXII.)

(*d*) COMMON CAROTID.—The common carotid artery is situated deeply in the neck and, in order to occlude it, pressure must be carefully applied in a backward and inward direction so as to compress the vessel against the transverse processes of the cervical vertebrae. During this procedure great care must be taken to avoid pressure upon the trachea (windpipe), which lies somewhat in front and to the inner side of the artery. The best point at which to apply pressure is about three fingers' breadth above the sterno-clavicular joint and just in front of the sterno-mastoid muscle. When compressing this artery it is advisable to kneel at the side of the patient and place the hand behind the neck with the thumb directed forwards over the pressure point, using the right thumb for the left carotid artery and vice versa. (Plate XXII.) When training, the ambulance pupil is advised only to locate the artery and not to practise its compression, as this procedure may have serious results.

2. ARTERIES OF THE UPPER LIMB—(a) SUBCLAVIAN.—The subclavian artery passes over the first rib and lies behind the clavicle. Pressure should be applied in a downward and inward direction immediately behind the middle of the clavicle so as to compress the artery against the upper surface of the first rib. In order to facilitate this procedure the clothes should be removed from the neck and upper part of the chest, the shoulder should be depressed so as to lower the clavicle and the head inclined towards the injured side ; in this way the artery and the first rib are rendered more accessible. Kneel opposite the shoulder of the wounded side, place the hands with the thumbs super-imposed and apply very firm pressure downwards and inwards against the first rib. If these directions are carefully carried out it should not be necessary to use a padded key or other instrument. (Plate XXI.)

(b) AXILLARY.—The axillary artery, the direct continuation of the subclavian, passes through the axilla to the arm, where it becomes the brachial artery. Owing to its situation the axillary artery is difficult to compress in the apex of the axilla, but in the lower part of this space the vessel may be compressed against the head or neck of the humerus by the application of digital pressure in an outward direction. When wounds of the axilla are associated with severe hæmorrhage digital pressure in the axilla is

usually impracticable ; in such cases it is better to control
the hæmorrhage either by compression of the subclavian
artery or by the method of forcible flexion.

(c) BRACHIAL.—The brachial artery runs along the inner
aspect of the arm and towards its lower end passes gradually forwards to lie in front of the elbow joint.   In severe
hæmorrhage from any part of the upper limb below the
middle of the arm the brachial artery should be compressed at once.   No time should be wasted in attempting
to control hæmorrhage, say from a wounded palmar arch,
by endeavouring to compress both the radial and ulnar
arteries at the wrist.   In order to apply digital pressure to
the brachial artery stand or kneel behind the patient ;
partially extend the elbow joint and support the forearm in
one hand ;   pass the fingers of the other hand round the
under aspect of the middle of the arm so that the four
fingers together rest over the artery and compress the
vessel firmly against the bone.   Owing to the frequency
with which the hand and forearm are wounded it is probable
that this vessel requires compression more often than all
the other vessels put together.   (Plate XX.)

3. ARTERIES OF THE LOWER LIMB—FEMORAL.—The
femoral artery is the direct continuation of the external
iliac.   It commences at the middle of the fold of the groin,
passes down the front of the thigh, inclines to the inner
and posterior aspect of the limb, where it becomes the
popliteal artery.   At its commencement, this artery passes
over the pubic bone, against which it can be easily and
efficiently compressed ;   lower down it cannot be satisfactorily compressed by digital pressure.   Therefore, in all
cases of hæmorrhage from the femoral artery, or from any
of its branches, the main vessel should immediately be
compressed at its commencement.

When applying digital pressure to the femoral artery lay
the patient on his back and kneel beside him facing his
head, place the superimposed thumbs exactly over the

G

pulsating vessel which can be felt in the middle of the fold of the groin and compress the artery directly downwards against the pubic bone. If the bleeding is coming from high up in the thigh, digital pressure must be maintained until a doctor arrives, relays of assistants being employed if necessary. If the hæmorrhage is coming from the lower part of the thigh or from the leg, a tourniquet should be applied to the thigh proximal to the wound. When assistants are unavailable and severe bleeding is occurring from the femoral artery or from its branches, forcible flexion at the groin or at the knee is the method of choice owing to the impossibility of applying a tourniquet and maintaining digital pressure simultaneously. (Plate XXIII.)

HAEMORRHAGE FROM VARICOSE VEINS

Veins are said to be varicose when, from changes in their walls and increased pressure within their lumen, they become dilated and tortuous. The skin overlying varicose veins tends to become stretched and thinned, so that the veins stand out as irregular swellings. Varicose veins are easily ruptured by a relatively slight knock or abrasion and, if the skin has become ulcerated, spontaneous rupture may occur. The condition most commonly affects the lower extremities. Haemorrhage from a ruptured varicose vein is a typical example of venous haemorrhage ; it may be extremely profuse, but it can be very simply controlled if the correct measures are promptly adopted.

TREATMENT.—The patient should immediately be made to lie down flat upon his back, and the affected limb elevated and supported in an almost vertical position. Any garters or other constricting bands above the bleeding point should be removed from the limb and the bleeding area thoroughly exposed. By this means alone the haemorrhage will be considerably diminished. A pad of aseptic cloth, or of any other clean dressing material, should then be placed over the bleeding point, and maintained in this position by a bandage firmly applied. It should rarely be necessary to apply direct digital pressure in order to arrest this variety of haemorrhage ; occasionally, however, indirect digital pressure may be applied over the vein on either side of the bleeding point. The latter method is preferable, because there is less danger of the wound becoming infected by contact with a dirty finger. Once the bleeding has been completely arrested, treatment for surgical shock may be administered if necessary, and the patient removed on a stretcher. Every case of this kind should be seen by a doctor at the earliest possible moment.

CHAPTER XI.

WOUNDS AND THEIR TREATMENT.

A WOUND is a forcible break in the continuity of any of the tissues of the body. Wounds are produced by external violence in contra-distinction to the processes of disease attended by the destruction of tissue. Certain wounds are of such a nature that the overlying skin or mucous membrane escapes; such wounds are spoken of variously as contusions or closed wounds. Owing to the application of the terms fracture and contusion to injuries of bone and deeper soft tissues respectively the term wound has come to mean a forcible break in the continuity of skin or mucous membrane together with subjacent soft tissues.

Wounds communicating with a surface of skin or mucous membrane are open wounds : where there is no break in these surfaces but contusion is present the injury is referred to as a closed wound : fractures are wounds in the truest sense of the term but these wounds are so specialized that entirely separate consideration is called for.

VARIETIES OF WOUNDS.

1. OPEN WOUNDS.

    (a) Incised wounds.
    (b) Lacerated wounds including abrasions.
    (c) Punctured wounds.
    (d) Gunshot wounds.

II. CLOSED WOUNDS OR CONTUSIONS.

III. CONTUSED OPEN WOUNDS.

1. (a) INCISED WOUNDS are breaks in the continuity of a skin or mucous surface without loss of tissue. These

wounds vary in degree from the slightest cut of the finger to the razor slash of the cut throat. They are produced by the cutting force of some sharp edge such as a knife, broken glass, thin sheet metal or other similar object.

An incised wound has sharp clean-cut edges which are drawn apart by the natural elasticity of the skin causing the wound to gape. The amount of bleeding depends upon the site of the wound and upon certain constitutional factors which are discussed in the chapter on haemorrhage. Incised wounds are attended by greater haemorrhage than accompanies any other type of wound because the blood vessels are cleanly severed and not crushed or torn. When an incised wound occurs in a region well supplied with blood vessels such as the face or scalp the bleeding is profuse. Incised wounds are less likely to be soiled and, on account of their free bleeding and uniform edges, are easily cleaned. Occasionally the appearance of an incised wound is closely simulated by the effect of a blow from a blunt instrument on skin stretched tightly over bone. Examples of such wounds are described in group III. Incised wounds are primarily dangerous on account of haemorrhage.

(b) LACERATED WOUNDS.—A lacerated wound is the solution in the continuity of skin or mucous surface accompanied by loss of tissue. The wound is produced by a tear from some relatively blunt instrument such as rough edges of metal or even of wood. The edges are irregular and serrated or ragged. The tendency for the wound to gape is less than in the case of an incised wound for the reason that bridges of skin and connective tissue escape injury and prevent complete separation of the edges. Bleeding is also less because blood vessels are resistant to a tearing force and because, for certain reasons, clotting occurs more readily in a torn than in an incised wound. Dirt is frequently ingrained into lacerated wounds at the moment of their occurrence and consequently the cleansing of such wounds is difficult and painful to the patient.

Lacerated wounds are dangerous on account of dirt and shock.

(c) PUNCTURED WOUNDS.—Punctured wounds are frequently termed penetrating wounds in virtue of the fact that their course implicates deeper tissues : even some internal organ or body cavity may be pierced. Owing to such penetration they are at once rendered the most serious type of wound : severe bleeding may occur into one of the body cavities or micro-organisms of disease may be carried deeply into the tissues. These wounds are produced by a stab from an instrument more or less sharp or pointed such as a dagger, a knife, a spike or a nail. They are sometimes referred to as stab-wounds. According to the degree of sharpness or bluntness of the instrument the surface appearance may be that of an incised or a contused wound. In contrast to the incised wound, where the depth is less than the length of the wound, the depth of the punctured wound is greater than its superficial extent. A pin prick in the finger is a form of punctured wound and the sting of a wasp or other insect may be similarly classified ; in such cases the danger arises not from the actual wound itself but from the septic disease-producing organisms or other poisonous substance which may be implanted in the tissues.

(d) GUNSHOT WOUNDS.—These wounds may be produced by the shot from a sport gun, an air-gun, a rifle or a revolver. Shot from an air-gun or a sport gun is generally lodged in the body after traversing the tissues for a varying distance whereas bullets from a rifle or a revolver are more penetrating and frequently traverse the entire thickness of the part. All gunshot wounds are of the order of punctured wounds and when produced by a rifle or revolver they are usually characterized by having two openings on the surface of the body—an aperture of entrance and an aperture of exit. In these cases the aperture or wound of exit is invariably larger than the aperture or wound of entrance. Gunshot wounds are always dangerous injuries and are especially grave when they occur in the vicinity of the head or of the body cavities : in most cases they are attended by haemorrhage and severe surgical shock.

II. CLOSED OR CONTUSED WOUNDS.—A contused wound is referred to as a contusion and is a form of injury affecting the soft tissues in such a manner that neither the skin nor the mucous membrane is broken. Contusion implies a crushing or tearing of the tissues beneath the skin without the damaged part being laid open on the surface. A contusion is usually produced by a blow from some blunt object such as a hammer or a fist or it may result from a fall. As the result of a contusion blood vessels are torn and bleeding occurs to a variable degree beneath the skin or mucous membrane. If the smaller vessels only are torn the blood spreads for a varying distance amongst the tissues and is said to be extravasated ; if a larger vessel is torn the blood collects in a mass locally and is said to form a haematoma or blood tumour. In either case the injured part very quickly becomes painful, swollen and discoloured. These effects are produced by the blood which accumulates and cannot escape from the tissues. The discoloration on the surface is frequently referred to as bruising and on this account such wounds are sometimes called " bruises." The discoloration or bruising on the surface may spread to a considerable distance from the original site of contusion. It is of interest to note that the bruising or discoloration is partly due to the colour changes in the blood pigments, which become altered when they are deprived of oxygen. A black-eye is an excellent example of a contusion, for this type of injury is especially evident where the lax soft tissues such as the eye-lids are affected. The danger of a contusion depends principally upon the part of the body affected : when it occurs over the abdomen the most serious results may follow, whereas a contusion of a limb may be of little significance. In a contusion there is little danger of disease organisms gaining access to the wound from without.

III. CONTUSED OPEN WOUNDS.—Such wounds resemble incised wounds or lacerations but their edges and the adjacent tissues are contused. They are generally produced by the forcible application of some blunt instrument to the soft tissues overlying a bony prominence. Bleeding is usually slight but it has to be remembered that the underlying bone may be fractured. In other respects they are similar to incised or lacerated wounds.

COMPLICATIONS AND DANGERS OF WOUNDS.

    I. Haemorrhage.
    II. Surgical Shock.
    III. Sepsis.
    IV. Disability.

I. HAEMORRHAGE or bleeding occurs in some degree with every wound. The ordinary amount of haemorrhage from a simple wound is inevitable and is beneficial rather than dangerous. When bleeding becomes so excessive as to cause weakness it constitutes an alarming complication and is a first-aid emergency. The amount of haemorrhage depends upon various factors, some of which are general or constitutional while others are local and peculiar to the site and nature of the wound. Constitutional factors have been considered under "Haemorrhage" but the local conditions modifying haemorrhage are more appropriately dealt with in the study of wounds. If a wound occurs in tissue which is richly supplied with blood, and especially if a vessel of even moderate size is severed, haemorrhage is correspondingly greater; if the main artery to a limb is cut the haemorrhage may be quickly fatal unless it is promptly arrested. The reader is reminded of the variations in haemorrhage which are dependent upon the actual nature of the wound, the incised and punctured types being much more dangerous in this respect.

II. SURGICAL SHOCK depends primarily upon the actual damage done to the body. It varies, therefore, with the severity of the violence and is modified by the vulnerability of the wounded part. To elucidate this further it may be stated that the more highly specialized the wounded part the greater the degree of shock. A contusion of the abdomen may be followed by severe collapse, as may a similar injury affecting the kidney or other vital organ, whereas a contusion of the buttock produces a negligible amount of shock. In any particular site the attendant surgical shock varies directly with the amount of actual tissue damaged ; thus an incised wound over the abdomen may be attended by practically no shock. The condition of surgical shock is aggravated by the amount of haemorrhage although haemorrhage is not the main factor in its production.

III. SEPSIS is the condition which results from the contamination of a wound by germs of disease. Germs are also referred to as micro-organisms or bacteria and, owing to their almost universal prevalence, the possibility of their entrance into any open wound must be considered. Since germs are present on the human skin and since any object likely to cause accidental wounding is also covered with germs, every open accidental wound must in the first instance contain germs. The infection of a wound by germs is soon followed by their multiplication and by a reaction on the part of the tissues manifested by the formation of pus or matter which is composed simply of dead leucocytes and organisms suspended in serum. Such a wound is termed a suppurating, festering, bealing or septic wound. The reaction of the tissues caused by the irritation of the germs is termed inflammation ; it is evidenced by the presence of four cardinal signs, heat, pain, redness and swelling. The heat is caused by the increased flow of blood to the inflamed part ; the pain is accounted for simply by the tension in the tissues ; the redness is due to the dilatation of the superficial vessels ; the swelling is produced partly by the increased amount of blood in the part and partly by the accumulation of fluid in the tissues. More will be learned of this later when the repair of wounds is considered.

Before the days of Pasteur and Lister suppuration was considered to be the inevitable sequel of every wound. The work of Pasteur in investigating the causes of fermentation and putrefaction led Lister to conceive the idea that suppuration might be due to germs of a nature resembling those which Pasteur described as causing those effects. The work of investigating how to combat those germs was carried out by Lister in Glasgow Royal Infirmary in the middle of last century. He discovered that certain substances had the power of destroying the germs of sepsis and to these substances the name antiseptics was given. Carbolic acid was the antiseptic which Lister used ; its existence was pointed out to Lister by Dr. Thomas Anderson, Professor of Chemistry in Glasgow. These epoch-making discoveries led to a radical change not only in general surgical practice, but also in the first-aid treatment of wounds. It led to the antiseptic method of treatment whereby all wounds were treated with strongly antiseptic lotions. This practice has never been superseded by any more recent method so far as first-aid treatment of wounds is concerned. It is of interest, however, to note that at a later period other methods were introduced to prevent the entrance of germs into wounds. It was discovered that heat could render instruments, dressings and lotions free from living organisms of sepsis ; instruments and other materials so rendered free from living organisms are termed aseptic or sterile ; the process by which asepsis is attained is known as sterilization. Modern surgery is primarily concerned with the exclusion of sources of infection and its method is a judicious mixture of aseptic and antiseptic principles.

IV. DISABILITY is to some extent an accompaniment of every wound. Pain and surgical shock produce general disability while certain local factors determine disability of the affected part. Among the local causes of disability the more important are the severance of nerve trunks causing paralysis and loss of sensation, division of a large blood vessel causing deprivation of blood and possibly subsequent gangrene or local death of the tissue, division of tendons or muscles resulting in loss of movement and deformity. While first-aid treatment cannot alleviate these immediate disabilities once they have occurred it is to be borne in mind that efficient first-aid treatment may prevent further damage and lighten the task of surgery.

REPAIR OF WOUNDS.

Before considering the treatment of wounds it is necessary to study briefly the fundamental principles of healing in a simple wound. In the case of an incised wound to which the access of organisms has been prevented healing occurs rapidly and with the minimum amount of permanent change in the tissues. Blood fills the gap and quickly becomes coagulated, the clot so formed sealing the wound, binding its edges together and preventing further hæmorrhage. White blood cells soon find their way into the clot and assist in its removal : at the same time other cells from the adjacent fibrous tissue multiply and migrate into the clot which they ultimately replace. With the formation of this fibrous tissue capillary vessels grow into the wound. In this way union of the wound edges occurs by the formation of a network of fibrous tissue and fine capillaries. Concurrently with these changes the surface cells of skin or mucous membrane shew signs of activity, multiply and cover over the space intervening between the edges of the wound. At a somewhat later stage the fibrous tissue contracts and compresses the capillary vessels so that in the course of time there remains only fibrous connective tissue or scar tissue. The ultimate appearance of the scar is white owing to the absence of blood vessels and there may be evidence of contraction of the affected part.

When a wound becomes infected with micro-organisms the course of healing is delayed and rendered much more complicated. The complications are due to the development of inflammation and resultant suppuration. If a wound becomes inflamed, in addition to the usual congestion of the surrounding capillaries, there occurs an accentuation of the features described in a simple wound. Thus the migration of leucocytes becomes so excessive to such a degree that pus is formed and discharged. Capillaries form a rich network of loops supported on a framework of young fibrous tissue ; such a velvety mass is termed proud flesh or granulation tissue. As a consequence of these processes the edges of the wound tend to separate and therefore the period of surface growth is necessarily prolonged. Due to these factors the subsequent deformity is much greater than in the case of an aseptic wound, where the formation of fibrous tissue is at a minimum.

THE TREATMENT OF WOUNDS.

Having briefly studied the characteristic features of the various types of wounds, their complications and dangers, and the factors concerned in their repair, the ambulance man is in a better position to understand the principles which have to be observed in the first-aid treatment of these emergencies. From what has already been said it will be evident that the following are the principles of treatment in order of importance :

(a) The arrest of haemorrhage.
(b) The treatment of surgical shock.
(c) The examination of the wound.
(d) The cleansing of the wound.
(e) The protection of the wound from further infection by the application of dressings.
(f) The support of the affected part.
(g) The removal of the patient.

(*a*) THE ARREST OF HAEMORRHAGE.—In a wound of any severity bleeding must be stopped before anything else is done. Rapidity of action is essential ; a moment's delay may be fatal. The various methods of treatment to be applied in the case of arterial or severe venous haemorrhage have been described under " Arrest of haemorrhage." When the haemorrhage is of the capillary variety it is to be remembered that the bleeding assists in the cleansing of the wound by washing out particles of dirt which might contain micro-organisms of infection. In these latter cases a moderate amount of oozing may be actually beneficial, and such bleeding can easily be controlled by the application of a dressing and firm bandage. Furthermore, it must be remembered that, in certain cases of wounding, especially in puncture wounds of the chest and of the abdomen, bleeding may be going on internally although none is evident on the external surface of the body ; in such cases appropriate measures must be adopted in order to diminish the haemorrhage so far as possible and to obtain medical aid at the earliest moment.

(*b*) THE TREATMENT OF SURGICAL SHOCK.—In cases of wounding, especially if accompanied by severe haemorrhage, surgical shock may supervene and necessitate urgent treatment. This has already been considered under " The General Principles of First Aid," and the methods advocated should be carried out in cases of wounding attended by shock. At the same time it should be remembered that while a patient is suffering from surgical shock there may be little evidence of haemorrhage unless a large vessel has been wounded. Therefore it is important to ensure that active bleeding has been controlled before the treatment for shock is instituted. A close watch should be kept for recurrence of haemorrhage during the period of reaction from surgical shock. The patient should be well covered up and kept warm, as soon as he can swallow he may be allowed to drink hot tea or coffee, and if these are unobtainable he should be encouraged to drink plenty of water.

(*c*) THE EXAMINATION OF THE WOUND.—Before proceeding to examine the wound an endeavour should be made, whenever possible, to find out how the wound was inflicted; in this way evidence may be obtained of a fracture or of some other serious injury requiring special consideration. Further, when the history or the circumstances of the accident suggest the possibility of contamination of the wound with road scrapings, manure or animal excreta, no matter how trivial the wound, this information should be carefully noted and any such case must receive immediate medical attention. The importance of this fact is stressed because the micro-organism which causes tetanus or " lockjaw " is frequently present in animal excreta or dung.

As soon as urgent haemorrhage has been controlled a brief examination of the wound should be carried out in order to discover so far as possible its nature and severity. This examination should be done by inspection alone, and sufficient clothing should be removed to expose the injured part. Some idea may then be formed as to the variety of the wound and its extent, special care being taken in the case of a wound of the punctured variety. If a punctured wound is suspected or is known to be present, the ambulance man must examine the patient further in order to discover the possible presence of the constitutional signs of internal haemorrhage. At this stage no handling of the wound or other interference is to be attempted.

(*d*) THE CLEANSING OF THE WOUND.—During this procedure it is important, firstly, to prevent the further contamination of the wound by contact with dirty hands, clothes or other septic material such as soiled handkerchiefs; secondly, to remove dirt from the wound. The method of cleansing a wound at the time of an accident will necessarily be modified by the conditions obtaining where the accident occurs. Therefore we shall briefly describe the method to be employed when the conditions are ideal and indicate later how to deal with some of the difficulties which may be encountered when the circumstances are less favourable. Assuming the best conditions, the hands should be quickly cleansed before the wound is touched. This can be done in a few seconds by scrubbing the hands in soap and water and bathing them in some antiseptic lotion such as lysol diluted in the proportion of two teaspoonfuls to the pint of water, carbolic lotion (1 part of carbolic acid to 40 parts of water) or methylated spirit. Attention is now directed to the wound. Gross dirt such as road scrapings, grass, mud, dung, or fragments of clothing may be removed by sponging, and any foreign bodies such as stones, glass or splinters of wood may be picked out so long as these are superficial and not firmly embedded in the tissues. In many cases this is all that is necessary. It should be remembered that the clotted blood is sterile and need not be removed from the vicinity of the wound unless it is intimately admixed with dirt. When further cleansing is considered necessary the edges of the wound should be gently sponged with some antiseptic solution such as diluted lysol, carbolic lotion (1 to 40), a weak solution of iodine (Liquor Iodi Mitis : B.P. 1932) or methylated spirit. A clean rag, fresh cotton wool or an unused handkerchief may be used for sponging. Such sponging materials are termed swabs. Some of the antiseptic used for cleansing the edges may be wrung out of a clean swab into the wound in order to complete the disinfection.

There are certain things which must be avoided in the treatment of wounds. Blood clot should not be removed or washed out, and the wound should on no account be opened up for cleansing or for any other purpose. In cleansing, wounds should not be rubbed with a swab owing to the danger of increasing haemorrhage or of further infection. It is better simply to dab the swab on the wound. If the case is especially urgent or if the facilities are not available, washing of the hands may be dispensed with altogether or they may be rapidly bathed in any available antiseptic lotion. In the absence of antiseptic lotions,

sterile water, *i.e.* water which has been boiled, or clean
tap or spring water may be used. Swabs and dressings
should be boiled if facilities permit. Soiled handkerchiefs
must never be employed for cleansing a wound. Finally,
we would strongly advise that, if circumstances are particularly unfavourable, it is better to dispense altogether
with the cleansing of the wound if this is likely to involve
any risk of further infection.

(e) THE PROTECTION OF THE WOUND BY THE APPLICA-
TION OF DRESSINGS.—The ideal dressing for a wound is
one free from germs of disease ; it may be antiseptic or
aseptic. Pieces of clean linen or cotton, handkerchief,
sheeting or towelling, in the absence of boracic lint, are
all suitable materials to use for a first dressing. Any
material which is used must either be rendered aseptic by
boiling or scorching, or antiseptic by immersion in an antiseptic solution such as those already mentioned. Boracic
lint is a dressing already antiseptic, and, if fresh, may be
used without any preliminary treatment apart from immersion in sterile water. Sterile dressings from sealed
packages, as recommended by the Home Office, may be
applied directly to the wound without any preliminary
immersion. Usually a dressing, of sufficient size to cover
the wound and to overlap it on all sides, is placed over
it, but where there is a large cavity in the wound the
dressing may be introduced into it. Over the dressing
there should be placed a piece of waterproof tissue sufficiently large to overlap the first dressing by about an
inch on all sides. The waterproof materials in common
use for this purpose are sheet gutta-percha tissue, jaconet
or oiled silk. When available, a layer of cotton wool or
Gamgee tissue should be placed over the waterproof tissue,
and finally the whole dressing should be fixed firmly in
position by a suitable bandage.

If suitable material cannot readily be procured, or facilities are unavailable for sterilization of the dressings, use
must be made of whatever covering is considered least

likely to cause infection. In this respect it may be mentioned that if the bleeding has completely stopped and blood clot has dried over the wound, nature has provided a most excellent form of dressing, and it is advisable, under those circumstances, to leave the wound exposed. The use of soiled handkerchiefs as first dressings for open wounds, the practice of applying a cobweb or the like are to be deprecated owing to the danger of causing sepsis.

(f) THE SUPPORT OF THE INJURED PART.—In any severe wound of the upper extremity it is advisable to apply a sling and, in the case of a severe wound affecting the lower extremity, it may be necessary to use splints to support and render the limb immobile.

(g) THE REMOVAL OF THE PATIENT.—Any case of wounding attended by a degree of surgical shock or haemorrhage should not be allowed to walk, but should be removed on a stretcher after a dressing has been applied and after suitable support to the injured part has been ensured.

WOUNDS IN SPECIAL SITUATIONS.

THE EYE.—The general principles of wound treatment are to be observed, but care must be taken to avoid the use of strong antiseptic solutions like iodine, carbolic and lysol.

The best dressing to apply is a piece of clean boracic lint soaked in water, or two or three drops of 10% argyrol solution may be introduced between the eye-lids. (Eye-drops as supplied under Order from the Home Office should similarly be introduced if available.)

THE EAR.—Wounds of the external ear call for no special form of treatment ; when the external ear has been almost cut off care should be taken to preserve it even if it be hanging only by a tag of skin. Strong antiseptics should not be used for such injuries. Special consideration of bleeding from the ear will be found in the chapter dealing with fractures of the skull.

THE MOUTH.—The same rule applies with regard to the use of strong antiseptic solutions as in the previous two instances. Wounds of the mouth are frequently complicated by the loss of teeth ; again teeth may simply be loosened or lying free in the mouth. In unconscious patients teeth lying free in the mouth should be searched for and preserved, since it is sometimes possible for them to survive after replacement by a skilled operator.

CUT-THROAT WOUNDS.—Here the great danger is hæmorrhage, which must be controlled by following the recognised methods. In these cases arterial bleeding never occurs alone because the large veins of the neck, being superficial, are more liable to injury. Accordingly, in the great majority of cases, the control of venous hæmorrhage by direct digital compression is the main concern of effective treatment. This not only arrests hæmorrhage but also prevents air from being sucked into the veins. Victims of cut-throat wounds often show a tendency to tear off their dressings or bandages ; this must be prevented by keeping a constant watch on the patient and, if necessary, tying his hands.

CHEST.—Wounds of the thorax deserve special consideration when they penetrate the pleura. This complication is attended by embarrassment to the breathing and it is advisable to have the patient's head and shoulders raised and supported.

ABDOMEN.—Wounds of the abdomen, when penetrating, are always of grave significance owing to the danger of septic infection and consequent peritonitis. Large wounds running transversely across the abdomen necessitate the patient lying on his back with the knees bent. The flexion of the thighs produced in this way effects relaxation of the abdominal muscles and prevents gaping of the wound. Extensive wounds running vertically require the patient lying with the legs and thighs straight for similar reasons. When the intestines protrude from an abdominal wound no attempt should be made to replace them. They should be covered with a sterile dressing soaked in warm water, warm boracic lotion or saline solution made by dissolving a teaspoonful of salt in a pint of warm water.

GUNSHOT WOUNDS.—Since gunshot wounds are essentially similar to other varieties of punctured wounds the same general principles of treatment should be observed. In all cases a second wound, the wound of exit, should be sought for and the affected part examined for fracture. In most cases haemorrhage and shock call for urgent treatment. With regard to the wound itself, a clean dressing should be applied but on no account should an ambulance man ever attempt to probe such a wound or to remove a bullet. In the case of a limb, splints should be applied if there is any suspicion of the existence of fracture. In every case a doctor should be summoned immediately and the patient removed on a stretcher to hospital.

POISONED WOUNDS.

DOG BITES.—Bites from dogs are dangerous principally on account of their liability to infection by germs and should therefore always be actively treated by strong antiseptics. Very occasionally, when a mad or rabid dog inflicts a wound, there is further danger of infection by the microbe of the disease known as rabies or hydrophobia. Since the symptoms of this infection do not show themselves for several weeks after the bite it is important to notify the police authorities when any dog attacks a person for no apparent reason. When any possibility of rabies exists a tourniquet should be applied between the heart and the wound and left in position and, until a doctor arrives, the ordinary antiseptic treatment should be followed.

SNAKE BITES.—These wounds are dangerous because of the possibility of their infection by snake venom. Further information regarding the nature and effects of this poison will be found in the chapter dealing with poisons. The treatment must be carried out at the earliest possible moment.

INSECT STINGS AND BITES.—The disagreeable effects of these minute wounds are caused by a form of chemical poison, formic acid, which is introduced into the tissue along with the sting. It should be remembered that insect stings and bites may also cause septic infection; therefore it is advisable to adopt antiseptic measures even in the absence of poisonous manifestations. If possible the sting should be expressed by means of a key or a piece of metal tubing and a dressing moistened with ammonia or baking soda applied to the part. Stings affecting the tongue or throat may endanger life by the rapid swelling of the soft tissues causing suffocation. In such cases a doctor should be summoned without waiting for signs of respiratory obstruction. See also chapter on poisoning.

CHAPTER XII.

THE RESPIRATORY SYSTEM.

ANATOMY OF THE RESPIRATORY SYSTEM.

THE series of passages through which air enters the lungs is known as the respiratory tract. This tract, together with the chest cavity and the essential respiratory tissue forming the great mass of the lungs, constitutes the respiratory system. Although the mouth is really a part of the alimentary tract, it is so closely associated with the first part of the respiratory tract and so important an adjunct to it, that it is convenient to describe a few of its anatomical points at this stage.

THE MOUTH is formed by the cheeks on either side, the palate above and the tongue below. Further description of this region is unnecessary except with regard to the palate, which forms the roof of the mouth and the floor of the nasal passages. The palate is divided into two parts : in front there is the hard palate, which is a rigid bony structure ; behind there is the soft palate, which is freely movable and composed mainly of muscle tissue. The soft palate is prolonged downwards posteriorly in the middle line as a small tongue-shaped portion of tissue called the uvula.

THE RESPIRATORY APPARATUS COMPRISES :

I. The Respiratory Tract, which is divisible into :

(a) The Nasal Passages.
(b) The Pharynx.
(c) The Larynx.
(d) The Trachea and Bronchi.

II. The Lungs.

III. The Chest Cavity.

I. The Respiratory Tract—

(a) The Nasal Passages are formed by two cavities separated from one another by a bony and cartilaginous septum in the middle line. Each cavity is partially subdivided from above downwards by three thin curved bony processes, the turbinated bones which project downwards and medially from the lateral walls. The cavities open on each side at the anterior nares or nostrils in front, while behind they communicate with the pharynx through the posterior nares.

(b) The Pharynx is the tubular cavity into which the nasal passages and the mouth open posteriorly. The line of division between the mouth and the pharynx is formed by the anterior pillars of the fauces, a pair of muscular folds stretching laterally and downwards from the uvula, above, to the back of the tongue below. Behind these folds are the tonsils, while behind the tonsils are two other similar folds, the posterior pillars of the fauces. Above the soft palate the posterior nares or back of the nose open into the pharynx. The walls of the cavity are surrounded by sheet-like muscles which are called the constrictor muscles of the pharynx. The roof of the pharynx is formed by the under surface of the body of the sphenoid bone anteriorly : posteriorly the basilar portion of the occipital bone roofs in the cavity. It is important to remember that the roof of the pharynx is formed by a part of the base of the skull. In each lateral wall, just above and behind the soft palate, there is the opening of a special tube called the auditory or Eustachian tube, which passes on each side upwards, backwards and outwards to the middle ear in the temporal bone. There is, therefore, a communication between the middle ear and the pharynx. Thus certain fractures of the skull which involve the petrous part of the temporal bone may be associated with the appearance of blood in the throat and mouth due to haemorrhage into the pharynx *via* the auditory tube. The posterior wall of the pharynx is constituted by the anterior surface of the cervical portion of the vertebral column. The lower end of the pharynx, the narrowest portion, is directly continuous with the oesophagus or gullet behind, and also communicates with the larynx in front.

(c) THE LARYNX is essentially the organ for the production of voice, and at the same time constitutes an important part of the respiratory tract. It forms a projection in front of the upper part of the neck in the middle line : above it communicates with the pharynx : below it is continuous with the trachea or windpipe. Its walls are composed mainly of flattened pieces of cartilage joined together by ligaments and moved by delicate muscles. Of the several cartilages forming the larynx three should be remembered. The thyroid cartilage, the largest and most important, consists of two flat plates or laminae joined together at an angle which is directed forwards in the middle line. It is placed above and in front, and forms the prominence of the Adam's apple in the adult male. The epiglottis is a leaf-like piece of yellow coloured cartilage attached by its stem to the notch at the upper end of the angle between the laminae of the thyroid cartilage. It lies just behind the root of the tongue. The cricoid cartilage is situated below the thyroid cartilage. It is shaped like a ring, and being wider behind than in front takes part in the formation of the lower posterior wall of the larynx. In the larynx there is a slit-like orifice formed by the vocal cords. Each vocal cord is formed by a band of elastic tissue, which projects from the side towards the middle line, and is attached in front to the angle of the thyroid cartilage and behind to a small conical cartilage poised on the back and upper surface of the cricoid cartilage.

(d) THE TRACHEA AND BRONCHI.—The trachea or windpipe is the downward continuation of the larynx. It is situated in front of the oesophagus or gullet, and is composed of a series of small hoop-like cartilages joined together by fibrous membrane so as to form a semi-rigid tube or airway. This tube is rounded towards the front and flattened behind, where the cartilaginous rings are imperfect. It commences above at the cricoid cartilage, passes downwards through the neck into the thorax, and ends below by dividing into the two bronchi.

The bronchi convey the air from the trachea to the lungs : the right lung is supplied by the right bronchus and the left lung by the left bronchus. In the substance of the lungs the bronchi divide up to form the bronchial tree.

In structure the bronchi resemble the trachea, but they are smaller and circular in cross section.

II. THE LUNGS, the essential organs of respiration, are two in number, situated within the cavity of the chest on either side of the heart. They are composed of soft spongy tissue, which floats in water in virtue of the enormous number of alveoli or minute air-filled sacs which they contain. Each lung is described as having an apex, a base, a costal surface and a medial surface. The apex is the rounded upper extremity of the lung, which occupies the highest part of the thorax and extends into the root of the neck for about one and a half inches above the first rib. The base is broad and concave and rests upon the upper convex surface of the diaphragm. The costal surface is in contact with the inner aspect of the ribs on the side wall of the chest, and is therefore convex and of considerable extent. The medial surface has an impression for the adjacent surface of the heart, with which it lies in contact : above and behind this area is a somewhat triangular depression called the hilum, where the bronchus and main pulmonary vessels enter and leave the organ. The two lungs are almost identical, but the right lung is slightly larger and has three lobes while the left lung has only two lobes. The surface of each lung is covered by a smooth moist, glistening membrane called the pleura. This pleural

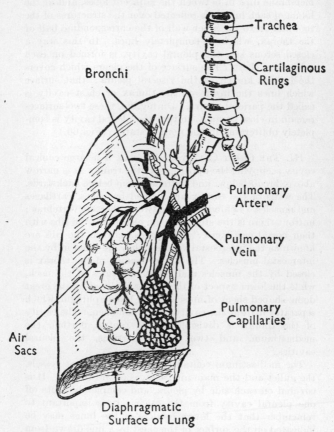

FIG. 60. DIAGRAMMATIC SCHEME OF RESPIRATORY SYSTEM.

membrane dips in between the adjacent lobes, and at the hilum of each lung it is reflected over the structures of the root and on to the inner wall of the corresponding half of the thorax, which it completely lines.   In this way a closed serous sac, the pleural cavity, is formed on each side of the chest.   The surface of the pleura which covers the lung is known as the visceral pleura : that surface which lines the inside of the thorax or chest cavity is called the parietal pleura.   During life, these two surfaces remain in close contact, so that the pleural cavity is completely obliterated in the normal state.   (Fig. 60.)

III. THE CHEST CAVITY OR THORAX is a large conical cavity occupying the upper part of the trunk.   It is narrow above, broad below, and flattened from before backwards. The walls of the thorax are formed by bones, cartilages and muscles.   Behind there are twelve thoracic vertebrae ; in front there is the sternum : on either side the ribs with their costal cartilages.   The spaces between the ribs are known as the intercostal spaces : they are filled in by the intercostal muscles.   The upper opening of the thorax is closed by the muscles and other structures of the neck, while the lower aspect of the thorax is closed by the great dome-shaped sheet of muscle called the diaphragm, which separates it from the cavity of the abdomen.   The cavity of the thorax is divisible into a central portion, the mediastinum, and two lateral portions, the pleural cavities.

The mediastinum contains the heart, the great vessels, the gullet and the main air passages of the thorax.   It is covered on each side by pleura, and completely shuts off one pleural cavity from the other.   It is important to remember that the lower borders of the lungs may be indicated on the surface of the chest by a line drawn from the sixth sterno-costal junction on either side in front, to the spine of the tenth thoracic vertebra behind.   This line is roughly horizontal.

PHYSIOLOGY OF THE RESPIRATORY SYSTEM.

Although a good deal has already been said with regard to the functioning of this system, it will be necessary here to assemble the facts systematically.

The primary object of the respiratory system is to supply the oxygen requirements of the body as a whole, and to get rid of the carbon dioxide which is a waste product of the activity of living tissue. The necessary oxygen is contained in the atmospheric air ; about one-fifth of the air we breathe is composed of oxygen, while the remainder is made up of nitrogen and other gases which have little or no part in the respiratory function.

We are constantly surrounded by an inexhaustible supply of atmospheric air containing the necessary oxygen. In the ordinary process of breathing we make use of this oxygen. Breathing is a rhythmical process ; each respiration or breath consists of two parts or phases. The act of breathing in is spoken of as inspiration, and breathing out is referred to as expiration. The whole respiratory act occurs with a frequency of about 18 per minute. Often it will be observed, however, that the respiratory rate is much increased. This may occur in emotional strain, in exercise, and in disease, particularly of the heart and lungs. Any condition whereby the oxygen want of the body is increased, as in exercise, or any condition tending to diminish the efficiency of the lungs, such as pneumonia, will increase the respiratory rate. Children usually breathe more rapidly than do adults.

The oxygenation and purification of the blood depends upon the bringing together of blood and oxygen into close proximity. This again depends on two factors : there must exist some sort of passage through which air may enter the body and come into close relationship with the blood in a capillary network, and there has to be some mechanism which will actively draw air through such a passage. The passage has been referred to before as the

respiratory tract, and mention has been made of its
anatomical structure.

Air enters the body in inspiration through the nostrils.
At the mouth of each nostril there are hairs, which are
directed downwards and inwards to act as a kind of sieve,
preventing gross foreign particles in the atmosphere from
entering the nose. In the cavities of the nose the inspired
air is warmed. This heating of the air depends upon the
extent of warm mucous membrane over which the air
passes. The area of mucous membrane is large, since it is
thrown into folds by the shelf-like projections of the
turbinated bones. Having passed through the cavities of
the nose, air enters the pharynx and is drawn into the
larynx and lower respiratory passages. In leaving the
pharynx it passes the epiglottis. This is a lid-like structure, the centre of which is composed of gristle. It serves
to prevent food entering the air passages, and in the act
of swallowing it covers over the opening into the larynx.
There is also another valve-like structure, which shuts
off the pharynx from the mouth in breathing. The soft
palate hangs like a curtain at the back of the mouth,
and thus a free passage of air from the posterior nares
into the windpipe is secured. In the larynx we find
a highly specialized structure in the form of the vocal
cords. These are seen as folds in the mucous membrane,
and they have elastic bands forming their core. By fine
muscular action the tension on the cords and the actual
length of the cords may be altered ; by the passage of air
throwing these structures into vibration we are able to
speak audibly. There is no point in discussing in detail
the questions of voice production, but it may be said that
the vowel sounds are produced by the expired air throwing
into vibration the vocal cords, and the consonants are
produced by the interruption of the stream of expired air
at certain levels above the larynx.

The larynx, trachea and bronchi are all of similar structure. The wall of the larynx is supported by special

cartilage plates forming the "Adam's apple." This structure is more prominent in the male than in the female. It is at this level that the vocal cords are situated. In the trachea there are incomplete bands of cartilage, which are referred to as the cartilaginous rings of the trachea. These cartilaginous masses are present also in the bronchi. Their purpose is simply to keep the air passages open and to provide a support for their walls. Lining the larynx, trachea and bronchi is a special type of mucous membrane. It is covered by microscopic hair-like structures called cilia. These cilia have an active movement, and they tend to sweep upwards against the stream of inspired air. The presence of glands just underneath the mucous membrane in these passages provides a secretion of mucus, which holds foreign particles from the inspired air in suspension. The mucus is driven upwards to the larynx by the activity of the cilia. In the larynx we have one of the most sensitive parts of the body : any foreign material will at once cause coughing or forced expiration, and the offending material is passed into the mouth and expectoration or spitting occurs. Another point is worthy of mention in connection with these lower air passages. The trachea and bronchi contain an amount of visceral muscle, which contracts to diminish the calibre of the air passages. The visceral muscle of the bronchi is believed to be thrown into spasm during an attack of asthma.

We have, so far, considered the main functions of the respiratory passages as they carry air down towards the lungs. It will be necessary now to show how the inspired air is permitted to come into close relationship with a blood capillary network. Some description of the great mass of lung tissue is therefore essential. Entering each lung we find a large bronchus, together with the pulmonary vessels. The point of entry on the medial aspect is spoken of as the hilum of the lung. Along with these structures there is a large amount of fibrous tissue, which forms a supporting framework for the essential tissues of

respiration.   The whole organ is covered by the serous
lining called the pleura.

Division of the bronchi, forming the bronchial tree,
occurs inside the substance of the organ until very fine
air passages are reached.   These very fine air passages open
out into what are termed air sacs, the walls of which are
beset with little box-like cavities called air cells or alveoli.
The number of air cells in one lung is enormous.   Air cells
are lined by a very thin membrane one cell thick.   The
whole object of having innumerable air cells lined by a
thin membrane is not far to seek.   Such an arrangement
exists solely to have a very large area of thin membrane
exposed to air.   On one side of the thin membrane we
have air, and on the other side we have capillary vessels.
So we find that there is a large surface of air separated
from blood merely by the thin membrane lining the alveoli
and by the walls of the capillaries through which the blood
flows.   These capillaries, of course, are derived from the
division and subdivision of the pulmonary arteries.   Actual
interchange between the gases of the air inside the lungs
and the gases inside the blood is carried on through the
membranes which separate the blood in the capillaries
from the alveolar air.   From the air in the alveoli, oxygen
is constantly being taken up into the blood, and carbon
dioxide is constantly being liberated from the blood into
alveolar air.   The lung capillaries reunite to form the
pulmonary veins, which return the re-oxygenated and
purified blood to the heart.

We have now to consider how air is drawn into the
lungs.   The essential mechanism of respiration depends
upon the variation in size of the chest cavity.   Such a
variation produced rhythmically will cause an inflow and
outflow of air from the air passages.   When the capacity
of the chest is increased in inspiration, air from the surrounding atmosphere is drawn into the lungs, and when
the cavity is diminished in expiration, air is driven out
from the lungs.   There is, therefore, during inspiration a

fall in pressure of air inside the lungs, and in expiration an increase in pressure : the consequence is that air will flow into and out of the lungs according to the rhythmic alterations in pressure, which are directly dependent on the alteration in the chest capacity.

During inspiration the volume of the chest cavity increases principally in two dimensions. The vertical dimensions of the chest increase, owing to the fact that the diaphragm tends to straighten itself out from its dome shape by the contraction of its muscular fibres. There is also at the same time an increase from front to back diameter of the thorax. This increase depends upon the sternum or breast-bone coming forwards and upwards. In inspiration not only does the diaphragm contract, but the intercostal muscles contract, and thus the ribs are drawn up. Since the ribs slope downwards and are fixed at their posterior ends, they will, in their movement upwards, describe an arc with their anterior ends, and thus the sternum will travel forwards and upwards. This movement would not in itself account for the increase in the air capacity of the lungs ; there must also be a corresponding increase in the volume of the lungs. Such an increase always attends inspiration, because the visceral and parietal surfaces of the pleura remain in close contact for certain physical reasons which need not be considered. In other words, the surface of the lung follows the chest wall in the movements of respiration ; this results, literally, in a pulling out of the lung tissue during inspiration and an opening up of the air spaces. The opposite movement of expiration occurs in virtue of two things : first, the relaxation of the muscles which were active in causing inspiration, and, second, the natural elastic rebound of the chest wall and of the lungs. It has been noted already that the chest wall, in virtue of its anatomical structure, is highly elastic, and it may be added here that in the lungs themselves there is abundance of elastic tissue, which allows the movements of respiration to be carried out without damage or prejudice to the essential organs of breathing.

To complete this section on respiration a little must be said with regard to the nervous control of respiration. The proper functioning of the respiratory mechanism is dependent upon the integrity of a small part of the nervous system, which is situated at the base of the brain and is referred to as the respiratory centre. The influences which act on the respiratory centre are numerous, and their manner of action is complex. When the respiratory centre is stimulated, from whatever influence, respiration is deepened and the exchange of gases is increased. When the respiratory centre is inhibited or checked, respiration ceases for the time being. The latter effect of inhibition is quite well illustrated in the mechanism of swallowing ; it is impossible to breathe and to swallow at one and the same time. One of the most important facts in human physiology is cited in order to illustrate the stimulation of the respiratory centre. The respiratory centre is stimulated most of all by an excess of carbon dioxide in the blood. When an individual is cyanosed or blue due to excess carbon dioxide in his blood, his breathing becomes rapid from a stimulation of his respiratory centre. A lack of oxygen in the blood is not such a powerful stimulant to respiration as is an excess of carbon dioxide. The combined effect of these two factors, but principally the effect of excess carbon dioxide in the blood, can be easily demonstrated. Let the reader hold his breath for as long as he can ; he will find that when he is compelled to breathe again his breathing is deep and rapid. If again he forces himself to breathe deeply and rapidly for a period of time, he will find that immediately afterwards his respirations will be slow and shallow. The first experiment is due to stimulation of the respiratory centre by excess of carbon dioxide in his blood, while the latter effect is due to his having washed out so much carbon dioxide that his respiratory centre is not stimulated.

CHAPTER XIII.

ASPHYXIA.

THE term asphyxia indicates an interference with the function of respiration and implies a depletion in the oxygen supply to the blood. There is cessation of the respiratory act and the co-existing insufficient oxygenation of the blood causes the apparent suspension of vital functions. In profound asphyxia the patient appears dead and, if not relieved immediately, will certainly die.

THE CAUSES OF ASPHYXIA.

These causes are divisible into two main groups.

A. The first group of causes includes a host of mechanical interferences which arise from outside the body and prevent air from entering the chest. These causes are purely of a mechanical nature.

B. The second group concerns those causes which arise from within the body and interfere with lung function. These causes are the result of disease and their ultimate mode of action may be either mechanical or nervous.

A. EXTERNAL CAUSES.

1. Foreign body in the mouth or air passages (choking).
2. Compression of the windpipe in
   - (*a*) Hanging.
   - (*b*) Strangulation.
   - (*c*) Throttling.
3. Smothering.
4. Foreign fluid in the air passages (drowning).

H

5. Foreign gas in the air passages (poison gases).
6. Rarefaction of the atmosphere (mountaineering and aeroplane sickness).
7. Fixation of the chest and abdomen by pressure.

   (a) Fall of debris in pit, quarry, or trench.
   (b) Hoist accidents, where a man is pinned under a hoist cage.
   (c) Pressure in crowds.
   (d) Overlying of infants.

8. Swelling of throat from burns, scalds and corrosions.

B. INTERNAL CAUSES.

1. MECHANICAL CAUSES.

   (a) Inhalation of vomited material in the unconscious.
   (b) Certain other causes arising from lung or chest disease.

2. NERVOUS CAUSES.

   (a) Poisoning of the respiratory centre by certain poisons.
   (b) Fixation of the chest muscles from strychnine poisoning.
   (c) Certain chronic diseases of the nervous system causing ultimately paralysis of the muscles of respiration.

GENERAL APPEARANCES IN ASPHYXIA.

When the respiratory function is suddenly interfered with there is immediate reaction on the part of the patient to overcome the cause of the asphyxia. This will evidence itself in a struggle for breath ; respiratory movements become violent ; the whole effort of the individual is to remove the cause of the asphyxia. If a case of asphyxia be seen early, therefore, the patient will be found to be restless ; there will be a struggle for breath ; the patient may tear at his throat ; owing to deficient oxygenation of the blood the face becomes livid ; the veins in the neck become engorged ; ultimately unconsciousness supervenes and the struggle is given up. This first stage of restlessness and violence may last from about three to five minutes ; it is followed by a second stage of paralysis of variable duration before the actual occurrence of death. During the second stage of asphyxia the patient is unconscious ; the respirations have ceased, but the heart continues to beat on although the pulse may not be felt at the wrist. In this stage the patient has given up the struggle and awaits death, which results from the rapid depletion of oxygen from the blood. The demand of the body tissues for oxygen in asphyxia still goes on although the source of its supply is cut off.

GENERAL TREATMENT OF CASES OF ASPHYXIA.

Certain general precepts may be formulated at the outset before giving particular instruction as to the treatment of the types of asphyxia arising from various causes. The first principle is to remove the cause of the asphyxia ; it will be seen that such a measure is possible in practically all the instances of the first group of causes, where some external influence is at play ; but, where some disease process causes asphyxia, this fundamental procedure is impossible. The second principle is to remove any conceivable hindrance to respiratory function. The asphyxiated patient must have no constricting clothing round his neck ; the clothing covering the chest must be loosened, even a tight belt round the abdomen should be slackened. In addition, the asphyxiated person is best treated in a current of fresh air. Carrying out these first two principles of treatment will be sufficient when the asphyxia has not advanced to the degree where the respiratory mechanism has been paralysed. Where respiration is feeble or has ceased

and the pulse is weak or absent artificial respiration must be
adopted. The methods about to be described must always
be considered as first-class emergency procedures. The
method selected in any case of asphyxia must be com-
menced at once, since asphyxia, with the possible exception
of haemorrhage, is the most urgent of all emergencies. Any
other first-aid measure, where artificial respiration is called
for, is therefore of a purely secondary character and must
always give place to the attempt to re-establish natural
breathing. It is evident that every second is of value and
that delay may mean loss of life. There is a danger after
resuscitation has so far been accomplished, that the patient
who has been breathing naturally for some time may
relapse ; it is therefore of paramount importance to keep
a close watch over the patient in order to be ready to re-
apply artificial respiration should the breathing fail ; on
no account must the patient be left alone until he has been
seen by a doctor, who will assess the general condition and
will give instructions as to further treatment.

I. Schäfer's Method.—This method is to be used in
almost every emergency of asphyxia and is certainly the
only method to be adopted in cases of drowning. The
patient is laid prone on the ground with the head turned
to one side. The ambulance man has two options with
regard to the position he may assume when administering
artificial respiration. He may either kneel beside the
patient or astride the buttocks ; in both instances he faces
the patient's head. Placing the hands over the small of
the patient's back, the thumbs pointing towards the
middle line and the palms and fingers embracing the
flanks, he proceeds to exert rhythmic compression on the
lower thorax. The whole action must be smooth and
regular and must imitate the normal act of respiration.
During the whole time of the procedure the hands

should not be moved away from the chest wall. No undue force is required. The act may be divided into three stages: first the state of compression, second the state of relaxation, and third a state of rest. The first stage represents natural expiration and the second inspiration, the third stage of rest gives the inspired air some time to act. The first stage is carried out by transmitting weight to the hands by leaning on the rigid arms, the second stage is accomplished by taking the weight off the hands and allowing the natural elastic recoil of the patient's chest wall to come into play. The third stage is purely passive. The three stages should be of about equal duration, the whole cycle being carried out at the rate of 12 per minute. There is absolutely no use in hurrying the procedure of artificial respiration; if it is performed rapidly the chances of resuscitation are diminished and the rescuer soon becomes exhausted. A second person assisting in the process of resuscitation should rub the limbs towards the heart in order to restore the circulation; he should also keep the patient as warm as possible, using any form of clothing which can be procured. In the event of a second person not being available the rescuer should, immediately after the re-establishment of respiration, pay attention to the stimulation of the circulation. It is necessary in cases where resuscitation is difficult and artificial respiration has to be carried out over a long period of time that those carrying out the procedure should work in relays. (Plate XXIV.)

II. SILVESTER'S METHOD.—This method has to be used only when, for any reason, it is undesirable to turn the patient on his face: for efficiency the method cannot be compared to that of Schäfer. Silvester's method consists in compressing the chest and attempting to expand it by manipulation of the patient's arms. The patient is laid flat on his back with a pillow under the shoulders, the ambulance man kneels at the head and faces the patient's feet. Grasping the patient's forearms just below the elbows with his hands the movements of inspiration are simulated by extending the patient's arms above the head and the movement of expiration by bringing the arms down and folding them across the chest, at the same time compressing the lower thorax. Thus the method of Silvester may be made to simulate the natural respiratory act ; extending the arms above the head causes air to enter the lungs, compression forces air out. The rhythm of the alternate movements should again be about 15 per minute. In this method there is a tendency for obstruction of the air passages to occur by the tongue falling back ; it is therefore necessary to pull the tongue forward. Since the tongue is difficult to hold a pin or safety pin may be run right through the substance of the tongue in order to secure sufficient control of the organ. The natural running out of fluid from the air passages is not permitted owing to the posture of the patient, hence its inapplicability to cases of drowning. The method of Silvester may be carried out by two people simultaneously, each grasping a forearm by the wrist and elbow and performing rhythmic alternate movements as described above ; such a procedure avoids fatigue on the part of the rescuer and permits of a more satisfactory excursion of the patient's chest wall. (Plate XXV.)

III. INFLATION METHOD.—This method consists of blowing into the lungs. Obstructing the nostrils to prevent escape of air, by gripping them between the finger and thumb and placing a handkerchief or a piece of gauze over the mouth, the rescuer expires forcibly into the patient's mouth and inflates the lungs. The natural act of expiration is simulated by the elastic recoil of an over-inflated chest when the pressure is taken away. The method is not applicable to cases of drowning or where breathing has been suspended for a long period of time.

In cases of asphyxia in children from causes other than drowning this method is the one of choice.

THE SYMPTOMS, SIGNS AND TREATMENT OF ASPHYXIA FROM PARTICULAR CAUSES.

1. FOREIGN BODY IN THE MOUTH OR AIR PASSAGES (CHOKING).

The evidence in the early stages are unmistakable. There is extreme distress on the part of the patient, whose whole movement and restlessness is expressive of the desire to expel the obstructing body. All are familiar with the excessive coughing which occurs when a small particle of food enters the larynx. The same kind of efforts are in evidence when a foreign body obstructs the entrance of air to the lungs. It is to be remembered that the obstruction is frequently merely partial and that the degree of asphyxia is purely relative. If the obstruction is complete there is rapid development of unconsciousness with cessation of respiratory movement. There are marked evidences of asphyxia, livid face, feeble or absent pulse and the eyes may protrude. Frequently information as to the nature of a foreign body which has been taken into the mouth can be obtained from those with the patient.

The treatment consists of removing the foreign body at once. Sometimes this may be effected simply by a thump on the back between the shoulder-blades. Children are often effectively treated by turning the child upside down and thumping the back. If such measures fail the patient's mouth should be opened and the fore-finger inserted; if a foreign body is felt the finger should be hooked round the obstructing object in order to remove it. All tight clothing about the neck should be quickly removed. Artificial respiration must be resorted to immediately if respiratory movements have become feeble or have ceased. The method to adopt is either that of Schäfer or of Silvester.

In all cases where artificial respiration has to be used a doctor must be summoned at once.

2. HANGING, STRANGULATION AND THROTTLING.

Hanging is the application of a constricting band round the neck, the constricting force applied to the band being the weight of the body. In judicial hanging death does not result from asphyxia but from a fracture-dislocation of the spine in the uppermost cervical region, the sudden-ness of death being due to the throwing out of action of the medulla oblongata. Strangulation is the application of a constricting band round the neck, the force of con-striction being supplied by someone tightening the band by twisting or pulling the ends. Throttling is the applica-tion of direct force over the windpipe, the constricting force being the fingers of an assailant. It is important to know, from the judicial point of view, which of the three has occurred. Hanging, nowadays, is practically always suicidal, strangulation and throttling are nearly always homicidal. In hanging, the victim is usually found sus-pended. In throttling and in strangulation, marks of violence are to be found on the neck ; in the former there is evidence of the force having been applied directly over the trachea in the mid line of the neck ; in the latter there is the mark of the constricting band and often the rope or other material which has been used will be found close by the patient.

In hanging and strangulation two things go to cause un-consciousness and death, the cutting off of the oxygen supply to the lungs and the suspension of the circulation to the brain through compression of the carotid arteries. There is another possible feature which has potent results, namely the compression of the great nerves which travel down in the neck to enter the thorax and supply the heart and lungs. In throttling the damage done is purely the result of asphyxia ; there are no other complicating factors at work.

The treatment in hanging is to cut the rope suspending the victim, taking the precaution that in so doing the person is not going to fall heavily to the ground and injure himself. Remove the constricting band from the neck and, if breathing is embarrassed or has ceased, commence artificial respiration. In strangulation, if the band still be in position remove it ; loosen all tight clothing and, if breathing is embarrassed or has ceased, commence artificial respiration. In throttling artificial respiration may have to be applied. In all three conditions, if the respiration is only slightly depressed, the application of smelling salts to the nostrils is an adequate first-aid measure.

3. SMOTHERING.

Smothering may be carried out with criminal intent. It is the prevention of the entrance of air into the lungs by the occlusion of the mouth and nose either by the hands of an assailant or by covering these orifices by some material which will effectively stop the entry of air. The method of occluding the nostrils and mouth by the use of the hands was resorted to by the notorious criminals Burke and Hare. Their practice had, from their point of view, a distinct advantage over the methods considered above in that no marks of violence were left on the body and consequently their crime was not easy to detect. Epileptics may smother themselves by turning over on to the face during unconsciousness following a fit. The treatment for smothering is to remove any material covering the face, loosen tight clothing and apply artificial respiration if necessary or use smelling salts if the respiration is only slightly depressed.

4. FOREIGN FLUID IN THE AIR PASSAGES (DROWNING).

The circumstances of any case of drowning are so obvious that little need be said on this particular score. There is one point, however, which must be made clear. Sometimes a dead body is thrown into water in order to conceal the crime of murder committed in some other way. If any doubt exists about the circumstances of a case where a body has been recovered from the water, the ambulance man must pay particular attention to the associated facts, as his evidence may be required in a court of law. The following points should be noted about accidental drowning. In the victim's tightly clenched hand there may be found twigs or seaweed, because the drowning man " clutches at a straw." When laying him on his face water will run out of the mouth and nostrils and more water will be expressed from the air passages when the first compression of the thorax is made in carrying out Schäfer's method of artificial respiration. It need hardly be said that a dead man thrown into water cannot grasp any object, nor can he inhale water into his lungs.

The treatment in cases of drowning is to place the patient on his face, raise the abdomen and permit the water to run out of the mouth and nose ; compress the thorax rhythmically according to Schäfer's method after having turned the head to one side. Schäfer's method is the only one applicable to cases of drowning. As people apparently drowned are chilled they must be kept as warm as possible and it is advisable to rub the hands and limbs in order to restore the circulation. This latter step may be conveniently carried out by a second person. It is also advisable to work in spells, and if two people are attempting to resuscitate a person apparently drowned they may exchange duties at appropriate intervals. After the victim has been so far resuscitated, it is probable that he may vomit a good deal of the water swallowed while he was immersed. It is recommended that further treatment should be given in the form of administering hot coffee or strong hot tea by the mouth once he is able to swallow.

5. FOREIGN GAS IN THE AIR PASSAGES (POISON GASES).

Carbon monoxide (coal gas, petrol gas fumes, and
choke damp in mines).
Carbon dioxide.
Acetylene.
Naphtha or benzene.
Sulphur dioxide.
Sulphuretted hydrogen (sewer gas).
Ammonia.
Chloroform and ether.
Hydrocyanic acid fumes.
Smoke in burning buildings.

CARBON MONOXIDE.—This gas is the main constituent of
coal gas, which is used for illuminating and heating purposes domestically. It is found in the vapour of petrol
and appears to be responsible for those deaths which occur
as the result of running a petrol engine within a confined,
ill-ventilated space. It may collect in some concentration
in close proximity to lime kilns and, further, it may collect
in mines in the form of choke damp. When pure it has no
smell and is an insidious poison. The smell of ordinary
coal gas is due to the presence of other gases which are
compounds of carbon and other elements and result from
the incineration of coal. The action of carbon monoxide
is unique because it forms with the haemoglobin of the
blood a very stable compound, carboxyhaemoglobin, which
cannot give off oxygen to the tissues of the body ; thus
the tissues become starved of oxygen and cease to function.
Carboxyhaemoglobin is a bright red pigment and imparts
to the blood a bright red colour. The appearances of a
case of carbon monoxide poisoning are not those of ordinary
asphyxia, since the blood is not livid from want of oxygen
but bright red owing to carboxyhaemoglobin. The lips and
face are also bright red from the presence of the pigment.

The treatment is to remove the patient from the atmosphere of coal gas, loosen tight clothing round the neck and

apply artificial respiration. Smelling salts may be applied to the nose and stimulants in the form of hot coffee may be given. The blood holds on to carbon monoxide for a long time and consequently the body has to make use of all the available normal haemoglobin. Every effort must be made to keep the circulation brisk and to insure free ventilation of the lungs.

CARBON DIOXIDE.—Carbon dioxide poisoning must be relatively uncommon. In crowded places any feeling of discomfort is not due to the excess of carbon dioxide in the air but to inability to lose heat by radiation from the skin. There is a rise in temperature of the atmospheric air and also the water vapour in the air is increased. Both of these factors operate to diminish loss of heat by radiation. Occasionally, where fermentation is going on in brewers' lofts, there may be a huge increase in the amount of carbon dioxide in the air. The result of inhaling such an atmosphere is that the individual will breathe much more deeply and more frequently. This effect is due to the fact that carbon dioxide is a stimulant to the respiration. By way of treatment it is usually sufficient to place the patient in the fresh air.

ACETYLENE.—Acetylene is used commercially in oxy-acetylene welding where a high temperature is required. It is used as an illuminant for cycle lamps and occasionally as an illuminating gas for country houses. The gas is a chemical compound of carbon and hydrogen and is therefore spoken of as a hydrocarbon. It is prepared by the interaction of water and carbide of calcium. The gas has not been responsible for cases of acute fatal poisoning, although inhalation of large quantities will cause asphyxia. There is no doubt that the constant inhalation of small quantities is prejudicial to health. The treatment is to remove the patient to the fresh air and, if necessary, to stimulate his respiration by smelling salts.

NAPHTHA, BENZOL, OR BENZENE.—This substance is a

liquid which owing to its volatile nature may cause symptoms of asphyxia by inhalation of the vapour. It is another gas belonging to the group of hydrocarbons. It is used commercially to dissolve waterproof material for the impregnation of fabrics. In drying it evaporates and may cause a fatal issue to those who may be so unfortunate as to inhale the vapour. The action of the gas manifests itself in the fairly rapid suspension of consciousness without much warning. The treatment is to remove the patient into the fresh air and to administer artificial respiration. Stimulants should be given in the form of hot coffee.

SULPHUR DIOXIDE AND SULPHURETTED HYDROGEN.—Sulphur dioxide and sulphuretted hydrogen are both very irritant gases. The former is seldom found outside the chemical laboratory, but the latter, although used extensively in chemical laboratories, is the poisonous constituent of sewer gas. Cases have occurred where men working in sewers have been fatally poisoned by the gas sulphuretted hydrogen. Apart from the intense irritation which these gases cause to the respiratory passages their poisonous effect is due to the action of the gas when absorbed into the blood. The sulphur forms a stable compound with the haemoglobin of the blood and so deprives the tissues of the body generally of oxygen. The usual methods of resuscitation form the active treatment for the condition.

AMMONIA.—Ammonia is used extensively in ice factories and bleaching works. When the vapour is inhaled it acts as a very strong irritant to the respiratory passages and causes much swelling of the membranes lining the nose, throat and upper air passages. The symptoms are choking and coughing with evidences of asphyxia. The treatment consists of the usual methods of resuscitation by artificial respiration and stimulation.

CHLOROFORM AND ETHER.—The fumes of these two substances are used to induce insensibility to pain during surgical operations. They are general anaesthetics. Sometimes individuals develop a liking for the fumes of chloroform and indulge in self administration of the substance. The action of chloroform is much more potent than that of ether and consequently in order to produce complete anaesthesia by the use of ether a special form of mask has to be used. It is, on the other hand, comparatively easy to produce profound unconsciousness by soaking a pad with chloroform and placing it over the mouth and nostrils. With either drug signs of asphyxia may develop and frequently evidence of failure of the heart's action may be present. Where the respiration is suspended, artificial respiration is necessary and, where the pulse is not palpable at the wrist, cloths wrung out of hot water should be applied over the heart. The patient must be kept warm, and when he can swallow hot coffee or tea may be given. Smelling salts may be useful to aid the other methods of resuscitation.

HYDROCYANIC ACID.—Reference is made to cyanide poisoning in the chapter on poisons. The gas is produced by the addition of an acid to a solution of cyanide. It is quickly lethal and has been fatal to people working carelessly with photographic solutions. The treatment is to administer artificial respiration and to give other stimulant treatment. For further particulars the chapter on poisons should be consulted.

SMOKE IN BURNING BUILDINGS.—Smoke in burning buildings may be powerfully asphyxiating. In addition to the carbon particles constituting the gross material of smoke, gases such as carbon monoxide and certain irritants are often present. In rescuing people from burning buildings, the rescuer should protect himself by wearing a mask of wet cloth or a smoke helmet when available. The treatment is to administer artificial respiration, and to overcome the shock which accompanies severe burns, by the administration of stimulants and by keeping the patient

warm. The actual dressing of burns is quite subsidiary to
the main work of resuscitation. Stimulants, it need hardly
be said, must not be given until the patient is able to
swallow.

6. RAREFACTION OF THE ATMOSPHERE (MOUNTAINEERING AND AEROPLANE SICKNESS).

Apart from the dizziness which certain people feel when
looking down from a height, a definite train of symptoms
may develop due to lack of oxygen when any normal person
ascends to a great height. The symptoms are much more
severe if a rapid ascent is made but those people who are
accustomed to high altitudes are not so liable to disturbance. Fainting, sickness and vomiting, dizziness with
ringing noises in the head and bleeding from the nose may
all be associated with an increased activity of the respiration. The treatment is to descend to a normal atmospheric
pressure and to stimulate the patient by hot drinks and
general heat.

Note.—There is an interesting counterpart to lack of
oxygen in a rarefied atmosphere. The opposite condition
occurs in caissons or diving bells such as are used for sink-
ing piers of bridges. Divers and miners when working at
great depths are subject to very high atmospheric pressures
and may complain of some discomfort. The pressure in a
caisson may reach 50 lbs. per square inch in contrast to
the normal pressure of 14 lbs. at sea level. Effects of high
atmospheric pressure are curious in that workmen find
muscular exertion extremely laborious, but usually there
is no emergency of illness when working in a high atmospheric pressure. The trouble arises when people are taken
out of a high pressure into the ordinary air. Bleeding from
the nose may occur ; the victim is dizzy, complains of
noises in the head, feels faint, and sometimes has curious
tingling sensations in the limbs. Paralysis may result
from this condition within a few hours and is due to the

formation of bubbles of nitrogen in the tissues of the central nervous system.

Treatment is of a highly specialised nature and is, in the main, preventive. With all caissons working at some depth special decompression chambers are in use. Workmen enter these chambers on coming up from the caisson, the pressure of the atmosphere in the chamber is raised to the level of that in the caisson and then gradual reduction is accomplished until the normal atmospheric pressure is reached. Should the reduction in pressure be too rapid, the workman will complain of the symptoms described above ; he speaks of them as the " bends." Recompression and gradual decompression should be carried out in these cases.

7. FIXATION OF THE CHEST AND ABDOMEN BY PRESSURE.

Fall of debris in a pit, quarry or trench or the fall of a hoist cage may pin a man so effectively as to render the movements of respiration impossible. Fixation of the thorax alone will not suspend the function of respiration, since the diaphragm can still act, but where both abdomen and chest are crushed, respiration is impossible. The treatment for such conditions after extracting the victim from the compressing mass is to administer artificial respiration. This type of asphyxia is often complicated by fractured ribs and consequently the method of inflation of the lungs may have to be attempted. The general condition arising from surgical shock and gross injuries may be treated in some cases concurrently with the administration of artificial respiration. Pressure in crowds has frequently been the cause of asphyxia in children and feeble adults. Such circumstances as are associated with the panic of a theatre fire are productive of the condition. The treatment is along the general lines indicated above. Overlying of infants is a punishable offence. An intoxicated mother may overlie an infant sleeping beside her, the weight of the body being sufficient to cause fatal asphyxia through fixation of the chest wall and abdomen. Seldom is the condition caught soon enough, but when the pulse may be felt artificial respiration must be carried out.

8. SWELLING OF THROAT FROM BURNS, SCALDS AND CORROSIVES.

There is a most alarming condition which may arise from swallowing scalding fluids or corrosive poisons or from inhaling steam. The mucous membrane of the throat and wind pipe, in response to the irritation, swells so as to occlude the channel and consequently the evidences of asphyxia are at once present. All degrees of asphyxia may be present according to the severity of the condition. There is great alarm and the patient has agonizing pain in the throat. A doctor must be summoned at once, since complete blocking may occur at any moment and the operation of tracheotomy may be required. In milder cases where the patient can swallow, the primary condition having been dealt with, demulcent drinks like milk and barley-water are often grateful. Where the condition is more severe and the respiration is noticeably embarrassed artificial respiration should be carried out in the hope of forcing air into the lungs.

B. INTERNAL CAUSES.

1. MECHANICAL CAUSES.

(a) *Inhalation of vomited material in the unconscious.*— Such a condition not infrequently arises in cases of profound intoxication from alcohol : it may occur in other cases of poisoning, such as from opium. The treatment here is to clear out the mouth and throat and to apply artificial respiration and other measures as in drowning. Such cases are often followed by severe acute infections of the lungs.

(b) *Lung or chest disease.*—In those conditions the patient has been ill for some considerable time. The progress of asphyxial signs and symptoms is slow and is usually under medical observation. Collapse of the lung, however, may occur quite suddenly when the patient is about his ordinary vocation.

2. NERVOUS CAUSES.

(a) Poisoning of the respiratory centre by certain poisons. The most notable of these is cyanide (prussic acid).

(b) Strychnine poisoning.—The reader is referred to the chapter on poisons.

(c) Nervous diseases.—Certain forms of nervous disorder terminate life by attacking the nerves, upon the integrity of which the action of the muscles of respiration depends. They do not concern the first-aid man because of the long train of symptoms which has preceded the fatal issue, and because the patient is usually under constant medical supervision.

CHAPTER XIV.

THE ALIMENTARY SYSTEM.

ANATOMY.—The food which we eat passes through a long tubular tract called the alimentary canal. In this canal the food is brought into contact with certain fluid substances, the digestive juices, which are secreted by special glandular organs and passed into the alimentary canal through tubular structures known as ducts. The alimentary canal, together with these associated glandular organs, constitutes the alimentary or digestive system.

THE ALIMENTARY SYSTEM COMPRISES :
- (a) The Mouth and Salivary Glands.
- (b) The Pharynx.
- (c) The Oesophagus or Gullet.
- (d) The Stomach.
- (e) The Small Intestine, Liver and Pancreas.
- (f) The Large Intestine.

THE ALIMENTARY CANAL commences at the mouth and ends at the anus, the lower orifice of the large intestine. The digestive tract is altogether about thirty feet long, and, while its structure in different parts varies, its cavity is lined by mucous membrane throughout and the walls of the tube are formed by muscle and membranous tissue.

(a) THE MOUTH has already been mentioned with reference to the respiratory system in a previous chapter, but it should be repeated that the mouth is essentially a part of the alimentary canal. In addition to the features already described, the mouth is furnished with two rows of teeth, there being normally sixteen in each jaw. The teeth have their roots embedded in the bone, which is covered by the mucous membrane to form the gums. Projecting forwards from the floor of the mouth there is a strong muscular organ, the tongue. It is somewhat conical in shape ; the broad base forms its root and gives attachment to the organ posteriorly, while the apex forms its tip and is freely movable anteriorly. Associated with the mouth there are three pairs of salivary glands, which pour their secretions, the saliva, into this cavity. The two largest glands are the parotids, which are situated on either side of the face in front of the ear, and each parotid gland is provided with a duct which opens into the mouth on the inside of the cheek. The submaxillary and sublingual glands are smaller in size, and are situated in the floor of the mouth, on to which they pour their secretions.

(b) THE PHARYNX has also been dealt with in a previous chapter. Here it is only necessary to mention that it has the double function of a food and air passage. It therefore forms part of the alimentary canal for the conveyance of food from the mouth to the oesophagus.

(c) THE OESOPHAGUS or Gullet is a muscular tube about nine or ten inches long. It commences at the lower end of the pharynx, extends vertically downwards in front of the vertebral column in the thoracic cavity, and passes through the diaphragm to enter the cavity of the abdomen. Immediately below the diaphragm the oesophagus ends in its communication with the stomach.

(d) THE STOMACH is a sort of bag-like structure or reservoir, in which the food remains for a time before being passed into the small intestine or bowel. The stomach is the most dilated part of the alimentary canal ; it is directly continuous above with the oesophagus and below with the duodenum, or the first part of the small intestine. The upper opening into the stomach is called the cardiac orifice : the lower opening or outlet is called the pylorus. Food enters the stomach at the cardiac orifice and leaves it by passing through the pylorus. Each orifice is guarded by a circular band of involuntary muscle termed a sphincter. The stomach is situated entirely within the abdominal cavity and mainly in its upper left quadrant. It is described as having a cardiac portion or body, which is the broad upper part, and a pyloric portion, which is

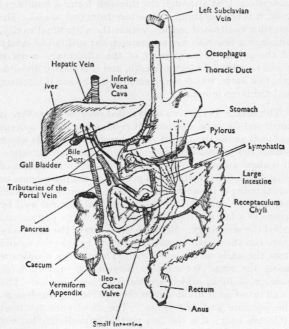

FIG. 61. DIAGRAMMATIC SCHEME OF THE ALIMENTARY SYSTEM.

the narrower or lower part, near the outlet. The walls of the stomach are mainly composed of layers of involuntary muscle; the cavity is lined by mucous membrane, and the organ is invested by a serous membrane, the peritoneum. The stomach is richly supplied with blood-vessels and lymphatics and nerves. (Fig. 61.)

(*e*) THE INTESTINE or Bowel is that portion of the alimentary canal which extends from the pylorus to the anus. It is a long tubular structure, the coils of which are sometimes called the " intestines," but it should be clearly understood that although the intestine forms a number of coils, it is one continuous structure from end to end. The intestine is situated mainly within the abdominal cavity, although a few coils are accommodated within the cavity of the pelvis. This portion of the alimentary canal is about twenty-eight feet in length, and it is clearly divisible into two parts, which are referred to as the small intestine and the large intestine.

THE SMALL INTESTINE is so called because its calibre is small and its walls are thin. It commences at the pylorus and ends at the ileo-caecal valve, a sphincter muscle which guards the junction of the small with the large intestine. It is about twenty-two feet long, and forms a succession of coils which are invested by a portion of the peritoneum or serous lining of the abdominal cavity. The coils of the small intestine are attached to the posterior abdominal wall by means of a fan-like double layer or fold of the peritoneum called the mesentery. Between the layers of the mesentery there run the blood-vessels, nerves and lymphatics to and from the walls of the intestine. The mucous membrane lining the small intestine is thrown into a very large number of folds, which are more or less circular. The small intestine is divided into three parts, the duodenum, the jejunum and the ileum. The duodenum is about 10 inches long ; it is the first portion immediately beyond the stomach, and is frequently the site of ulcer formation. The jejunum and ileum are respectively the second and third parts of the small intestine. They require no special description.

THE LIVER is the largest of the abdominal organs associated with the alimentary canal. It is situated mainly in the upper right quadrant of the abdomen, and is slung from the lower surface of the diaphragm by ligaments formed from folds of the peritoneum which invests the organ. Its functions and structure are complicated, but here it may be mentioned that it is responsible for the manufacture of bile, which is poured into the duodenum through the bile duct. On the under surface of the liver, at a point corresponding to the tip of the ninth costal cartilage, is the gall-bladder, which communicates with the bile duct and contains a small amount of bile. It is important to recognise that the liver is supplied by blood from two different sources. In addition to the arterial supply of blood from the aorta through the hepatic arteries, all the blood leaving the abdominal portion of the alimentary canal passes to the liver through the portal vein. This latter circulation of blood is known as the portal system.

THE PANCREAS is a small glandular organ which produces two quite different kinds of secretion. Firstly, there is the digestive secretion or pancreatic juice, which is poured into the duodenum through the pancreatic duct. Secondly, there is the internal secretion, which is poured directly into the blood. This organ is situated on the posterior wall of the upper abdomen; it is somewhat comma-shaped, and lies transversely across the spinal column, with its head to the right and its tail towards the left.

THE LARGE INTESTINE extends from the lower end of the ileum to the anus. Its structure is essentially similar to that of the small intestine, but it may be distinguished by certain characteristic features : it has a greater calibre ; its walls are thicker and sacculated ; the outermost layer of muscle is arranged in three distinct bands, which are clearly visible through the transparent serous peritoneal membrane. Further, the large intestine is more closely attached to the posterior abdominal wall and only parts of it have a mesentery. It is not arranged in coils, but for the most part it forms one great arch which embraces the coils of the small intestine. The large intestine is altogether about six feet in length, and may be described as having three distinct regions : the caecum, the colon and the rectum. The caecum is simply the first and most dilated portion of the large intestine. It forms a large pouch immediately below the ileo-caecal valve, where the terminal part of the small intestine joins the large intestine at right angles. The caecum is situated in the right lower quadrant of the abdomen, just above the outer half of the fold of the groin. The appendix is an elongated worm-like structure arising from the medial and lower aspect of the caecum. It varies considerably in size, but is most commonly about three or four inches long and about as thick as a large earth-worm ; its narrow cavity normally communicates with that of the caecum. It is of interest to note that acute inflammation of this small structure gives rise to the urgent and all too common disease known as appendicitis. The colon has three parts, which are referred to as the ascending, transverse, and descending colons, according to their direction. The ascending colon is the upward continuation of the caecum on the right side of the abdomen. When the colon reaches the under surface of the liver it takes a right-angled turn to the left into the transverse colon. This right-angled bend forms the hepatic flexure. The transverse colon is suspended in a festoon from the posterior abdominal wall by a relatively long mesentery. It extends from the hepatic flexure on the right side to a similar angular bend on the left side of the abdomen just below the spleen. This bend is termed the splenic flexure, and at this point the transverse colon becomes continuous with the descending colon. From the lower border of the transverse colon there hangs an apron-like structure called the omentum which, composed of fat between layers of peritoneum, acts as a means of protection to the intestines. The descending colon commences at the splenic flexure and passes down the left side of the abdomen to enter the pelvis, where it becomes continuous with the rectum. The lower portion of the descending colon forms an " S "-shaped loop, usually referred to as the sigmoid colon. The rectum is the lowest portion of the alimentary tract, and is situated entirely within the pelvis. It opens to the exterior through the anus, a circular orifice guarded by a muscular ring, the anal sphincter.

PHYSIOLOGY.

In order to appreciate the functioning of the alimentary system it is necessary to have some knowledge of the composition of the food which constitutes the everyday diet of man. It consists essentially of three main types of substance—protein, carbohydrate and fat. In addition to these materials it is necessary that certain minerals must be consumed : iron, potassium, sodium, calcium and magnesium. These substances are not taken into the body as such, but they are combined chemically with certain elements to form salts which are contained in the ordinary diet. Other substances called vitamins, of which little is definitely known, are essential to the maintenance of health.

PROTEINS are complex in their chemical structure, and are formed by the combination of carbon, oxygen, nitrogen, hydrogen and sulphur. They are found in greatest proportion in meats such as beef, mutton, chicken, fish, etc. The white of an egg contains a protein called albumen. It should be remembered that if one takes any protein it cannot be split up by any physical process into particles of carbon, nitrogen, and so on ; a protein is a chemical compound which presents a very different appearance from the separate elements which go to make it up.

CARBOHYDRATES consist of chemical combinations of carbon, hydrogen and oxygen in certain proportions. These substances are the sugars and starches of the vegetable world, and are therefore found in abundance in potatoes, fruits, cereals, bread, etc.

FATS, like carbohydrates, are chemical compounds of carbon, hydrogen and oxygen, but in different proportions. They exist in butter, cream, cheese, the fat of meat, and in vegetable oils.

While it is usual to speak of a diet as being a carbohydrate, protein or fat diet, it should be remembered that these terms are merely relative when used in this connection, and that every ordinary diet is a combination of all three primary elements of food. A carbohydrate diet is, therefore, one which is rich in that particular substance.

Food is required for the supply of energy to maintain vital processes. This is accomplished by the breaking down of food by means of a process of burning. Burning is simply a chemical action which occurs with the liberation of heat. The three primary substances of food are all burned and yield heat in the process. From this heat the energy of the body is derived, as in the case of coal in the furnace. In all three instances the ultimate products of burning are carbon dioxide and water, both of which are excreted, as we have already seen. The process of burning is a gradual one, and is manifested by the breaking down of complex materials into simpler substances.

This process of breaking down is generally spoken of as katabolism. There is another process, however, going on in the body, referred to as anabolism, which is the reverse of katabolism, and is the building up of chemical substances, from the simpler to the more complex. These two processes occur at one and the same time, and are together spoken of as metabolism, which is really the total chemical activity of the organism.

PROTEIN is essential for the replacement of similar substances which are used up in the wear and tear of the body. They are necessary for the repair of broken-down tissue, such as results from muscular action. In addition to this function they liberate a certain amount of heat. We do not store protein in the body but we store carbohydrate and fat.

CARBOHYDRATE is readily used by the body, since it is easily burned to give energy in the form of heat. It is stored in various situations in the form of animal starch—glycogen—which store of supply may be utilised when easily available energy is demanded by the body.

FAT is broken down like carbohydrate and protein with the evolution of heat. The storage of fat is exemplified in the laying down of fat underneath the skin, particularly in the region of the abdomen. It should be noted that carbohydrate may be converted into fat and stored as such.

MINERAL SUBSTANCES.—These substances are found in the earth, and are not the products of the chemical processes of life as are the three principles of diet, protein, carbohydrate and fat. In addition to their being found in the mineral world, they are also found in living things, but they arrive there directly from the soil. As an example of the part played by minerals, it has been proved that a certain amount of iron is necessary to maintain life. Some iron may be found in certain drinking waters, but we take iron into the system through eating the flesh of animals living on plants which in turn have taken their store of iron from the soil. We may also consume iron as it is presented to us in a diet consisting of vegetables. There are many mineral substances which it is necessary to consume, but it is not advisable to burden the mind with any detailed information on the subject. It should, however, be noticed that these mineral elements enter into combination with certain other elements to form salts, such as chlorides, carbonates and sulphates, and that these salts play a most important rôle in the human mechanism. In the body there is a tremendous amount of water, which carries these salts in solution, and it is necessary that these body fluids should have certain fairly constant concentrations of salts in order that the mechanism may function normally.

WATER.—Water plays a most important part in the human economy. By means of water it is possible for solid substances to be carried from one part of the body to another. It is a suitable vehicle for the excretion of waste products also, and, consequently, it is most important that the supply of water should be adequate. This is provided for by the quantities of water which we drink in the ordinary way and by the large proportion of water in every diet. It is possible to go without food for two or three weeks, but it is impossible to go without water for even a few days.

VITAMINS.—Much which has been written with regard to the nature of vitamins is purely hypothetical. Their absence from the diet is said to produce certain diseases, such as scurvy and rickets. These substances are found in fresh foods of animal and vegetable origin, such as meat, butter and fresh fruit. Some vitamins are easily destroyed by the heat of cooking.

Our daily diet is comprehensive enough to include all the elements which are necessary for the maintenance of life: the proteins for repair and replacement of tissue, fats and carbohydrates for the storage of energy, calcium for the building up of bone, iron for the maintenance of the colouring matter of the blood, water, salts and vitamins for vital functions.

It is necessary to refer briefly to the energy-giving value of food. Proteins, carbohydrates and fats have each a definite heat-yielding or caloric value. The reader cannot be expected to memorize the measurement of these values, but in these days it may be of interest to make some reference to what is termed the caloric value of food. In some American restaurants the caloric value of each delicacy on the menu is noted, so that any customer may consume wittingly so many calories of food. The calorie is the unit of heat ; and every ounce of carbohydrate or other principle in the process of metabolism yields a constant number of calories or units of heat. According to the age and size of the individual, there are certain minimum requirements of heat units as presented to us in the form of food. If the individual performs work, he will require more calories according to the amount of work he performs—so that the lumberman of Canada may consume four times as many calories as the man of sedentary occupation. The appetite of the healthy man is a good ready-reckoner of caloric requirement.

Let us now enquire into the state of affairs existing in the human body enabling us to utilize efficiently the diet of everyday life.

Digestion is the process whereby food is broken up mechanically and chemically, in order that it may be rendered absorbable by the blood.

CHEWING.—It is quite obvious that a meal of meat, steak and whole potatoes cannot be used straight away to supply the needs of the body. Food must be presented in a broken-up condition. The teeth have different shapes and positions according to their different functions, and therefore those teeth which we use for biting are situated in the front part of the mouth, and are shaped so that their free biting edges are comparatively sharp. They are called the incisor teeth, because they literally incise the food which we consume. This incised food is taken on to the surface of the tongue, and is presented by the movements of that organ to the premolars and molars, which have flat tops and are used to grind up the food into small particles. The process of biting and chewing is referred to as mastication. While the process of grinding is going on, the food becomes intimately mixed up with the saliva or secretion of the salivary glands. This is the first of the digestive juices, and it plays quite an important part in the process. The main functions of the saliva are to form a basis for the particles of dry food, cementing them together to form what is termed a bolus, or ball, and to break up complex carbohydrates into simpler materials. In the saliva there is a special digestive ferment called ptyalin, which acts on the starchy part of food and ultimately breaks it down into simpler carbohydrates like sugars. After the food has been thoroughly mixed up with the saliva, bolus formation occurs largely through the movements of the tongue, which, by its action, initiates the act of swallowing. The bolus is passed over the back of the tongue and over the epiglottis to the posterior pharyngeal wall, where swallowing occurs.

The bolus next enters the oesophagus, which, by its muscular action, passes the food into the stomach. When the bolus enters the stomach, the digestion of carbohydrate ceases on the surface of the bolus, but the further digestion of carbohydrate is permitted to proceed in the centre of the bolus, since the ptyalin which is mixed up with food is not in contact with the secretions of the stomach. When the bolus is broken up by the digestive ferments and the stomach movements, all carbohydrate digestion is stopped. The secretion of the stomach, the gastric juice, is strongly acid owing to the presence of hydrochloric acid (spirits of salt). This juice is secreted by certain specialised gland-ular cells at the cardiac end of the stomach. Functionally the secretion of hydrochloric acid must be regarded as a means of preparing the protein part of the meal for further digestion, and, consequently, we find a ferment at the pyloric end of the stomach having this function of break-ing down protein ; it is termed pepsin. As has been learned already, the wall of the stomach is largely made up of visceral muscle. In virtue of its action two things happen : firstly, the food is intimately mixed up with the secretion of the organ, and, secondly, the contractions of the muscle are of such an ordered nature as to cause food to be passed constantly in one direction. This is accom-plished by a wave of contraction succeeding a wave of relaxation, so that food is pushed by the contracted band of muscle into the relaxed area. This kind of action is termed peristalsis, and is characteristic of the muscular functioning of the whole tube making up the alimentary canal. In addition to this there are specialised kinds of muscular activity, which are exemplified at the entrance to and the exit from the stomach. These orifices are guarded by thickened muscle bands called sphincters. When the bolus of food reaches the lower end of the oesophagus, the cardiac sphincter of the stomach relaxes and the food is allowed to pass into the stomach ; again, when digestion has proceeded a certain length, the pylorus relaxes and peristalsis pushes the stomach contents—now called chyme—into the duodenum, which is the first part of the small intestine. Into the duodenum there are poured certain very important digestive juices which come from the liver and the pancreas. Bile, secreted by the liver cells, is ultimately conveyed by the common bile duct to the duodenum. There is an important accessory to this mechanism, namely the gall-bladder, which opens into the common bile duct. In the gall-bladder thin bile excreted by the liver is concentrated until it becomes quite viscid. In this state it is poured into the duodenum. The pancreas is a composite gland, which has a duct opening along with the common bile duct on to the duodenal surface : its chief secretion is known as trypsin.

Let us consider the bile and the pancreatic juice together. They act on the three main principles of diet. In reaction the juice is alkaline. Protein has been prepared by the action of hydrochloric acid, and has been broken down a little by the action of pepsin. There now occurs a further breaking down of protein, so that absorption into the blood of comparatively simple substances may occur. It will be remembered that the carbohydrates are incompletely digested in the mouth, and the action of the stomach juices is to stop carbohydrate digestion ; in the duodenal contents there is necessarily a substance which will cause the starches to split up into simple substances, until sugars of the order of simplicity of glucose are obtained and made ready for absorption ; thus the work started by ptyalin in the mouth is completed. So far no mention has been made of the fats. These substances are also split up, and are absorbed as globules not directly into the blood stream, but in a rather complicated fashion into the lymphatics. The fat absorption is rendered easy by the presence of bile, which makes the fat into an emulsion. This digestive process of fat, carbohydrate and protein is continued and completed by the action of the ferments coming from the glands in the mucous membrane of the small intestine—the succus entericus. Further description would be merely repetition of the function of the duodenal juices.

The problem of absorption has been left to the present, since there is little absorption from the stomach, and since the bulk of absorption of nutriment takes place from the small intestine. Absorption of nutriment depends on the existence of a blood capillary network in close relationship to the material to be absorbed. For this purpose there is a special apparatus—the portal circulation—which not only supplies the intestines, but also goes through the liver. From the abdominal aorta certain vessels of large calibre arise ; these go to the stomach and intestines, where they break up into a network of capillaries, which reunite to form the portal vein. The portal vein breaks up in the liver to form small sinusoids or channels—the sinusoids of the liver—and the liver seizes what it requires in the way of food from the blood circulating through the sinusoids before the other organs, as it were, get a chance. Here we have quite a unique state of affairs : the arteries going to the alimentary tract in the abdomen break up to form a capillary network, and then there is a reunion of capillaries to form the portal vein and a further capillary network through the division and subdivision of the portal vein in the liver. There is, however, another blood supply to the liver, coming directly from the aorta, so that the liver is supplied—as in the ordinary systemic circulation—with oxygenated blood which has not gone through a capillary network. It should be remembered that both the portal circulation and the circulation of systemic blood through the liver have a common route of egress through the hepatic vein into the inferior vena cava. Having followed the above description of the portal circulation, the reader will at once appreciate that all blood coming from the stomach and intestines passes through the liver before it reaches the right side of the heart. It is the portal circulation which is responsible for the absorption of nutriment in its ultimate form from the alimentary canal. Only two kinds of food, however, are absorbed into the portal circulation in this way : these are the end products of the digestion of protein and carbohydrate. Carbohydrate in the form of glucose is kept at a fairly constant concentration in the blood, and when this level tends to rise the liver fastens on to the excess of glucose and converts it into glycogen or animal starch, in which form it is stored in the liver cells. This mechanism is disturbed in the condition called diabetes.

Fat after being split up by the digestive juices is absorbed in the form of fat globules. It is a fundamental principle in nature that, where a substance has to be absorbed into a living organism, the surface area through which absorption takes place is large. This principle was demonstrated in the lung, where it was shown how extensive the area of flattened epithelium lining the air cells is. In the case of the alimentary tract we not only have a large surface area for absorption in virtue of the length of the canal, but in the small intestine there are finger-like processes of mucous membrane, the villi, which project from the inner surface of the bowel and so increase the area of the absorbing membrane.

Each villus has a capillary plexus of blood-vessels, into which the elementary substances from protein and

ι

carbohydrate digestion are taken, and lymph channels
called lacteals, into which the globules of fat find their way.
The fatty fluid contained in the lacteals is termed chyle.
The lacteals by intermediate lymphatics communicate
with the receptaculum chyli, which is a small lymph sac
situated on the upper lumbar vertebrae. This sac gives
rise to a duct—the thoracic duct—which travels through
the chest and enters the left subclavian vein at the root
of the neck. In this way, from lacteal to receptaculum
chyli to thoracic duct to subclavian vein, is fat absorbed
into the blood stream.

We have now learned something of the breaking down
and absorption of food-stuffs. All the material which we
take into our bodies cannot be digested so that everything
is absorbed, and consequently from the small intestine
there is passed on to the large intestine, through the ileo-
caecal valve, the ash of diet. This waste material is quite
fluid when it passes from small to large intestine, and the
subsequent changes in its consistency are due to the
absorption of water through the lining membrane of the
great bowel. The ultimate state of the ash is in the form
of the faeces or excreta from the alimentary tract. In
chronic constipation, where the ash has lain in the large
bowel for a period of time far in excess of normal, the
faeces are hardened and contain little water owing to the
continued absorption of water by the large intestine.
When sufficient material has reached the lowermost
regions of the large bowel the desire to get rid of the waste
material arises. If the individual obeys the call of nature,
he goes to stool, relaxes the anal sphincter, and defaecation
occurs. It is neglect of the regular call to defaecation
which is responsible for the misery of chronic constipation.

CHAPTER XV.

THE EXCRETORY SYSTEM.

In this chapter we shall have to consider those organs which are directly concerned with ridding the body of waste products. In the course of former description it has been seen that the large intestine and the lungs are excretory organs. The former gets rid of the residue of food, but the blood also passes a certain amount of waste material into the large bowel, and thus active excretion as well as passive excretion is characteristic of the action of the large intestine. The lungs get rid of carbon dioxide—the waste of metabolic processes, of a certain amount of moisture, and of volatile substances in the nature of acid poisons which may form in disease. There are, in addition to these excretory organs, the liver, the kidneys and the skin. The functions of the liver were dealt with in the chapter on digestion, and only a further word is necessary. Bile pigment, which is formed by the breaking down of haemoglobin, is really of the nature of an excretion, but the bile possesses so many characters which render it an important part of the digestive mechanism that the excretory aspect of the liver is frequently overlooked.

THE KIDNEYS.—These organs are bean-shaped, and lie one on each side of the vertebral column in the upper abdomen. The upper pole of each kidney is approximately at the level of the eleventh rib. They are enveloped in fat which protects them from injury. On the medial side of each kidney a sac-like membranous structure is to be observed—the pelvis of the kidney ; from this sac arises the ureter, a thin tube which runs down one on

each side of the vertebral column to reach the urinary
bladder in the pelvis. Each kidney has a multitude of fine
tubules, which lead into the pelvis of the kidney and pour
the excretion of urine into that structure. From the pelvis
of the kidney urine passes down the ureter into the bladder,
where it lies until the desire for micturition or passing
urine arises and the individual goes to pass water. The
actual act of micturition is the result of a contraction
of the muscular wall of the bladder and the relaxation of
a sphincter which guards the exit of the urethra from the
bladder. The urethra is the tube which leads from the
bladder to the exterior. (Fig. 62.)

Having considered the actual method of passing urine,
let us return to study the mechanism whereby the urine
is manufactured in the kidney. As has been pointed out,
each kidney contains an enormous number of tubules.
These tubules arise from an expansion of the tube into a
capsule which encircles a tuft of blood-vessels. The blood-
vessel tufts are formed by the branches of the renal artery,
which enters the kidney near the pelvis of the kidney.
Thus we find a system of blood-vessels in close relationship
to a small cavity which prolongs itself into a tubule. In
virtue of their close relationship, fluid is filtered from the
blood into the capsule surrounding the capillary tuft of
blood-vessels. As the fluid passes along the tubules from
the capsules, alterations in its concentration and composition take place, until finally the ultimate product,
urine, is poured into the kidney pelvis. This method of getting rid of waste products is an important one ; anything
wrong with the mechanism is always of serious import.

The normal amount of urine passed during twenty-four
hours by the healthy adult is 50 ounces. In conditions
like diabetes the amount of urine passed in twenty-four
hours is much increased. After ordinary exercise the
urinary output is diminished owing to the loss of water
by the sweat glands and the loss of water vapour by the
lungs. The drinking of much fluid in the ordinary course

of events will cause a corresponding increase in the output of urine. Certain substances like caffeine, the stimulant

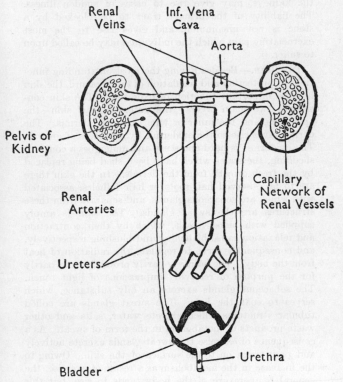

Renal Veins

Inf. Vena Cava

Aorta

Pelvis of Kidney

Renal Arteries

Capillary Network of Renal Vessels

Ureters

Bladder

Urethra

FIG. 62. DIAGRAMMATIC SCHEME OF THE URINARY SYSTEM.

constituent of tea and coffee, cause an increase in the urinary output.

It is advisable to remember that the kidneys play an important rôle in the human mechanism. Any disturbance of the urinary functions may be attended by serious consequences. Bright's disease, a condition affecting the kidneys, may give rise to cases of sudden illness. The liability of the urinary tract to be blocked by a stone is not uncommon, and gives rise to the most excruciating pain which the individual may be called upon to suffer.

THE SKIN.—Besides having the most outstanding functions of protection and regulation of temperature, the skin has the important function of excretion. The skin consists of two main layers: the outer or scarf skin—the epidermis, and the inner or true skin—the dermis. The dermis gives rise to the epidermis by a process of growth. The epidermis is hard and scaly and undergoes a constant shedding, the scales which have been shed being replaced by the fresh growth from the dermis. In the skin there are to be observed hair-roots or hair follicles, associated with which are sebaceous glands, and separate from these structures are the sweat glands. The skin is amply supplied with blood-vessels, which by their contraction and relaxation cause blanching and blushing respectively, and consequently serve to regulate the radiation of heat from the body. The hairs are partly protective and partly for the purpose of receiving impressions of light touch. The sebaceous glands excrete an oily substance, which serves to coat the hair. The sweat glands are coiled tubular structures which excrete water, salts and other waste products of metabolism in the form of sweat. As a consequence of exercise the sweat glands excrete actively and pour sweat on to the surface of the skin. Owing to the increase in the metabolism as a result of exercise, the general temperature of the body tends to rise, but this rise is prevented from becoming too great by the evaporation of moisture on the skin and the consequent reduction in the surface temperature. It is interesting to note that, when the excretion of urine is interfered with, the physician attempts to eliminate the waste products of the body by adopting measures to make the patient sweat copiously. From this fact it will be seen that the skin forms a very important excretory organ. It will also be clear that it is important to keep the skin clean by washing away the sweat and the scales which it constantly sheds.

CHAPTER XVI.

POISONING.

A POISON is a substance which is capable of destroying life, either by its direct local chemical action or by its effect on the vital organs when absorbed into the body. This definition will exclude such agencies as heat and electricity.

When a poison acts locally it may produce either complete destruction of the living tissue with which it comes into contact, or it may irritate the tissue. In the first instance there is localized death of tissue or necrosis ; in the second instance the irritation causes inflammation of the tissue. The ultimate result of necrosis is that the dead tissue separates off, leaving a raw surface or ulcer which will heal provided the patient survives and the cause of damage is removed. In the second case the inflammation will die down, and a normal condition will be restored once the irritating cause ceases to act ; if the irritation be continued the condition lapses into one of chronic inflammation. To contrast these various results further, it may be remarked that where necrosis results the tissue is killed and ceases to function.

Inflammation which is the result of irritation may cause at the start over-action of the tissue irritated ; chronic inflammation is attended by suspension of function, because the tendency is for overgrowth of fibrous tissue to occur ; this in turn crowds out the originally active tissue and causes its functional impairment.

When a poison acts generally or systemically it does so in virtue of the fact that it is absorbed into the blood stream. The action may be completely general or it may be quite selective, choosing some particular organ on which to exert its pernicious influence. In this way we find that some poisons may have a predilection for the tissue of the brain ; others have a preference for the heart. We must now enquire how these substances may reach the blood. From a study of physiology it will be remembered that substances find their way into the circulating blood mainly by two routes : from the alimentary canal through swallowing and from the lungs through inhalation. People may accidentally poison themselves by swallowing some nocuous substance ; or when they desire to commit suicide they deliberately swallow a poison. This method of poisoning does not, however, cover all the cases ; many suicides prefer to inhale a poisonous gas ; for example, coal-gas, which accounts for the great majority of suicidal deaths from inhalation. Poisons may get into the blood stream in ways other than through the alimentary canal and lungs. Sometimes a poison may be injected · into the loose tissue just below the skin. It is absorbed from this site by the blood, and usually acts much more quickly than if swallowed and absorbed from the alimentary canal. Sometimes a poison may be absorbed from a wound ; the arrow wounds in primitive warfare were often fatal, not because of the actual damage to the superficial tissues, but because of the poison on the point. Rarely, poison is absorbed through the skin when a poisonous substance is constantly applied to it.

From the foregoing a classification of the various types of poison may be made, but as we proceed it will be evident that any classification of poisons is bound to be unsatisfactory since many poisons act in more than one way. A poison may irritate the mucous lining of the alimentary canal, and produce remoter effects on the brain or heart when absorbed into the blood. It has been found more convenient to deal with the inhalation of poison gas under the heading of asphyxia. The classification of poisons is most satisfactorily derived from a consideration of how the poisons act, rather than from reference to the actual nature of the poison. One may speak, however, of poisons of mineral origin and of organic origin ; the latter class of poison being derived almost entirely from the vegetable kingdom.   Before proceeding with the classification of poisons, it should be noted that there are developed in the body poisons which are the result of activity on the part of micro-organisms or germs.   These poisons are elaborated in the course of infectious disease and in festering wounds, where the fundamental cause in both instances is infection by germs.   These poisons do not call for any consideration here, since our original definition does not allow for poisonous substances developed in the body, but there is one type of poison, the result of germ activity, which must be mentioned, because it is taken into the body and absorbed with pernicious effects : this is the poison of bad food, giving rise to ptomaine poisoning.   This poison is manufactured by germs attacking food which has not been properly treated for preservation.   Ptomaine poisoning is a rare condition.

CLASSIFICATION OF POISONS.
CORROSIVES.

   Acids :

   Sulphuric Acid (Vitriol).
   Nitric Acid (Aqua fortis).
   Hydrochloric Acid (Spirits of Salt).
   Carbolic Acid (Phenol).
   Oxalic Acid.
   Acetic Acid.

   Alkalis :

   Caustic Soda.
   Caustic Potash.
   Caustic Ammonia.

   Corrosive Salts :

   Silver Nitrate.
   Oxalate of Potash (Salts of Sorrel).

Irritants.

>Any of the corrosive poisons in dilution.
>Salts of Heavy Metals :
>>Mercuric Chloride.
>>Copper Sulphate.
>>Zinc Sulphate.
>>Arsenical Salts.
>>Antimony Tartarate.
>>Tin Chloride.
>>Lead Acetate.
>Iodine.
>Phosphorus.
>Croton Oil.

Narcotics.

>Opium.
>Belladonna (Deadly Nightshade).
>Alcohol.
>General Anaesthetics.
>Prussic Acid.
>Cocaine.

Systemic.

>Digitalis (Foxglove).
>Laburnum.
>Yew.
>Privet.
>Aconite (Monk's-hood).
>Conium (Hemlock).
>Strychnine.
>Snake Venom.
>Potassium Chlorate.
>Coal-gas and other poison gases.

The above classification is merely an attempt to present the subject of poisons in a clear fashion. The classification may be justified in that it deals with the action of the

poisons. The classification which divides poisons into
gaseous, mineral, vegetable and animal is not satisfactory
for the purposes of first aid. Our classification does not
use the word narcotico-irritant, because of the extreme
vagueness of the term, and because of the great variety of
drugs and poisons which may be classed under this particular heading. The use of such a term as systemic will
be justified to the reader by what follows. Before dealing
with the individual classes of poison, it will be well to
make some general remarks about the circumstances of a
case of poisoning.

When an individual, previously healthy, becomes suddenly ill, poisoning must be considered as a possibility.
The suspicions are strengthened when two or three people
become suddenly ill. The actual poison used may or may
not be apparent. In cases of accidental poisoning the
nature of the poison has often to be judged from the
symptoms presented. In suicidal poisoning a bottle
may be found containing remains of the poison used.
Evidences may be got from finding poison in the patient's
pocket. In cases of gaseous poisoning the circumstances
of the case will make the cause apparent. Destruction
of the lining membrane of the mouth will lead one to
suspect the use of a corrosive. Excessive vomiting will
imply the use of an irritant. Coma or unconsciousness
will result from the use of narcotics. The results of
the use of systemic poisons are so varied that no
definite indication can be given to recognise this group
as a whole.

The aims of the ambulance man in a case of poisoning
will be to stop the action of the poison by removing it,
and to neutralise the poison which he cannot remove. The
first procedure may mean the removal of the patient from
an atmosphere of poison gas or the administration of an
emetic to cause vomiting, which will ensure the rapid
elimination of the poison from the stomach. The neutralisation of the poison remaining may be brought about in

two ways according to the nature of the poison. If the poison is an acid it may be neutralised by the administration of an alkali and *vice versa*. If the poison is a narcotic it may be neutralised by the administration of a stimulant, and poisoning by a stimulant may be neutralised by the administration of a narcotic. These curative substances are termed antidotes. Neutralisation by the conversion of a strong acid into an innocuous substance is the result of the administration of a chemical antidote. Stimulation of the body by the administration of a substance when a narcotic poison has been taken involves the use of a physiological antidote. The chemical antidote acts by neutralising the actual substance taken; the physiological antidote acts by causing the body to respond in the fashion opposite to the effect produced by the poison. The poisoned person is usually collapsed and suffering from shock. The measures adopted in the treatment of shock from other causes should be carried out in cases of poisoning. Poisoning is a grave condition; the subsequent amount of detailed description is proportionate to the seriousness of the condition and to the usefulness of appropriate first-aid treatment.

CORROSIVE POISONS.

ACIDS.—Corrosive poisons are poisons which corrode. These substances are very potent chemically, and many of them will dissolve metals such as iron, lead and zinc. The first three in the series are the most powerful acids known, and all must be handled with care. They are termed the mineral acids. Sulphuric acid is a heavy, syrupy liquid which mixes with water, causing much evolution of heat. Nitric acid in the forms usually obtained gives off pungent brown fumes. Hydrochloric acid gives off white pungent fumes, which have the characteristic smell of the gas chlorine. These three acids are not very commonly used as poisons, but the evidences of their use are unmistakable. Cases have occurred where sulphuric acid has been thrown in the face of an individual, leaving the most disastrous disfiguration to the features as a result of the corrosive action of the acid. Vitriol-throwing constitutes a very grave criminal offence. Hydrochloric acid is used by plumbers as spirits of salt. Nitric acid is not in common commercial use.

Carbolic, oxalic and acetic acids are non-mineral acids of great importance. They are corrosives in the same fashion as the mineral acids. Carbolic acid or phenol is in very common use throughout the country as an antiseptic. Other forms of the acid are to be found in lysol, which is a very common means of poisoning, in creosote paints, and in many other antiseptic preparations. Pure phenol is seldom used as a poison, but it is most commonly swallowed in solution in water or in a soapy fluid. Lysol is a phenol preparation dissolved in a soapy liquid. The smell of carbolic soap is familiar to all, and is characteristic of all the poisons derived from carbolic acid. Oxalic acid is of common use in shoemaking, brass finishing and polishing, bookbinding and straw hat making. It is derived from plants ; many vegetables in everyday use contain oxalic acid in very small quantity, but not in sufficient amount to cause grave symptoms. Acetic acid when diluted with water is commonly used as vinegar ; when in concentrated form it is spoken of as glacial acetic acid, and is a powerful corrosive poison.

ALKALIS.—Of the alkaline corrosives, the one in most common use is ammonia, which is employed in laundries for washing. Poisoning by ammonia, caustic soda and caustic potash is not common. These substances are not quite so powerful in their action as the mineral acids ; when highly concentrated they may cause much destruction to cloth fabrics. Even fairly dilute solutions of these alkalis, on coming in contact with the skin, give the feeling of a soapy solution. This feeling is extremely characteristic of these poisons.

CORROSIVE SALTS.—Only two salts are given in the classification. These are both very poisonous substances. They cause corrosion in much the same way as the other corrosives. Silver nitrate, often known as lunar caustic, is in crystalline form, and is used frequently to remove warts, or to apply to ulcers. When dissolved in water it acts as a corrosive poison. Oxalate of potash or salts of sorrel is a favourite household substance for removing rust stains from clothing. It is as poisonous as oxalic acid, from which it is derived.

GENERAL APPEARANCES IN CASES OF CORROSIVE POISONING.—The lips are usually burned by the local action of the poison, which destroys the mucous membrane lining the mouth. There may be considerable swelling of the tongue, the pharynx, and of the tissues surrounding the mouth and throat. Usually the mind is clear, except in the case of carbolic poisoning. There is extreme difficulty in breathing, owing to the great swelling of the tissues of the throat. Death in these cases may be due to asphyxia from the swelling of tissues round about the larnyx and pharynx, to shock or to perforation of the stomach through the corrosive action on the stomach wall. It will be observed that the patient is cold and collapsed, and shows all the evidences of profound surgical shock. There is continual retching and vomiting of bloody material, the natural reaction of the body to rid itself of the poison. The patient when able to speak complains of agonising, burning pain in the mouth and throat ; he suffers from extreme weakness and intense thirst. The onset of these symptoms and signs is immediate after the swallowing of the poison. It is most important to know whether alkali or acid has been used. In poisoning by the mineral acids the destruction of tissue is much more extreme. Nitric, hydrochloric and carbolic acids have characteristic odours, ammonia is easily recognised by its smell : the caustic alkalis of potash and soda have no smell, but a soapy feeling which is characteristic.

TREATMENT OF CASES OF CORROSIVE POISONING.—
Administer a chemical antidote. In the case of sulphuric,
hydrochloric and nitric acid poisoning the chemical antidote is an alkali. Several alkalis may be used, but sodium
bicarbonate or baking soda is by far the most readily
available, and is one of the most satisfactory. On no
account must one attempt to get rid of any of the corrosive
poisons by the administration of an emetic, because infinite damage may result from its use. Substances like
magnesia and chalk on coming in contact with the mineral
acids neutralise their action, and scrapings of room wall
plaster may have to be used in the absence of baking soda.
The relief to the patient after the administration of an alkali
is immediate. Unfortunately the administration of a
simple alkali does not suffice for all the corrosive poisons.
The caustic alkalis must be neutralised by the administration of weak acid. Vinegar is the most appropriate substance for this purpose. Usually the symptoms are not
quite as urgent. The treatment of poisoning by ammonia
must be slightly different from the treatment of caustic
soda and potash poisoning, because of the fact that, owing
to the extremely volatile nature of the poison, asphyxia is
an important manifestation of the condition. Artificial
respiration may have to be carried out. The special instances of poisoning by oxalic acid, potash oxalate and
carbolic acid all demand attention. If baking soda be administered to an individual poisoned by oxalic acid or
potassium oxalate, sodium oxalate is formed and absorbed
into the blood to exert an extremely poisonous action. If,
on the other hand, chalk is given, calcium oxalate is formed ;
this substance is insoluble, and consequently it cannot be
absorbed, but remains harmless in the alimentary canal.
Chalk is therefore the best antidote to oxalic acid or
oxalate poisoning. Carbolic acid poisoning is rather different from any yet considered. In virtue of the fact that
it is rapidly absorbed, the suspension of consciousness is
an early feature of the condition, and often the patient is

quite unconscious before the ambulance man arrives. He will therefore have no means of getting first-hand information, and will have to rely on his sense of smell to diagnose the condition. There are two very appropriate measures in dealing with carbolic acid poisoning : the administration of Epsom salts and the giving of alcohol. Both of these substances have a direct effect on the poison.

In every case of poisoning by means of corrosives there is considerable pain and irritation in the mouth, throat and gullet. Very often the patient will be eased by the administration of demulcent drinks such as milk, gruel, white of egg and milk. The giving of such demulcents, which are soothing to the patient, must never be the first mode of treatment, but should always follow the primary chemical neutralisation of the poison. Again, severe pain in the abdomen may be treated by the application of heat over the stomach. Shock, which is constantly present in all these cases, must be treated by keeping the body warm.

THE IRRITANT POISONS.

These substances are mostly of mineral origin, and are chemical compounds of metallic substances. They are mostly salts of the heavy metals, and in the classification the most important example of each is quoted. They act by causing irritation and inflammation of the alimentary canal. The salts of mercury are extremely poisonous when swallowed. They are very commonly used as disinfectants, mercuric chloride or corrosive sublimate being the most common of the mercurial disinfectants. Corrosive sublimate exists as a white crystalline salt, and may be mistaken for calomel, another salt of mercury which is used in medicine as a purge. Although the substance is named corrosive sublimate, it has got the poisonous effects of an irritant rather than of a corrosive. Copper sulphate is a blue crystalline substance, and is commonly known as blue-stone ; certain types of electric cell contain copper sulphate solution. Zinc sulphate is commonly used to impregnate fabrics. The salts of arsenic are found in certain weed-killers ; an outbreak of arsenical poisoning occurred in England some time ago owing to the presence of arsenical salts in beer ; certain rat poisons contain arsenic, and arsenic paste is used by taxidermists.

Of the other poisons mentioned under the heading of irritant poisons the most important are iodine, lead acetate, and phosphorus. Iodine in solution is much used as an antiseptic. Lead is in common commercial use as white and red lead, and not infrequently those who work with these substances become subject to chronic lead poisoning. Acute symptoms of irritant poisoning are certain to develop on swallowing iodine and lead salts in sufficient quantity. Phosphorus poisoning is not very common, although children sucking heads of matches may contract it. Croton oil is administered medically in very small doses ; poisoning results from careless use of the drug.

THE GENERAL APPEARANCES IN CASES OF IRRITANT POISONING.—The signs and symptoms are not so early in their onset as in the case of corrosive poisoning. Since their main action is that of irritation, there will be much reaction on the part of the stomach to counteract this irritation. Many of these substances cause much pouring out of mucus from the glands associated with the upper part of the digestive canal. In this way the poison is much diluted, and consequently its action is diminished. The extreme irritation causes an intense increase in the flow of blood to the lining of the alimentary canal. The consequence is that blood is shed from the mucous surfaces, and blood will therefore appear in the vomit. This tremendous congestion causes discomfort, while the associated retching is attended by violent contraction of the muscular walls of the stomach and much pain results. Retching and vomiting are merely attempts by the body to rid itself of the irritant poison. If the case be observed later, the continued irritation causing increased activity of the intestine will evidence itself in painful diarrhoea and even the passing of blood with the faeces.

To summarize these effects : In irritant poisoning there is continuous painful retching and vomiting, severe abdominal pain and, later, diarrhoea. The vomited material frequently contains blood. After some time the pulse becomes feeble and rapid, the body becomes cold and clammy, cramps in the limbs occur, and finally death may supervene from the shock associated with the condition or as a result of poisonous effects produced by absorption. The shock produced by irritant poisons is not of immediate onset as in cases of corrosive poisoning ; it is rather the result of the action of the irritant over some period of time—one or two hours in cases of acute poisoning. Usually the mind is clear until profound collapse is in evidence.

In all the instances of irritant poisoning quoted above two distinct sets of symptoms may arise. The symptoms which have been noted above are those of acute poisoning where large doses of the poison have been swallowed, but one may find that cases of irritant poisoning assume a chronic nature due to the taking of a poison over a long period of time. In the latter case we are not concerned with the condition produced, since the symptoms are not those of sudden illness.

TREATMENT OF CASES OF IRRITANT POISONING.—The first procedure is to get rid of the poison. This means the administration of an emetic. Fortunately, in most instances of irritant poisoning vomiting occurs as one of the natural reactions to the poison. The administration of an emetic should be resorted to whenever it is known that a person has swallowed an irritant poison, whether the individual shows definite signs of poisoning or not. Irritation of the back of the throat by the forefinger will cause vomiting in many cases, but it is usually desirable to supplement this by the administration of an emetic.

The emetics in most common use are :

I. Large draughts of tepid water.

II. *Mustard.*—One tablespoonful of the flour of mustard to half a pint of tepid water—a tumblerful.

III. *Common Salt.*—Two tablespoonfuls in half a pint of warm water.

After the stomach has been thoroughly emptied, while waiting for the doctor, it is safe to give raw eggs or white of egg. This measure gives most irritant poisons something on which to act. The administration of tannin in the form of strong tea is also a protective measure. The patient must be kept warm, and stimulants may have to be resorted to in cases of collapse. Severe pain in the abdomen may be treated by the application of heat. In the case of lead poisoning, Epsom salts may be used with great advantage.

IODINE POISONING.—The action of iodine when swallowed is typically that of an irritant; when quantities of the strong solution are consumed there may follow corrosive effects. The most notable appearances are dark brown staining of the lining of the mouth and marked swelling of the tongue ; the smell of iodine is usually present to give the diagnosis. Vomiting, burning pain in the mouth and throat and a feeling of constriction about the neck are the most prominent symptoms. Iodine in itself when taken in sufficient doses acts as an emetic. Treatment in the form of administration of soft starchy food like arrowroot or cornflour should be resorted to rather than the giving of an emetic. As anyone suffering from acute iodine poisoning is severely shocked the usual treatment for shock must be administered.

In phosphorus poisoning on no account must any oily substance be given, since oil dissolves phosphorus and renders it absorbable. The effects of phosphorus when absorbed into the body are particularly fatal.

CROTON OIL is the most purgative drug known, and symptoms of vomiting and drastic diarrhoea with blood and mucus in the stools may appear within a very short time of swallowing the oil. Treatment consists in keeping the patient warm and in administering white of egg.

NARCOTIC POISONS.

Under this heading are included those substances which when taken into the body cause primarily an impairment of the action of the nervous system. Their action may cause early suspension of consciousness, or may interfere so seriously with the brain function as to cause wild delirium. While the other poisonous groups may have ultimate effects on the nervous system, it is not to be thought that these effects are primary as in the case of the narcotic poisons. The first of the narcotics is opium, a vegetable product, in extensive use in medical practice. Opium or its derivatives are found in laudanum, morphia, and its salts, and in certain cough mixtures, which, however, cannot now be obtained without a medical prescription. Opium is one of the greatest and most useful drugs in medicine. It has given welcome relief to countless sufferers by inducing sleep and banishing pain, but it has also wrecked the lives of thousands by the formation of a drug habit which is far stronger than alcohol addiction. Opium-smoking in China has caused terrific impairment to the usefulness of the natives as members of the community. The most notable example of the opium habit in an Englishman is to be found in De Quincey, who has written his confessions, and to whom the reader is referred for a cultured account of opium addiction. Cases of addiction to opium or morphine are not by any means uncommon in this country. They usually occur in people who have access to drugs, and in spite of any measure taken to deprive the addict of his drug the *habitué* will attempt to circumvent such precautions by every possible means ; nothing is too desperate for him : he will lie, he will steal, or he will commit graver criminal offences in order to obtain the drug. Fortunately the law has become so stringent in the matter of the sale of opium that it is hardly possible for the ordinary citizen to become an opium addict.

The source of belladonna is the deadly nightshade, a plant common in this country ; it bears tempting-looking black berries at seed time. Belladonna and its derivatives are quite commonly used in medicine. The active constituent of the drug belladonna is atropine, which is frequently used to cause dilation of the pupils. Poisoning may be caused by mistaking a solution of belladonna or atropine for some less nocuous drug. It sometimes is used by women who desire to improve their attractiveness by having large pupils, and in this way some cases of belladonna poisoning have arisen. It is from this practice that the name belladonna (beautiful woman) is derived.

The distribution of alcohol is well known. It occurs in various percentages in all forms of intoxicating liquor. The actual alcohol in these beverages is ethyl alcohol, and its abuse gives rise to all degrees of poisoning from slight " tipsiness " to profound unconsciousness and collapse. Methyl alcohol, the use of which is very general domestically, is sometimes taken as an intoxicant, and is used illegally by the unscrupulous to enhance the action of ethyl alcohol. In spite of the addition of poisonous material to methylated spirits, drinking this type of liquor seems to continue, but in a rather less degree than formerly.

The general anaesthetics are chloroform and ether. The vapour of these two liquids is inhaled in order to produce a profound action on the nervous system. Liquid chloroform is not often consumed as a poison, but some people get " drunk " on ether by swallowing the liquid.

Prussic acid is one of the most potent poisons, and is known chemically as hydrocyanic acid. The salts which are formed through a chemical combination of the metals with the acid are the cyanides. They are just as poisonous as the acid when taken into the body. It has to be remembered that, if an acid is added to a cyanide, prussic acid may be given off and inhaled in the gaseous form. Since cyanides are of very common use in photography, this reaction is by no means unimportant. Prussic acid is contained in laurel and in oil of bitter almonds, rendering those two sources very poisonous.

COCAINE.—Forms of this drug are in very common use in medicine. Dentists use derivatives of the drug in order to accomplish painless extraction of teeth. Seldom do dentists use pure cocaine nowadays. The cocaine habit is more pernicious than the alcohol habit; but again the law has prevented the habit from assuming large proportions.

GENERAL APPEARANCES AND TREATMENT OF POISONING BY NARCOTICS.

OPIUM.—The drug may be found on the patient. Sometimes a hypodermic syringe may have been used to inject morphine. In the less profound stages of morphine or opium poisoning the patient is stuporose, and when roused can converse coherently but languidly. In more marked cases the patient cannot be roused; the pupils are small and contracted, the skin is cold and clammy, the respirations shallow and infrequent, the pulse weak and irregular. In children it is not infrequent to find convulsions immediately preceding death. The treatment of opium poisoning where the drug has been swallowed is to give an emetic. In the deeply unconscious patient the emetic may not be effective and, consequently, other measures must be adopted. The administration of potassium permanganate is very effective as an antidote, as this substance converts the active constituent morphine into a harmless compound. The best form in which to administer potassium permanganate is in solution in water, as much permanganate as will cover a sixpence dissolved in a tumblerful of water. Coincident with the above treatment, if the patient is not already unconscious every effort must be made to keep him awake by flicking the body with wet towels; if unconsciousness has supervened strenuous attempts, even of a rough nature, must be made to arouse him. Heat must be applied to the body; if the patient can swallow, hot coffee should be given; the inhalation of smelling salts through the nostrils is a useful measure in stimulating respiration, which is so liable to fail in cases of this kind.

In cases where morphine has been injected by a hypodermic syringe, the above treatment is inapplicable so far as the administration of an emetic is concerned, but the methods of keeping the patient awake, applying heat to the body and administering hot drinks must be carried out.

BELLADONNA.—The effect of belladonna is very different from that of opium. It produces a disturbance of brain function, which is often manifested by alternating phases of delirium and unconsciousness. Delirium is a condition where there is irrational muttering accompanied by purposeless movement of the limbs and general restlessness. Occasionally the patient may become wildly excited. The ambulance man must hold himself in readiness to deal with these emergencies. In belladonna poisoning the pupils are dilated, and do not respond to stimulation by light. The tongue and mouth are extremely dry, and if the patient is not deeply under the influence of the drug he complains of excessive thirst. Treatment of the condition is mainly stimulating after an emetic has been administered. The patient should be kept warm, hot tea and coffee may be administered and smelling salts applied to the nostrils.

ALCOHOL.—It is generally agreed that from the very first the action of alcohol is to cause paralysis of nerve centres. Those higher faculties which have come to man in the later stages of development are of an inhibitory nature, and prevent him from acting as a purely instinctive creature. He is consequently a respectable member of a civilized community. Alcohol in moderate doses removes the influence of those higher centres and this is evidenced by his readiness to express himself, the controlling influence of reserve having gone. In the earlier stages of intoxication there may be very little sign of any impairment of reason. Later his reason becomes interfered with and there is no rationality in his speech, which becomes thick owing to upset of the finely co-ordinate mechanism of speech. Sensibility becomes correspondingly diminished, and it may be possible to demonstrate that the intoxicated person has no appreciation of pain, the capability of appreciating more highly developed sensations than the fundamental sensation of pain having long been lost. These phenomena are accompanied by further evidence of inco-ordination of the nervous mechanism. The sense of balance goes, his power of co-ordinate movement is paralysed, and ultimately he falls dead drunk to the ground. In this ultimate state only the most fundamental centres of his nervous system have not been touched by the paralytic influence of alcohol those centres which control his breathing and the action of the heart. It is rare that so much alcohol is taken as to suspend even these last-mentioned functions. Another effect of alcohol is to produce a dilatation of the blood-vessels of the skin. This occurs with moderate doses of the substance, and the dilatation of superficial blood-vessels causes such a radiation of heat from the body that it is unsafe to go out into very cold weather after having consumed even a moderate amount of liquor. Death from exposure is liable to occur when a very drunk person lies out in the cold overnight.

There is a condition found quite frequently which is due to the consumption of alcohol—delirium tremens. In this state there is excitement amounting to actual mania. The individual is violent as the result of fear. Fear is produced by the onset of hallucinations of a terrifying nature. The patient sees all sorts of things which have no basis in reality ; highly coloured animals, particularly repulsive animals such as snakes. The onset of such symptoms may be quite sudden, and is the result of large doses of alcohol.

There is one point of extreme importance, which has been left until now in order that its importance may be emphasised. Alcoholic coma may be distinguished from unconsciousness due to other causes by the condition of the pupils. If an alcoholic has been lying undisturbed under the influence of liquor for about half an hour his pupils will be found to be contracted. When he is disturbed by someone trying to rouse him the pupils become gradually dilated. It must never be assumed that because a man is unconscious and his breath smells of liquor he is in a condition of alcoholic coma. Such an assumption may cause a man with a fractured skull or apoplexy to spend a night in a police cell when he requires hospital attention.

The treatment for alcoholic coma is first to empty the stomach by the use of an emetic or by irritating the back of the throat. Further measures, if the patient can swallow, are the administration of Epsom salts and hot coffee. The body must be kept warm, and the emergencies of mania and tendencies to violence must be controlled. Smelling salts may be used in cases of collapse with great advantage.

GENERAL ANAESTHETICS.—Chloroform and ether have precisely the same type of action on the nervous system as has alcohol. The reaction is, however, much more rapid and much more profound. In the case of ether swallowing, symptoms of intoxication come on at once and pass off much more quickly than those of alcohol. It is possible to become drunk on ether several times in one day and to have lucid intervals between the bouts of intoxication. The treatment is the same as that for alcoholic coma, except when the anaesthetic has been inhaled.

PRUSSIC ACID.—After swallowing prussic acid or any of the cyanides the onset of symptoms is rapid. There is transitory burning pain in the mouth and throat, vomiting and collapse. Unconsciousness supervenes rapidly and convulsions occur ; the limbs are thrown out rigidly and the neck and trunk arched strongly backwards. The pupils become fully dilated, and death supervenes in a short period of time. The cause of death in prussic acid poisoning appears to be paralysis of the respiration. The treatment is to administer an emetic at once. Condy's Fluid may be given immediately after emptying the stomach. Since the poison acts mainly on the respiration to produce death, artificial respiration should be carried out with a view to eliminating the poison which is excreted by the lungs. If a person can be kept breathing for an hour after taking prussic acid he will recover. The inhalation of strong prussic acid is liable to cause immediate death.

COCAINE.—Apart from the usual purpose for which cocaine is used, that of paralysing those nerve endings which receive the impression of pain, there is a definite action on the central nervous system. The first effect of cocaine is stimulating ; it causes a feeling of well-being and general pleasure. If taken in sufficient dose the effect is depressing and coma results. Generally the onset of unconsciousness is accompanied by convulsions. The pupils are moderately dilated. Cocaine seems to kill by acting on the vital centres of the heart and respiration in the medulla. The treatment is to empty the stomach by an emetic if the emetic will work, which is doubtful owing to the anaesthetic action of cocaine on the lining of the stomach. Stimulants should be given, ammonia or smelling salts by inhalation, hot coffee or tea by the mouth. The patient must be kept warm, and artificial respiration may have to be resorted to when the respiration fails.

THE SYSTEMIC POISONS.

This class has been devised in order to include poisons which have some particular action on the internal organs. Many of them may cause symptoms which would be described as irritant or narcotic, but their main action is on some internal mechanism other than the brain itself or the alimentary tract. They may act directly on the heart or blood, or they may cause some grave disturbance when inhaled, through irritation of the air passages, and so produce asphyxia. Owing to the variety of these poisons, each will be dealt with separately.

DIGITALIS is obtained from the plant foxglove, and is used extensively in medicine in many forms of heart disorder. The onset of signs and symptoms from over-dosage is slow ; the pulse may fall to 35 or less and may become totally irregular. The patient becomes restless, develops air hunger, and coma may supervene. There is usually some nausea and vomiting in the earlier stages. The treatment is mainly to keep the patient warm until the arrival of a doctor. Should a child have swallowed some foxglove, give an emetic. In cases where the terminal stages have been reached smelling salts are useful.

LABURNUM, YEW AND PRIVET POISONING.—The laburnum tree is familiar to everyone owing to its extensive distribution in our gardens and woods. The drooping tassels of yellow flowers catch the eye and may attract children. These flowers fade and leave pods filled with seed. When either flowers or seeds are consumed very marked symptoms of poisoning arise. First among the symptoms is vomiting with abdominal discomfort ; the patient becomes exceedingly restless and coma may supervene. Convulsions occur before the onset of death. The poison is first an irritant and then a narcotic.

The treatment consists in emptying the stomach by using an emetic and keeping the patient warm.

The yew tree is also common in our woods and gardens. Its red berries are sometimes consumed by children, with disastrous result. The symptoms and signs of yew poisoning are those of irritation and the treatment is that for an irritant poisoning.

Privet hedges bear purple berries which, when consumed, cause irritant poisoning.

The treatment is that of irritant poisoning.

ACONITE.—This poison is to be found in the plant monk's-hood. It is not commonly used in medicine, but it is a constituent of A.B.C. liniment. Cases have been recorded where swallowing this liniment has had a fatal issue. The symptoms and signs are, first, a generalized prickling or burning sensation, followed by a general blunting of sensation. This is quite characteristic of the condition. The nature of the action on the heart is not clear. There is, however, rapid weakening of the heart's action and consciousness is lost. If a child should swallow monk's-hood, give an emetic, keep the child warm and send for a doctor, who will complete the stimulant treatment.

CONIUM.—This poison is contained in hemlock, which grows everywhere in hedgerows and fields. It has a white flower which spreads out like an umbrella. The use of conium as a drug has been given up. In earlier times a decoction of hemlock was administered to criminals under sentence of death, so certain is the action of the poison. Plato has written an account of the death of Socrates, who took the poison. The substance acts by causing slow paralysis of the muscles of the body. Curiously the lower extremities become paralysed first ; the paralysis spreads to the arms and throat ; finally the diaphragm and chest muscles become paralysed and death results, the mind remaining clear until the end.

The treatment of conium poisoning is to administer an emetic immediately after the poison has been swallowed.

With failing respiration, stimulation by the application of smelling salts may be tried, and artificial respiration may have to be undertaken. The patient must be kept warm, and stimulated by hot drinks when he is able to swallow.

STRYCHNINE.—This drug is one of the most potent in medicine ; it is of vegetable origin and has an extremely bitter taste. It is derived from the nux vomica bean and is much used as a tonic in the form of tincture of nux vomica. The natural habitat of the plant from which strychnine comes is India, and poisoning by swallowing the beans occurs from time to time in that country. Strychnine itself is a white crystalline powder. It has been taken in mistake for other drugs, such as salicylic acid, which is of extreme value in the treatment of rheumatism. The drug strychnine has often been classified as a narcotico-irritant, but as consciousness in a case of strychnine poisoning remains clear until the end, the drug is by no means a narcotic. After consuming a poisonous dose of strychnine vomiting may occur, absorption of the drug causes spasm of voluntary muscle, the limbs become rigid, convulsions occur, the jaws are clenched, the body arches strongly back, the spasm becomes so severe that pain in the muscles causes much distress. Any stimulation of the body causes increase of symptoms. The patient shows actual fear of being interfered with. Voices become painful to hear and, ultimately, death results, partly from the exhaustion of prolonged muscular contraction and from fixation of the muscles of respiration. The first-aid treatment is to keep the patient as quiet as possible. In a severe case an emetic cannot be administered owing to the spasm of the jaw muscles, and it is usually necessary for the doctor in attendance to administer chloroform in order to overcome the spasms and convulsions.

CHLORATE OF POTASH is much esteemed as a curative measure in sore throat. The tablets containing the salt are sold by druggists. Over-dosage has caused death.

The poison is rapidly absorbed from the alimentary canal, and exerts a lethal influence through destruction of the oxygen-carrying power of the blood. The normal pigment haemoglobin is changed into an inactive allied pigment which does not function. Symptoms do not usually arise immediately after swallowing the poison, but some little time afterwards. Stimulation by the ordinary methods may be tried, the patient being kept warm until the arrival of a doctor.

SNAKE VENOM.—Poisonous snakes are not common in Great Britain, but occasionally one hears of poisoning having occurred through a bite by the small poisonous viper, which is still found in this country. In India the cobra causes much death, and from poison bites the annual death-roll is 20,000.

In cobra poisoning the symptoms do not set in until the elapse of an hour or two, death occurring in about six hours. The poison acts mainly on the spinal cord and brain, sickness and vomiting preceding convulsions and paralysis of the limbs. The respiratory system is the last to be thrown out of action. There is marked destruction of blood cells.

The Daboya or Russell's Viper occurs in India, and its venom acts mainly on the blood cells, the capillaries and the heart ; death may occur quite rapidly or after the lapse of a few days.

The patient should be removed to a place where the appropriate anti-serum for the venom may be administered. The anti-serum is a product from an animal's blood ; the animal having been treated by small doses of the venom of the snake. In this way thousands of lives have been saved.

The viper which is found in this country is hardly poisonous in cold weather, but in warm weather it may cause symptoms of paralysis and lowered temperature.

The treatment is to apply a tourniquet above the wound if the bite has occurred in a limb and suck out the venom ;

potassium permanganate may then be applied to the wound.

POISONING BY INSECTS' STINGS.—All degrees of poisoning may be found in stings from insects, from the discomfort of a flea-bite to death in a person over-susceptible to wasp or bee poison. Even ordinary flea-bites may, in a susceptible person, cause remarkable symptoms, excessive swelling and itch being the most prominent. In the case of an individual who is over-sensitive to wasp poison, unconsciousness, cyanosis, weak fluttering pulse, irregular spasmodic breathing and even death may result. The treatment of stings is to remove the sting and to apply locally weak ammonia or baking soda moistened with water. General stimulant treatment has to be carried out according to the general condition of the patient.

FOOD POISONING.

Ptomaines are elaborated in decomposing food. The bacteria or germs which attack food cause the food to become tainted owing to the development of poisons, which when taken into the body cause upset of the digestion, vomiting and diarrhoea. The ptomaines may cause poisonous effects on the heart and brain, but most of them merely cause some digestive upset. Ptomaine poisoning is not very common, but when tainted food has been swallowed an emetic should be given. The condition is not to be confused with the intense inflammation in the alimentary tract which arises from eating infected mussels and other shell-fish. This condition arises from the presence of a germ which actually attacks man. Another form of food poisoning is botulism, where the germ attacks decomposing meat and causes marked paralysis when infected meat is swallowed. The paralytic agent seems to select the muscles of the eyes, face and throat, and causes death in a short period of time.

POISONING BY MUSSELS AND SHELL-FISH.—The symptoms arising from the eating of these foods are of an irritant nature and vomiting may arise. Very often most curious symptoms arise, such as swelling of the face and limbs, breathlessness and general collapse. Huge wheals may appear on the skin and give rise to a generalized nettle rash. It is only when profound collapse occurs with these conditions that it is necessary to carry out active treatment. The stomach should be emptied by an emetic and hot drinks should be given, the body being kept warm.

POISONING BY FUNGI.—Not infrequently people suffer from symptoms due to eating poisonous mushrooms. These are collected and may be cooked alone or with innocuous mushrooms, which are generally appreciated as a delicacy. The symptoms are usually evident some hours after consuming the mushrooms, and are ushered in by vomiting ; collapse, severe abdominal pain, cold sweating and excruciating headache follow. The stomach should be emptied by the use of an emetic. A dilute solution of permanganate of potash may be given. The patient must be kept warm.

K

CHAPTER XVII.

THE NERVOUS SYSTEM.

ALTHOUGH the first-aid student cannot be expected to have an intimate acquaintance with the anatomy and physiology of the nervous system, it is necessary that he should know something of the main features of its anatomy and of the principal facts concerning its physiology. As the anatomical features are so closely bound up with the physiology of the nervous system, this chapter will deal with both aspects together.

The brain and spinal cord which is continuous with the brain are situated in a cavity which is mainly composed of bone. The brain occupies the inside of the skull, while the spinal cord lies in that tubular cavity which is formed by the bony arches of the vertebrae, together with the tough ligaments between the individual arches. The skull and vertebral canal form an efficient protective covering to the brain and spinal cord. There are, however, other protective structures. The dura mater is a tough membrane which lines both the cranial cavity and the vertebral canal. It is a tough sheath, which forms a covering to the brain and spinal cord. Inside the dura mater are two other membranous sheaths, the arachnoid mater and the pia mater. The latter is closely applied to the surface of the brain and spinal cord, while the former lies between the dura mater and the pia mater. Between the arachnoid mater and pia mater there is to be found a quantity of clear fluid, the cerebro-spinal fluid. This acts as a water cushion to the brain and spinal cord, so that when the body receives a sudden jar this fluid damps down the transmission of the injuring force, and thus prevents injury to the delicate structure of the brain and spinal cord. It is worthy of mention at this point that when an individual fractures his skull, the dura mater and the arachnoid may be torn and cerebro-spinal fluid may escape.

So far mention has been made only of the brain and spinal cord. Together, these structures form what is termed the central nervous system, and for the purposes of elucidation of the nervous action it will be necessary to make a differentiation between the various parts of the nervous system in man. We have first of all the central nervous system, comprising the brain and spinal cord. From these structures nerves arise and pass out of the cranial and vertebral cavities ; these nerves are known as the peripheral nerves, and together they make up the peripheral nervous system. Individually these nerves serve to convey impulses to and away from the central nervous system.

We have a further set of nerves which together are termed the sympathetic or autonomic nervous system. This last set of nerves has a more or less independent existence, and is concerned mainly with the control of the internal organs, such as the heart, lungs, intestines, and so on.

We shall now proceed to deal with the individual parts of the human nervous system.

THE CENTRAL NERVOUS SYSTEM.

When we open the human skull and expose the brain, we see that it is shaped somewhat like a huge walnut. It has well-marked depressions on its surface ; the larger of these are called fissures and the smaller are termed sulci. The elevated areas between the sulci are called convolutions. It is well known that the pattern of the convolutions on the surface of the human brain is much more complicated than that of any other animal. This complicated pattern, together with the fact that, in proportion to the size of the body, the human brain is larger than any other animal's brain, is the direct consequence of the extraordinary development of the faculties of man. The next point which we observe is that the brain occupies practically the whole of the cranial cavity, and that we cannot take out the brain from this cavity without cutting through nerves which arise from the lower aspect of the brain, and without cutting through the upper end of the spinal cord which is directly continuous with the substance of the brain itself. Suppose that we have the whole brain removed from the cranial cavity, we note that there is a great mass of nervous tissue with a convoluted surface ; it occupies the vault of the skull and the anterior and middle fossae of the base. This main mass of nervous tissue is called the cerebrum or great brain. It is divided into two equal parts, a right and a left, by the longitudinal fissure ; these halves are termed the cerebral hemispheres. On the under surface of the cerebrum towards its posterior end there may be observed two small hemispherical structures which occupy the posterior fossae of the skull. These together form the cerebellum or little brain. Arising from the central region of the base of the cerebrum there are columns of nervous tissue, which run directly down to the spinal cord and make the cerebrum and spinal cord continuous. These columns are modified at various levels inside the cranial cavity to form, just as they leave the cerebrum, the cerebral peduncles or mid-brain, and below, just before leaving the cranial cavity by the foramen magnum, the medulla oblongata or hind brain. We may look on the central nervous system, then, as being composed of the brain stem and certain accessory structures. We have highest up and most anteriorly the cerebrum or fore brain, then the peduncles or mid-brain, then the hind brain or medulla oblongata, and finally in the same stem the spinal cord. The accessory structures are the cerebellum and a band of tissue which bridges the interval between the two halves of the cerebellum by running in front of the brain stem. This bridge of tissue is the Pons Varolii. (Fig, 63.)

Having dealt with the main anatomical features, let us now consider each of these structures in some more detail.

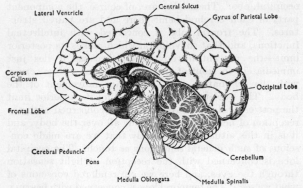

FIG. 63.—LONGITUDINAL SECTION THROUGH THE BRAIN IN THE MIDDLE LINE.

THE CEREBRUM.—This is the fore brain, and it must be considered as the anatomical expression of the highest activities of man. It is relatively of enormous size, and it is concerned with the reception and the transmission of nervous impulses. Here is the actual place where we are made conscious of what is happening in our environment. Examination shows those fissures which we have already noted : the longitudinal fissure dividing the cerebrum into the cerebral hemispheres ; the Sylvian fissure, one on each side, arising from that level, which divides the anterior from the middle fossae, and running horizontally to end before reaching the posterior part of the cerebrum ; the central or Rolandic fissure, one on each side, arising from the vertex and running downwards and slightly forwards, but ending before reaching the level of the

Sylvian fissure. Lying in front of the central fissure of Rolando is the frontal lobe of the brain; behind the central fissure and above the Sylvian fissure is the parietal lobe; below the Sylvian fissure is the temporal lobe; and behind the termination of the Sylvian fissure is the occipital lobe. These lobes are, of course, the component parts of each cerebral hemisphere and are paired structures. The frontal lobe is concerned with intellectual functions, and that convolution which makes its posterior limit—the precentral convolution, because it lies just immediately in front of the central fissure—is concerned with the crigination of all voluntary movement of the body. The parietal lobe has bounding its anterior limit the post-central convolution, which is concerned with the reception of nervous impulses from all over the body, and it is in this situation apparently that we are made conscious of such general sensations as touch. The occipital lobe is concerned with the reception of light sensation through the eyes, and here we are rendered conscious of what we see. The temporal lobe is concerned with hearing.

Let us imagine that we have now cut into the substance of the brain. At a first glance we notice a marked difference between the substance which immediately forms the surface and the tissue which makes up the great bulk of the interior. The superficial substance is dark in colour and is composed of grey matter, while the interior is composed of white matter. These appearances are due to the arrangement of the nerve cells which go to make up the whole of the nervous system. Each nerve cell has a cell body and certain long processes arising from the cell body, nerve fibres. (Fig. 64.) When cell bodies are aggregated together grey matter is formed, and when nerve fibres are found in bulk white matter is formed. The integrity of nerve fibres which conduct nervous impulses away from and to the cell body depends upon the integrity of the cell body from which the fibre arises. When a nerve cell in the cerebrum is injured the nerve fibre arising from it ceases to conduct nervous impulses. The layer of grey matter covering the whole of the cerebrum is termed the cerebral cortex. Cortex is a term which means bark; the bark of tree is the cortex of the tree. It is necessary in a brief fashion to give some information about the fibres which arise from the cells of the cerebral cortex. In the precentral convolution or motor area of the brain, the cells of the cortex give rise to fibres which run down through the brain stem, through mid-brain, medulla and spinal cord, where they come into close connection with the cells of the grey matter of the cord. The cells of the grey matter of the spinal cord in turn give rise to other fibres, which leave the spinal cord to run in the peripheral nervous system to the muscles which are under control of the will. One of the most important points in this study of the nervous system is to remember that when the fibres from the motor area reach the level of the medulla in the brain stem they cross to the opposite side, so that the cells of the right motor area of the cerebral cortex are responsible for voluntary movement of the left side of the body. An individual who survives an injury to the right cerebral cortex has frequently some paralysis of the left side of his body. The fibres which are concerned with the transmission of impulses to cause muscular action are termed motor fibres. Let us now consider those fibres which are concerned with the mechanism of sensation. In the skin, muscles and tendons there are to be found minute

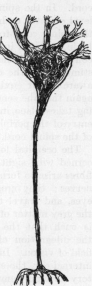

FIG. 64.

structures, nerve endings, which are responsible for the reception of impulses giving rise ultimately to such sensations as those of pain, touch, position of the limbs in space. From these nerve endings arise sensory fibres, which run in the peripheral nerves towards the spinal cord. In the spinal cord fresh fibres arise, either at the level of entry or higher up, and these fibres travel up in the spinal cord to the medulla oblongata and the mid-brain, and end in the cells of the post-central or sensory convolution of the cerebrum. In this way do we receive stimuli from the outside world and are ultimately made aware of our environment. It is to be remembered here again that the sensory paths are also crossed : the crossing takes place in the spinal cord, either at the level of entry of the peripheral nerves or in the uppermost reaches of the spinal cord.

The occipital lobes are, as has been pointed out, con-cerned with sight. From the retina of each eye nerve fibres arise to form the optic nerves—these are peripheral nerves ; they cross partially, soon after they leave the eyes, and travel through the cerebrum until they reach the grey matter of the occipital cortex. The arrangement is such that the left occipital cortex is responsible for the integration of what we see on the right half of the field of vision. In the same way fibres which arise in the internal ear, the special organ of hearing, go to the audi-tory cortex or temporal cortex of the opposite side. Apart from the areas of the cerebral cortex which are set aside for the actual reception of special sensation, such as hear-ing and sight, there are adjacent areas which are concerned with the storage of the memory of such sensations. This is possible through the existence of nerve fibres termed associative fibres, which connect the various parts of the cerebral cortex. By means of these fibres communications between the various parts of the cerebral cortex exist, so that we are able to associate the sensations and memories of what we hear with what we see or have seen and *vice versa.* In a like fashion there are similar fibres connecting the two cerebral hemispheres, so that we can perform co-ordinate movements of both sides of the body. The fibres which connect the cerebral hemispheres are to be found in the depths of the longitudinal fissures, and they are observed to be aggregated together into a structure termed the corpus callosum. The final important point which it is necessary to make concerning the cerebrum arises from the fact that the majority of people are right-handed. Greater development both anatomically and physiologically is to be expected naturally in the left cerebral hemisphere of right-handed people. Such is, indeed, the case to an amazing degree, for not only is the anatomical structure larger, but, from the point of view of function, the higher processes of speech, reading, and the understanding of spoken words are dependent upon the integrity of the left cerebral cortex in right-handed people. In left-handed people the opposite is true.

Further description of the cerebrum is unnecessary to the first-aid student ; should he, however, see a brain dissected, he will note the presence of a space in the centre of each cerebral hemisphere. These are the lateral ventricles of the brain, and they contain cerebro-spinal fluid. He will also notice large masses of grey matter in the centre ; they are the basal ganglia, but much obscurity still characterizes our knowledge of these structures, so that any description of them is quite unnecessary.

THE CEREBELLUM.—Only the briefest description of this organ is necessary. It has no activity to arouse any conscious disturbance, nor does it initiate any voluntary movement. Its connections are complicated, but it should be remembered that it is mainly concerned with balance and the maintenance of muscular tone. The connections of the cerebellum are with the special organs of balance in the petrous temporal bone and with the spinal cord. Impulses coming from both sources are received by the cerebellum, are integrated there, and are sent out to have a direct influence on the motor tracts. In this way it is possible to maintain balance automatically and unconsciously.

THE PONS VAROLII is simply the corpus callosum of the cerebellum, and is concerned in the co-ordination of the action of the two sides of the cerebellum.

THE MID-BRAIN.—The main interest in the mid-brain is the fact that it serves as a conducting structure, and also that from it nerves arise which are concerned with the movements of the eyes.

THE HIND BRAIN OR MEDULLA OBLONGATA.—This is the most fundamental part of the central nervous system. Here lie the pieces of grey matter which are concerned with the control of vital functions such as breathing, regulation of temperature and the control of the heart's action. These points are of the greatest importance in the consideration of injuries to the skull, because, as can be readily imagined, any injury to the posterior fossae of the skull is much more likely to prove fatal than a similar injury further forward. It has to be remembered that running through the medulla oblongata are fibres which communicate between brain and spinal cord.

THE SPINAL CORD.—The spinal cord is not co-extensive with the whole length of the vertebral canal, but stops short about the level of the first lumbar vertebra. Its anatomical features are easily summed up in that this structure contains a central core of grey matter of a peculiar shape, having two horns directed posteriorly and two anteriorly, the dorsal and ventral horns respectively. The rest of the spinal cord is composed of white matter, which consists of fibres conducting impulses from the spinal cord to the brain and from brain to spinal cord. In this white matter there are also associative fibres which connect one part of the spinal cord with another. Arising from the spinal cord are a series of nerves, the peripheral spinal nerves, and these we notice have each two roots of origin. The anterior or motor root arises from the anterior horn cells, while the posterior root or sensory root is connected with the posterior horn of grey matter. The two roots join a short distance from the cord, and run out as a single nerve trunk through an intervertebral foramen.

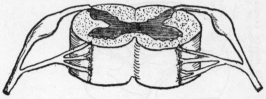

FIG. 65.

These spinal nerves are numbered according to the particular level at which the nerve arises. A diagram is given of what is termed a spinal segment, which is that region of the spinal cord giving origin to a pair of spinal nerves—that is, from each spinal segment a right and a left spinal nerve arises. It can be seen from the above description that the spinal nerves are mixed—partly motor and partly sensory. (Figs. 65 and 66.)

THE PERIPHERAL NERVOUS SYSTEM.

These nerves all arise from the brain and spinal cord and run through the body generally. They have the function of conducting impulses to and away from the the central nervous system. Some of these peripheral nerves are of great importance; the optic, auditory and other nerves of special sense give the human being a knowledge of his environment, the great motor nerves of the body enable him to perform muscular work, and peripheral nerves, which go to vital organs such as the heart and lungs, are of the first order of importance.

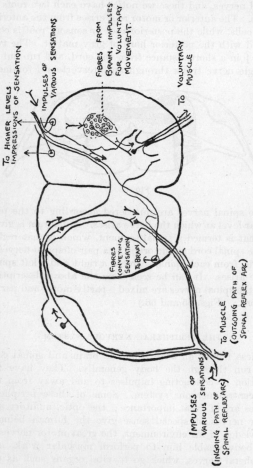

FIBRES FROM BRAIN, IMPULSES FOR VOLUNTARY MOVEMENT

TO VOLUNTARY MUSCLE

IMPULSES OF VARIOUS SENSATIONS

TO HIGHER LEVELS IMPRESSIONS OF SENSATION

FIBRES CONVEYING SENSATION TO BRAIN

TO MUSCLE (OUTGOING PATH OF SPINAL REFLEX ARC)

IMPULSES OF VARIOUS SENSATIONS (INGOING PATH OF SPINAL REFLEX ARC)

FIG. 66.

Before leaving the consideration of the central and peripheral nervous system, there are one or two points which must be mentioned with regard to the functioning of the nervous system. When a series of sensory impulses reaches the central nervous system, they are conducted to the cerebrum, where they are integrated, consciousness is disturbed, and as a result some definite action is forthcoming due to the ultimate stimulation of the motor cortex. This sort of action is dependent upon the existence of the associative fibres of the cerebrum. But for definite motor responses to result from sensory stimulation, it is not necessary that these stimuli should reach as high a level as the cerebrum, and consciousness is therefore not necessarily involved. The ordinary balance which we maintain is due to sensory impulses reaching the cerebellum, and, after integration there, finding egress in motor tracts closely associated with the main motor tracts coming down from the brain. Again, in the spinal cord associative fibres may simply short circuit the long routes taken by sensory impulses and a motor response is obtained, the impulse never having risen above the segment of the spinal cord which it enters. This last type of action is referred to as a spinal reflex. It is best exemplified by tapping the patellar tendon ; this is attended by extension of the leg, and the reflex path involved is simply the sensory fibres and the motor fibres in the peripheral nerve trunks and the associative fibres in the spinal cord. In this way we can look on muscular activity as being the expression of nervous activity at one of three levels, spinal, cerebellar or cerebral. The reflexes of the body are numerous, and are all analogous to the spinal reflex. When an individual looks at a bright light the pupils of his eyes contract ; if he looks at a near object the pupils again contract ; these are spoken of as the light and accommodation reflexes respectively. These reflexes as seen in the pupils are important from the point of view of first-aid, as has been demonstrated in the consideration of poisoning.

THE SYMPATHETIC NERVOUS SYSTEM.

This system still constitutes one of the most difficult problems of human physiology. Running down each side of the vertebral column may be seen a chain of nerve fibres with small knots of nervous tissue at intervals. These nerves communicate with the spinal nerves, and send off branches which form plexuses or networks. The ultimate goal of these nerve fibres is the viscera of the abdominal and thoracic cavities. The blood-vessels of the body are also supplied by those nerves. Together with peripheral nerves from the central nervous system, to which their action is opposed, they serve to control the functioning of the internal organs. Not much can be said further, but with regard to the function of these sympathetic nerves it may be stated that when the body is put under some stress requiring the expenditure of considerable muscular energy, such as in flight from danger, the sympathetic system is stimulated generally, and the organs of the body respond in such a way as to meet the sudden demand.

CHAPTER XVIII.

STATES OF INSENSIBILITY.

INSENSIBILITY means a condition in which the individual is incapable of appreciating any feeling. It is always due ultimately to a failure on the part of the brain to receive stimuli from the outside world. Words such as unconsciousness and coma are practically synonymous with insensibility, and there is no point in making any differentiation between those terms, since such would be arbitrary. There are various degrees of insensibility, from a general blunting of sensation in surgical injury to the profound unconsciousness which immediately precedes death due to cerebral compression. The causes of insensibility are also various ; and, while a suspension of some part of brain function is the rule in every case, the underlying causes differ. These causes may be situated in the brain or in some other organ, or they may be the result of the introduction of some poison into the body.

The causes of insensibility are :

I. Injury to :
    (a) Head ;
    (b) Body, causing surgical shock.
    (c) Blood-vessels, causing haemorrhage.

II. Diseases of the Nervous System.
    (a) Apoplexy.
    (b) Epilepsy.
    (c) Hysteria.

III. Poisoning by Drugs.
        Alcohol, opium, chloroform, ether, etc.

IV. Poisoning from Disease.
      (a) Diabetes.
      (b) Uraemia.

V. Anything causing diminution in the Blood Supply to the Brain.
      (a) Fainting (Syncope).
      (b) Heart Disease.

VI. Anything causing prolonged cutting off of the Oxygen Supply to the Blood (Asphyxia).
      (a) Exposure to Poisonous Gases.
      (b) Drowning.
      (c) Throttling and Strangulation.

VII. Heat Apoplexy.

VIII. Infantile Convulsions.

I. INJURY.

(a) *To Head.*—The insensibility due to head injury has been dealt with under the complications of fracture of the skull.

(b) *To Body generally.*—Insensibility due to injury to the body is in reality due to associated surgical shock. The insensibility is not deep, and is manifested usually by an indifference on the part of the patient, who is not so responsive to painful stimuli.

(c) *Haemorrhage.*—Haemorrhage may be so severe as to cause suspension of consciousness ; this may be due to fainting because of impairment of the heart's function from lack of blood.

II. DISEASES OF THE NERVOUS SYSTEM.

(a) *Apoplexy.*—Very often loss of consciousness arises from some catastrophe in the brain substance. The origin of such a disturbance lies in the blood-vessels of the brain, which are frequently the seat of disease processes. Such blood-vessel disease may be associated with a high blood pressure, and when the process of disease causes a weakening in the vessel wall the vessel may rupture, and haemorrhage will occur into the substance of the brain. The gush of blood tears up the tissues of the brain, causing such a great disturbance of function that unconsciousness supervenes immediately. The patient's condition is recognized by the presence of complete unconsciousness ; the pupils may be unequal and fixed, and the limbs are observed to be limp and flaccid. Sometimes it is possible to detect a difference between the two sides of the body ; when such is the case, the apoplexy has occurred on the side of the brain opposite to the more flaccid limbs. The breathing is stertorous, or snoring, due to paralysis of the palate. The reflexes are abolished. The pulse is full and bounding, like that found in cerebral compression. When the apoplexy is in the Pons Varolii the temperature may rise to 107° or to 110° F. It is rare to find apoplexy in a young person.

In some instances a brain vessel may become blocked, due either to disease of the vessel or to some solid material let loose in the circulation coming from the heart lining or from the lungs. These causes need not concern us further, since they are manifested by such signs as described above.

(b) *Epilepsy*.—In this disease unconsciousness is the accompaniment to a remarkable series of manifestations of brain disturbance. The epileptic may have been feeling out of sorts. He suddenly emits a cry, the warning cry of the epileptic seizure or fit, he falls to the ground unconscious, the limbs become rigid, breathing ceases, the face becomes livid, the rigidity is soon followed by an exhausting generalized convulsion during which spasmodic, noisy breathing re-establishes itself gradually, foaming occurs at the mouth, the patient may bite his tongue, he may pass urine and faeces ; the twitchings become less frequent and breathing—deeper than any other form of abnormally deep breathing—commences. When breathing is fully re-established and convulsions have ceased, the face resumes its normal complexion and the patient falls into a profound sleep. Such is the series of events in the epileptic seizure; the warning cry, the tonic or rigid stage, the clonic or convulsive stage, and finally the state of sleep. During the whole fit the patient is unconscious, the pupils are dilated and fixed, and during the tonic stage the eyes and head are turned to one side. Sometimes one fit may be succeeded rapidly by another, and thus the individual is said to be in the epileptic state, or status epilepticus.

(c) *Hysteria.*—This condition is peculiar in that unconsciousness occurs without evidences of gross abnormality. The type of individual is quite characteristic. The patient is usually a female, and the exciting cause is frequently slight. There is a tendency for the individual to lose consciousness in propitious circumstances, and, curiously enough, many cases of supposed fainting in women occur when there is a man conveniently at hand to receive the burden. The circumstances of the case are usually sufficient to make the diagnosis clear, but it is important that hysteria should not be mistaken for one of the serious conditions described above. In hysteria there may be an imitation of epilepsy or of fainting, but the careful observer will find that the imitation does not conform to the true picture. Whenever there is any doubt, it is safe to consider the case as some real malady.

III. Poisoning by Drugs.

To deal here with the effect of drugs and poisons is much too extensive a subject, and consequently a chapter is devoted to this study.

IV. Poisoning from Disease.

(a) *Diabetes.*—In this condition there is an upset in the internal secretion of the pancreas, and the consequence is that there is an upset in the utilization of sugar by the body. For reasons which are not clear, inability of the body to utilize sugar is accompanied by an incomplete breaking down of fat. These products of the metabolism of fat are very poisonous, and they do not exist in the normal person, who breaks up fat into carbon dioxide and water. The poisons are acid and volatile, and consequently can be smelt in the breath, which has a " fruity " odour. Respiration is stimulated by these poisons, and therefore one of the main accompaniments to the unconsciousness of diabetes is air hunger ; the patient gasps for breath. It is, of course, only in certain phases of the disease that unconsciousness supervenes in diabetes. In the less severe phases the patient may be only drowsy, but nevertheless able to go about his work. Unconsciousness may come on so suddenly as to be recognized as an emergency of disease.

When first seen the following points are usually noted : the patient may be roused slightly with difficulty or he may be completely unconscious ; his breath has the smell of an orchard, he gasps for breath and the reflexes are usually intact.

(b) *Uraemia.*—This is a manifestation of disease of the kidneys. They are thrown out of action, and the onset of uraemia is the consequence of the retention of poisonous substances. This failure is associated with a diminution in the output of urine ; indeed the kidneys may entirely fail to function. The diagnosis is usually made by the doctor, but its onset may be sudden enough to demand the attention of the ambulance pupil. The breath may perhaps smell of urine, and the individual may have fits which resemble superficially those of epilepsy. The patient may show some of the other signs of kidney disease, dropsy or puffiness of the skin. The pupils are usually small, but they react to light. There is also present in uraemia a disturbance of the respiratory function. This may take the form either of deep breathing or of Cheyne-Stokes respiration. In the latter the breathing varies in such a manner that periods of deep respiration alternate with periods of very shallow or suspended respiration.

V. ANYTHING CAUSING DIMINUTION IN THE BLOOD SUPPLY TO THE BRAIN.

(a) *Fainting.*—This is quite a common condition, and is the result of some stress put on the body. Sometimes, after severe exertion, lack of sleep or lack of nourishment, some slight additional strain will cause a temporary cessation of the heart's function and fainting results. Severe emotional strain, such as hearing some piece of distressing news or the sight of something very repulsive, is a potent cause of the condition. Many cases of unconsciousness in injury are due to this cause—an individual may receive a very slight injury such as a cut finger, and as a result consciousness is suspended owing to the interference with the heart's action, because of the distressing sight of blood causing the emotion of fear. People faint frequently from sudden grief or fear, rarely through excessive joy. There are individuals who faint more readily than others. Neurotic or highly-strung women are very prone to faint when in a situation of difficulty. Indeed, there is, in many cases, only a fine dividing line between true fainting and the faint of hysteria. True fainting is characterized by absence of pulse at the wrist ; the pulse, as the patient recovers, reappears and gradually becomes stronger. There is suspension of respiration also and extreme pallor of the face. The limbs are cold and clammy. Often cold sweat bathes the skin. Frequently the student at his first operation faints, and the evidences of imminent fainting are often so manifest that an assistant may tell the student to leave the operating theatre before fainting. The signs are the extreme pallor of fairly sudden onset, the pulse weakens, the individual feels nauseated, and may hear strange ringing in the ears : he faints, and falls to the ground unconscious. Often the losing of consciousness is not unattended by such pleasurable sensation as floating through the air. Consciousness returns, not without some nausea or feeling of sickness, the patient feels chilled and moist, and only gradually does he recover his normal condition. Often the condition of fainting may be referred to as syncope.

(b) *Heart Disease.*—When an individual has some disease process attacking the heart, the liability to loss of consciousness from failure of the heart's function increases. The contributory causes are those which have been mentioned in connection with fainting. The symptoms are similar, but the history of the case will show something of the impairment of the heart. The individual will probably have been complaining of breathlessness on exertion for a considerable period of time ; palpitation and fatigue are also prominent among the symptoms of heart disease. Owing to the difficulty of the heart's action there is impaired oxidation of the blood, and consequently this type of patient is likely to be habitually of a livid complexion, the lips are blue and the cheeks a dusky red. These symptoms of breathlessness and lividity do not persist in the faint ; they are replaced by a depression in the respiration and by extreme pallor.

VI. ANYTHING CAUSING PROLONGED CUTTING OFF OF THE OXYGEN SUPPLY TO THE BRAIN.—The justification for this separate heading is that while fainting implies a diminished supply of blood to the *brain*, in most of the conditions to be mentioned the primary cause is that the supply of oxygen to the *lungs* is cut off.

(a) *Exposure to Poisonous Gases.*—The gas is so irritating to the lining membranes of the respiratory passages that the individual's respiration is suspended ; or it may be that the inhaled gas is absorbed into the blood and substitutes itself for oxygen.

(b) *Drowning.*—In drowning oxygen is excluded from the air passages by the presence of water.

(c) *Throttling and Strangulation.*—In throttling direct pressure is applied over the windpipe so that the victim cannot breathe ; in strangulation compression of the carotid arteries and the main nerves of the neck plays a part in the causation of unconsciousness, in addition to the cutting off of the oxygen supply to the lungs.

In all three instances the evidences are those of asphyxia or suffocation : the onset of unconsciousness is rapid, the pupils are usually dilated, and if unconsciousness is profound the reflexes are abolished.

VII. HEAT APOPLEXY.—When the atmosphere is moist and hot the potentiality of the body for losing heat is much diminished, since the physical conditions are against loss of heat by evaporation. It does not necessarily follow that the person has to be exposed to the direct rays of a scorching sun in order to suffer from this complaint. An overheated moist atmosphere in the stokehold of a ship is often the cause of heat apoplexy. The condition may manifest itself in sudden collapse ; the patient suddenly becomes unconscious ; the pulse is feeble and rapid ; the skin is bathed in sweat. The temperature may shortly start to rise and ultimately reach 107° to 109°. All cases do not commence without warning in this way. Some have premonitory symptoms, in that they become weary, restless and drowsy. Delirium may precede the onset of unconsciousness.

EXAMINATION OF THE UNCONSCIOUS PATIENT.

To draw up a system of general rules in the examination of an unconscious patient is almost impossible. So much depends upon the circumstances and upon what has previously occurred. There may be certain things obvious which make the diagnosis of the condition certain, and it is the simultaneous association of different observations which in many cases makes the conclusion obvious. If an unconscious man smells of carbolic and shows evidences of burning of the mucous membrane of the mouth, there is no reason to consider the possibility of his suffering from angina pectoris. It is rare to find that the obvious is far misleading.

The following points may be followed in examination :

I. PULSE.—A fast, weak pulse is found in fainting, asphyxia, concussion, surgical shock, diabetic coma, and in narcotic or irritant poisoning.

A bounding pulse is found in laceration of the brain, apoplexy, epilepsy and uraemia.

A very slow bounding pulse is found in compression of the brain.

II. RESPIRATION.—Observation of the breathing may be of some use in arriving at a conclusion. In those conditions attended by a racing, weak. pulse, respiration is usually shallow. It is well to remember the extreme deep breathing in epilepsy, the air hunger in diabetes, the Cheyne-Stokes respiration in uraemia and in cerebral compression. Breathing is often noisy, according to the condition of the patient. Where there is paralysis of the soft palate stertorous breathing is the rule, and this is seen in cases of cerebral injury and in apoplexy. The spasm of the larynx in epilepsy causes the first respirations to be noisy : this is observed in inspiration which is attended by a " whoop."

III. GENERAL CONDITION OF THE MUSCLES AND OF THE REFLEXES.—The unconscious person is usually lying limp, but in certain conditions the general musculature of the body may be in a state of spasm : twitching of muscle may be part of the generalized convulsions of uraemia, epilepsy or strychnine poisoning, or it may be evidence of cerebral irritation. In the other conditions the skeletal muscles are relaxed, except in hysteria, where they may either be in spasm or in relaxation. In those cases where unconsciousness is profound the knee jerks and ocular reflexes are diminished or abolished. This is the invariable rule in cerebral compression, in apoplexy, and in deep coma from diabetes or uraemia. The reflexes are only slightly diminished where the insensibility is of moderate degree, such as is found in conditions of poisoning, either by drugs or by disease, where the onset is relatively slow.

IV. CONDITIONS OF THE EYES AND PUPILS.

(a) Deviation of the eyes to one side may be found in apoplexy and in epilepsy.

(b) Condition of the conjunctival reflex. This is elicited by touching the conjunctiva or the covering of the white of the eye. Reflexly, in the normal person the eye is closed. This reflex is abolished whenever consciousness is sufficiently suspended. It is absent in cerebral compression, in many cases of apoplexy, and wherever coma is profound.

(c) Dilated pupils are found in epilepsy, in certain cases of poisoning by drugs, in cerebral compression, in fainting and in hysteria as a rule.

Contracted pupils are found in certain cases of poisoning, and in apoplexy into the Pons Varolii.

Unequal pupils are found in apoplexy, and in cerebral injury and in glass or artificial eye.

(d) Condition of pupillary reflexes. These reflexes are elicited by noting the reaction of the pupil when light is allowed to fall on the eye. The eyelid is raised, and the normal reaction of the pupil when light is thus allowed to enter the pupil is that the pupil contracts or becomes smaller. The presence of this reflex again depends upon the depth of unconsciousness. The intact reflex is found in most cases of early coma from poisoning, where the outset of symptoms has been slow, in uraemia and diabetic coma. In cerebral compression the pupils are fixed, as in most cases of apoplexy and in the tonic and clonic stages of epilepsy.

The further examination of the patient must be guided by the circumstances of the case. Poisoning will have its associated signs : smell of the drug or poison. the discovery of the poison, and so on (see chapter on poisoning).

Confirmation of suspected heart disease, uraemia or epilepsy may be obtained by judicious enquiry.

TREATMENT OF CASES OF INSENSIBILITY.

I. INSENSIBILITY FROM INJURY.—See sections on Head Injury, Surgical Shock and Haemorrhage for treatment of these conditions.

II. DISEASES OF THE NERVOUS SYSTEM.

(a) *Apoplexy*.—This condition calls for very little in the way of first-aid treatment. The main thing in treatment is to keep the air passages clear. Remove any artificial teeth, keep the head to one side and, if breathing is very difficult, press behind the angle of the jaw to keep the jaw forward and so facilitate breathing. The head should be slightly raised, and must be kept to one side since mucus may collect in the throat and cause much embarrassment to the respiration. All tight clothing must be loosened at the neck. The body should be kept warm with rugs and hot-water bottles. On no account whatever must any stimulant be given to the apoplectic.

(b) *Epilepsy*.—In this condition two things are essential. The patient must have air and he must be prevented from doing himself injury. Insert a wedge between the teeth—a key with a handkerchief wrapped round it does well—to prevent the patient from biting his tongue and to permit of access of air to the respiratory passages. Loosen all tight clothing round the neck. The more urgent thing must be done first—the air passages must be kept clear. If, for example, during the fit the epileptic breaks his artificial teeth, there is no point in fumbling about the neck to loosen the collar : the first and most urgent thing to be done is to make sure that the respiratory passages are clear. Attention to the epileptic during a seizure is of great importance ; often they show a tendency to turn on to the face ; epileptics have been drowned in water a few inches deep : others have been asphyxiated by turning over on to a soft pillow. The movements of the body during the convulsive stage must be controlled and guided in order to prevent the patient from doing himself bodily injury. Often, after recovery from an epileptic fit, the patient is not responsible for his actions. He may do himself or some other person injury, as the result of virtually insane impulse. The epileptic has not recovered until he is quite rational. This peculiar state, which is characterized by resistance and temper on the part of the patient, is quite characteristic of the disease, and the fact of its persistence must be borne in mind. Should the epileptic remain in this condition, he must not be left alone until he is under capable care and the responsibility is removed from the ambulance man. It must also be remembered that the epileptic may have fit after fit in rapid succession. Here it may be necessary to remove the patient during the epileptic state to his home or to hospital. There is no first-aid treatment other than has been indicated above. The patient must be watched constantly. Do not attempt to administer anything to a person in an epileptic fit.

(c) *Hysteria.*—The best advice here is to treat the more serious condition which is simulated by the patient. It will never do any harm. If the ambulance man is certain of the condition being hysteria, then he must not speak harshly to the individual. In so far as there is some disturbance, it must be attributed to a cause ; if this cause is not physical, it is then psychological : and psychological errors are not corrected by harshness.

All cases of insensibility, from whatever cause, must either be seen by a doctor or taken to hospital. It is the duty of every ambulance man to make arrangements for a doctor being brought to a case. There is no doubt that strict adherence to this rule will always leave him satisfied that he has done his duty.

III. POISONING BY DRUGS.—The treatment for these

conditions of insensibility is considered under the headings in the appropriate chapter on poisoning.

IV. POISONING BY DISEASE.

(a) *Diabetic Coma.*—From the point of view of first-aid there is little to be done, since the treatment of this condition is a matter for skilled practice. The patient must have his respiration embarrassed in no way by tight clothing or by anything in the mouth. If the patient is able to swallow and can be roused from coma, there is no harm in giving large amounts of tepid water. The patient must be kept warm by the usual means.

(b) *Uraemic Coma.*—From the first-aid point of view the treatment here is precisely the same as in diabetic coma, except that copious draughts of water must not be given. The ambulance man should not give any case of coma water to drink, unless he knows that the condition is one of diabetic coma, and then only if the patient is able to swallow.

V. ANYTHING CAUSING DIMINUTION IN THE BLOOD SUPPLY TO THE BRAIN.

(a) *Fainting.*—In this condition it is necessary to insure the free access of air to the lungs. Cold water may be thrown on the face and smelling salts applied to the nostrils. Sometimes fainting may be very effectively treated by raising the lower limbs. The head may be lowered. In crowded places, such as a theatre, it may be inconvenient to lay the patient flat ; in these cases putting the head between the knees is often a most effective measure. The limbs may be rubbed from the distal to the proximal parts, in order to restore the circulation by driving back blood to the heart. The body must be kept warm.

(b) *Heart Disease.*—In old people, and in heart disease when fainting occurs, the lower extremities should not be raised, since too great a strain may be thrown on an enfeebled heart, but the individual must be kept flat on the back. In all cases the body must be kept warm.

VI. ASPHYXIA.—The treatment of asphyxia is dealt with in the chapter on Asphyxia and Drowning.

VII. HEAT APOPLEXY.—In order to prevent heat apoplexy careful attention must be paid to keeping the atmosphere at an equable temperature ; good ventilation is absolutely necessary. People liable to be exposed to high temperatures should not over-eat ; if they are to be exposed to bright sunshine, the back of the neck and head must be protected from the direct rays of the sun. The treatment of heat apoplexy is to lay the patient in a draught of air, and to reduce his temperature by cold water or by ice if ice be available.

VIII. INFANTILE CONVULSIONS.—A typical convulsion in a child is of sudden onset, manifesting itself in rigidity and clonic jerking of muscle, interference with the rhythm of breathing, clenching of the jaws, sometimes foaming at the mouth and often cyanosis in the face. Any convulsion or fit is an emergency and must not be treated lightly. Children react to processes of disease by going into a fit, whereas in the adult a similar disease process would result in shivering and fever. Teething, indigestion from irritating food, worms, rickets, infectious disease, anything producing asphyxia all cause convulsions in the child. Apart from the causes enumerated of prime import is the presence of epilepsy which may simulate convulsions from any other cause.

The duty of the first aid attendant is to determine if any gross cause such as obstruction to respiration is at fault. If such an obvious cause is present—remove it. Where there is no obvious cause, the assumption is made that the child is suffering from some disease productive of convulsions and a doctor should be summoned. While awaiting the arrival of the doctor the child should be immersed in a bath of hot water and watched carefully.

CHAPTER XIX.

BURNS, SCALDS, FROST-BITE AND ELECTRIC SHOCK.

A burn may be defined as an injury produced by heat on a localised part of the body. In the widest sense of the term this definition will scarcely suffice, because injuries produced by strong acids and alkalis are technically referred to as burns.

A scald is an injury produced by the effect of heat from moist vapour or liquid. There is no essential difference between a burn and a scald, but to make some distinction is convenient. With a moderate degree of heat, as in an overheated room, the body reacts in virtue of its heat regulating mechanism by dilatation of the superficial vessels, thus causing a generalised flush in the skin and increasing the loss of heat from the body. With more intense degrees of localised heat, as in sitting in front of a bright fire, the parts of the body exposed to direct heat become intensely red and do not immediately recover their normal appearance when removed from exposure to heat. A further example of this is to be found in the persistent redness after the application of a poultice ; in such cases the capillaries of the skin remain engorged for a variable period of time. Blistering of the skin is a sequel to the application of a still more intense heat : thus too hot a poultice is often attended by blistering. When blistering occurs there is destruction of the more superficial layers of the skin ; more severe degrees of burning are associated with an amount of tissue destruction in proportion to the intensity and duration of the heat application. In this way the extent of damage may vary from simple reddening of skin to the most serious destruction of muscle, blood-

vessels and even bone. With the most severe burns charring occurs, the destroyed tissues presenting a black appearance owing to the production of charcoal.

The injuries caused by burning produce not only local
tissue damage but also remote or constitutional effects.
In burns from heat of sufficient intensity to cause blistering,
but not so severe as to cause charring, the constitutional
disturbance varies in direct proportion to the surface area
of skin affected. This general rule is modified by the
situation of the burn in that burns over the thorax,
abdomen and cranium are relatively much more dangerous
than burns which only affect the extremities. Burns
associated with charring and destruction of the deeper
tissues are serious on account of the increased danger of
infection and inevitable subsequent deformity. Following
immediately upon the burn the constitutional effects are
those of profound surgical shock. The later effects of burns,
namely, toxaemia, septic infection and deformity, do not
directly concern the ambulance man except in so far as
he may be able to minimise them by intelligent first-aid
treatment.

CAUSES OF BURNS AND SCALDS.—Burns may be produced
by heat from many different sources. The more common
burns are those produced by contact with actual flames,
hot metals, hot-water bottles, poultices, boiling water,
steam, molten metal, or tar and boiling oil. Frequently
severe burning results from the clothes catching fire.
The heat produced by forms of energy other than actual
combustion is equally effective in causing burning injuries.
Examples of these sources are the heat produced by the
passage of an electric current through the body and the
heat produced by friction, as in " brush burns " resulting
from contact with a rapidly revolving buff, shaft or
wheel. The corrosive effect of strong acids or alkalis on
the tissues causes burning with negligible evolution of heat.

SYMPTOMS AND SIGNS OF BURNS AND SCALDS.—A good

deal has already been said in the introductory paragraph of this chapter concerning both the local and remote effects of burns.   For the sake of clarity the symptoms and signs will now be briefly reviewed :

SYMPTOMS.—1. Intense local burning pain.
2. Loss of function of the affected part.
3. Faintness and nausea.

SIGNS.—These depend upon the severity and the circumstances of the burn.

1. Redness of the affected area.
2. Blistering.
3. Swelling.
4. Charring.
5. General signs of surgical shock.

TREATMENT.—Obviously the first step in the emergency treatment of a burning accident is to remove the source of heat from the patient or *vice versa*.   In cases where the clothes have caught fire and are still burning the patient should immediately be pulled to the ground and wrapped in any available blanket, rug or large piece of clothing such as an overcoat in order to smother the flames.   People whose clothes have caught fire are often wildly excited and run about, thus assisting combustion by the creation of draughts.   Such people may have to be forcibly knocked down in order to control them.   Where surgical shock is manifest the most important treatment is that of counteracting this general condition.   In all cases of severe burning the patient must be kept warm ; hot coffee may be given to drink if the patient is conscious.   With regard to the local treatment of burns where damage is considerable, any further activity on the part of the ambulance man is to be discouraged.   The treatment of extensive burns is a matter for skilled technique and requires the conveniences of a well-equipped hospital ; therefore immediate arrangements for removal to such an institution must be made.

LOCAL TREATMENT.—In cases of relatively slight burning, and in cases of severe burning where facilities for skilled treatment are not readily available, the local condition must be treated. The clothing over the affected part should be carefully removed according to the principles laid down in the chapter on the treatment of fractures.

When clothing is adhering to a burned skin surface it is dangerous and painful to remove it forcibly ; in these cases the cloth should be cut around the margin of the burned area. The ultimate removal of the adherent material is effected by bathing the part and soaking the cloth with some mild antiseptic lotion, preferably boracic lotion. In the actual removal of the clothing care must be taken to avoid bursting the blisters.

In those cases of very extensive burning where skilled aid is unavailable it is occasionally helpful to immerse the patient or the affected part in a warm bath at body temperature ; the bath should be kept slightly antiseptic by the addition of a sufficient quantity of boracic acid (about 3 to 4 ounces to an average sized bathful of water, or a teaspoonful to the pint for smaller quantities). This procedure is particularly useful in the case of children.

It is essential that the burn should be covered, as exposure to air increases pain and shock. So far as the actual dressing of the burn is concerned the old practice of using oily dressings is to be condemned, since it encourages septic infection. Strips of lint or some other aseptic material should be soaked in one of the following antiseptics : (1) picric acid lotion, (2) acriflavine lotion, (3) sodium bicarbonate solution.

The methods of preparing these lotions will be found in Appendix III.

Having gently covered the wound with strips of dressing material in this way the whole area should be covered with a layer of cotton wool and the dressing fixed in position by means of a bandage loosely applied.

Burns due to the action of a corrosive acid are treated

by the application of lint or strips of lint soaked in a solution of baking soda (one teaspoonful to one pint of water), whereas those due to burning with corrosive alkali are best treated by the application of some mildly acid solution such as household vinegar.

Should the appropriate acid or alkali solution be unavailable the burned part should immediately be bathed in pure water.

Burns due to electricity should be treated on the same lines as other burns.

BURNS IN SPECIAL SITUATIONS

THE THROAT AND LARYNX.—These burns are always very serious, since great swelling of the mucous membrane and other soft tissues of the throat may rapidly occur and cause suffocation. Burns of the throat are generally of the nature of scalds and are most commonly produced by drinking excessively hot fluids or corrosive solutions such as strong acids or alkalis ; occasionally the throat is severely burned by accidentally swallowing hot potatoes or other food : more rarely children scald their throats by attempting to drink from the spout of a boiling kettle.

The symptoms are severe burning pain, difficulty in swallowing and in breathing, and surgical shock. The signs revealed by examination of the throat are those usually associated with burns.

TREATMENT.—This will depend to some extent upon the cause and severity of the burn. In severe cases send immediately for a doctor, since, at any moment, it may become urgently necessary to perform the surgical operation of tracheotomy, which is the making of an opening into the windpipe for the relief of suffocation. While awaiting the doctor's arrival elevate the patient's head and shoulders, keep him quiet, and carry out the treatment for shock. If the burn has been caused by a corrosive fluid the appropriate antidote (see poisoning) must be administered

L

immediately to neutralise the effects of the acid or alkali; water may be given to drink in order to dilute the corrosive. Pieces of cloth wrung out of cold or warm water should be placed around the neck and upper chest, as this will minimise the swelling inside the throat. In minor cases, when the symptoms are not severe and only slight discomfort is experienced, the only treatment necessary is to give the patient a drink of some bland fluid such as milk. It should be remembered that the swelling of the throat and larynx may not become evident for some time after the burning. It is therefore necessary to keep these patients under observation until all chance of danger has gone. Whenever a patient is able to swallow ice, ice drinks or ice cream may be administered.

BURNS OF THE EYE BY ACIDS, ALKALIS AND QUICKLIME.

These accidents are always very serious and necessitate immediate action.

The eye should be immersed or bathed in water and the corrosive substance washed out. In the absence of an eye bath or when an egg cup, which does very well when a proper eye bath is unobtainable, the whole face should be immersed in water and the patient instructed to open and close his eyes. If the nature of the burning fluid is known, an appropriate fluid may be used to neutralize the effect of the acid or alkali. In the case of an acid a weak solution of washing soda or baking soda, one teaspoonful to the pint of water, may be employed; in the case of an alkali a solution of vinegar, one tablespoonful to a cupful of water, will be found effective. If the burn is caused by quicklime the eye should at once be washed out with cold or tepid water, after which the lids should be everted, and any visible particles brushed away. To relieve the intense pain and irritation which follow burns of the eye from such causes a drop or two of castor oil should be inserted between the lids and a clean pad and bandage applied to exclude air and limit movement.   Burns of the eye due to scalding fluids, red hot sparks or even flames should be treated promptly by similar measures.   It should be noted that burns of the eye produced by alkali are more serious than those produced by acids since the action of the alkali is likely to be more prolonged.

FROST-BITE.—This condition results from the action of extreme cold upon the tissues ; it is rarely met with in this country.   The most distal parts—fingers, toes, nose and ears—are most commonly affected.   When a part of the body is frozen by the direct effect of cold the process is almost painless ; the part becomes pale and waxy owing to constriction of the vessels but the tissues are not immediately destroyed.   The survival of the frozen tissue depends to some extent on the duration of exposure and also very largely on the slowness with which gradual thawing may be accomplished.   When the frozen tissues commence to thaw the blood-vessels dilate and the part becomes swollen and extremely painful as if it were intensely inflamed.   The more gradual the thawing the less pain and reaction will occur and the greater will be the chance of survival ; injudicious treatment by rapid application of heat may cause the loss of a limb.

TREATMENT.—Remove the clothing over the affected part with extreme care, since irreparable damage may be done during this procedure.   Gently rub the parts with snow or ice-cold water and endeavour to warm the tissues with the heat of the hands alone.   Never allow warm water to be used nor allow exposure to the heat of a fire or hot-water bottle.   Wrap the parts in a thick layer of cotton wool and elevate them on a soft pillow ; in this way swelling may be reduced.   Attend to the general condition, keep the rest of the body well covered up, and apply stimulant treatment as for surgical shock.

One of the most potent contributory factors in the causation of frost-bite is wearing tight clothing—gloves, socks and boots. People who are subjected to extreme degrees of cold should not only attend to the warmth of their clothing but should wear loose-fitting garments.

ELECTRIC SHOCK.

In these days there is increasing danger from accidents by electric shock. There is an ever-growing demand for electricity as a source of power and illumination. Huge schemes are at present in progress to give the great majority of the population the advantages of electricity. Unfortunately such an advance is not an unmixed blessing because of the danger to life when intense currents of electricity pass through the body. Everyone should be aware of these dangers, and the first-aid man in particular should familiarise himself, not only with the manner in which these currents may injure, but also with some of the more fundamental principles which appear to govern electricity, in order that he may treat cases of electric shock efficiently, and, further, that he may not submit himself to any risk. It is essential, in order to gain some appreciation of the problem, that some of these fundamentals should be briefly stated.

No one can define electricity and, consequently, much of the explanation of its nature is based on analogy. Suppose two tanks at different levels, the higher tank being filled with water. These tanks may be taken as representing the positive and negative poles of a simple electric battery. No water or current flows from the higher level to the lower level or from the positive to the negative pole when no pipe or wire connects them. Suppose a pipe of a certain diameter is put between the tanks and a wire between the two poles of the battery. Water immediately commences to flow through the pipe from the higher to the lower level, and electricity begins to flow through the wire from the pole of higher electrical potential, to use the technical term, to the pole of lower potential. The intensity of the flow of water, like the intensity of the current of electricity, depends upon two factors, the difference in height or of electrical potential, and the diameter or resistance of the pipe or of the resistance of the wire respectively. The difference in level of the tanks is analogous to the difference in electrical potential which is measured in volts, the resistance of the pipe to the flow—the narrower the pipe the greater the resistance—is analogous to the resistance of the wire which is measured in ohms.

In order that an electrical current may flow it has to form what is termed a closed circuit. Thus a connection has to be established between a high and a low potential. In the circuit there may be an electric lamp or a motor to drive some machine ; no matter what may be in the circuit there has to be a return from the lamp or motor back to the negative pole. This may be accomplished either by connecting the interposed apparatus with the negative pole by means of a wire, or the negative pole may be connected with the earth, and the machine may also be earthed. In the latter way the current reaches the negative pole by flowing through the earth. This point is of extreme practical significance ; since the electric cable conveying supply to a house comes from the mains positive pole it is a " live wire " and may be earthed by someone touching it, the return current of domestic supply being through the earth.

Before going on to discuss the problem further some mention must be made of resistance. The lower the resistance the greater is the intensity of the current. Substances which have a low resistance or conduct electricity well are known as good conductors. Metals are notably good conductors, moisture over an object renders it a good conductor ; vulcanite, ebony, dry wood, rubber, dry wool are very poor conductors of electricity and are termed insulators. The dry skin of the body is a poor conductor, sweat and moisture increasing its conductivity immensely, but the rest of the tissues of the body are fairly good conductors.

Some general rules about electrical shocks may now be formulated. As a general principle anyone who proposes to work with the wiring of a house or any piece of electrical apparatus connected to the mains supply should first of all see that the current is switched off at the mains. This measure would prevent much pain and many fatalities which occur domestically from electric shock. Coming into contact with an exposed live wire and shortening the current to earth is dangerous in proportion to the conductivity of the connection between the body and the earth. Thus it is dangerous to work with electric irons or electric toasters in the neighbourhood of a kitchen sink where there is the risk of coming into contact with a live wire, particularly if the skin is wet and if contact is established with the sink which is well earthed through lead pipes. Furthermore, owing to the same danger, such practices as listening to wireless, using ear-phones connected to a set driven from the "mains" while in a hot bath, are to be discouraged. From what has been said it will be seen that it is not the voltage passing through the body which is dangerous, but the danger is proportional to the number of ampères which pass through the body. It is possible to touch a live wire carrying a high voltage provided the body is insulated from the earth. Thus it is safe to handle high tension wires while wearing special rubber gloves or standing on some insulating material. There are, of course, certain very high voltage currents which can hardly be insulated ; the most notable example of such a current is that of a discharge of lightning, where the difference in potential between the thunder-cloud and the earth is of the order of 1,000,000,000 volts.

The discharge of electricity from a lightning-flash occurs in one-thousandth of a second, and the intensity of the current is comparable with one of 50,000 ampères. There is enough energy in a single flash of lightning to raise a weight of 500 tons through a height of $1\frac{1}{3}$rd miles. These huge charges of electricity are not necessary to kill. A fatal result may follow touching any live wire with the usual domestic current of 250 volts, provided the circumstances for the earthing of the current are favourable. It does not follow that a person struck by lightning is killed, because he may get only a very small part of the current through his body. The current of a lightning-flash travels through the air, which has a high resistance ; it takes the easiest route to earth, which is often through a tree or a lightning conductor on a tower. It is probably safer to be in a place which is efficiently protected with lightning-conductors than in the open during a thunder-storm.

The country is now being supplied with alternating current : this plan has great economic advantages, for reasons which cannot be explained here. The alternating current is conveyed by aerial wires over the whole countryside. Such currents are at extremely high voltages, 33,000 and 66,000 volts ; they are much more dangerous than ordinary direct currents, where the current flows steadily from the high potential to the low one. An alternating current changes the direction of its flow regularly and frequently, the usual frequency of the alternation being 50 times per second. The usual domestic alternating current is about 200 to 250 volts of 50 cycles or alternations per second. These voltages are transformed from the high voltages of 33,000 or more volts. Alternating current is much more dangerous since the effect derived from an electric shock is momentary, occurring when the circuit is completed : a similar effect is obtained when the circuit is broken. When a 50-cycle current passes through the body the sensation of the electric shock is continuous. A very high frequency current of 5000 cycles may be passed through the body without any result except a rise in temperature ; in such frequencies 1,000,000 volts may be passed through the body with safety.

The effect of electric currents passing through the body is to cause the muscles to be thrown into painful spasm. Effects may be produced on the central nervous system: the respiratory centre may be paralysed and the heart's action may be stopped provided the current's intensity is sufficiently great. There is always profound collapse simulating surgical shock after a severe electric shock.

In injury from lightning, arborescent or branching marks may appear on the skin and, either with strong currents or with lightning, severe burning often occurs.

The first principle in treatment of electric shock is to remove the conductor from the patient or the patient from the conductor. The conductor may be grasped in the hand covered with a rubber glove, wool cap, felt hat or several thicknesses of newspaper. Extraordinary care has to be taken by the first-aid man not to receive a shock, because two people suffering from the result of electric shock is always a worse circumstance than one. The patient earthing a live conductor may be pushed off by a broom handle or may be safely removed if the rescuer be standing on an insulator. Further treatment is to administer artificial respiration if it be called for. It is usually hopeless to obtain resuscitation when the patient's pulse cannot be felt at the wrist, but, if at all possible, cloths wrung out of boiling water may be applied over the heart. When breathing has been established it is necessary to treat surgical shock by keeping the patient warm and administering hot coffee or tea once he is able to swallow. Surgical wounds and burns are purely a secondary consideration. It is needless to say that, where emergency treatment is required, a doctor must be summoned.

CHAPTER XX.

MISCELLANEOUS.

FOREIGN BODIES IN THE EYE.

A LARGE variety of foreign bodies may find their way into the eye : usually they are very small particles of matter such as sand, dust, grit, fine cinders, metal splinters, seed and even minute insects. These particles, no matter how small, cause an intense degree of irritation and may set up acute inflammation if they are left in the eye for any length of time. Fortunately, in the majority of cases, the foreign body in the eye is found lying loosely under the lids and can be removed without much difficulty. In other cases, however, when the foreign body is sharp and gritty and when it strikes the eye with considerable force, it becomes firmly embedded in the tissues of the eyeball and may cause serious damage.

TREATMENT.—This will depend upon whether or not the foreign body is embedded in the eye ; in all cases the patient should be prevented from rubbing the eye, as this increases the irritation.

1. WHEN THE FOREIGN BODY IS LYING LOOSELY UNDER THE EYELIDS.—An attempt should be made to pull the upper lid down over the lower lid so that the inner surface of the upper lid may be brushed by the lashes of the lower lid. The upper lid is seized between the fore finger and thumb of one hand and pulled downwards and slightly outwards while the lower lid is pushed upwards by the index finger of the other hand. This procedure can often be carried out by the patient himself if he simply grasps the

lashes of the upper lid and pulls it downwards over the lower lid.

Another method of removing foreign bodies from under the upper eye-lid is to evert the lid. This may be done by the following method : Place the patient in a chair facing the light and stand behind him. Take an ordinary match or some similar object, place it across the upper eyelid about half an inch from the margin and ask the patient to look downwards. Now grasp the eyelashes of the upper lid in the other hand and gently evert the lid over the match. In this way the under surface of the upper lid can be inspected and the foreign body removed by brushing gently with a moist piece of linen. As soon as the foreign body has been removed the upper lid should be returned to its former position by gently turning it forwards. If it is thought that the foreign body lies under the lower lid this region may be inspected by pulling the lid downwards with one finger. In this way a good exposure will be obtained and the foreign body, if present, can easily be brushed out with a small piece of moist linen. Subsequent irritation may be relieved by bathing the eye with warm boracic lotion or cold tea and inserting a drop of castor oil.

2. WHEN THE FOREIGN BODY IS EMBEDDED IN THE TISSUES OF THE EYE.—Never attempt to remove the foreign body but send for, or take the patient to, a doctor as soon as possible. Warn the patient not to rub the eye and for his temporary relief place two or three drops of castor or olive oil in the eye : if the lids are held firmly closed by spasm of the muscles, evert the lower lid while putting in the oil. A pad of any clean moist dressing material should be placed over the affected eye and bandaged in position to limit the movement of the eyelids.

FOREIGN BODIES IN THE NOSE.

A foreign body in the nose is seldom likely to cause any harm unless it is sharp, such as a pin or a piece of glass.

In most cases it is best to do nothing until a doctor sees the patient. The only danger in delay is that a foreign body may be sniffed backwards into the pharynx and swallowed. Foreign bodies in the nose are most commonly met with in children and usually consist of buttons, peas, ends of crayons or pencils, glass beads or even pins. Often the irritation causes sneezing and this may result in dislodgment.

TREATMENT.—If a portion of the foreign body is protruding from the nostril an attempt may be made to withdraw it, but if there is much resistance it is better to leave it alone. Under no circumstances should instruments be used by an unskilled person to remove a foreign body from the nose. Provided it is known that the foreign body has no sharp cutting edges the patient may be encouraged to attempt to expel the foreign body by occluding the free nostril and blowing the nose or sneezing. To prevent excitement he should be reassured as much as possible. If it should happen that the foreign body slips backwards and is swallowed, a large meal consisting of food such as bread and potatoes should be given and a doctor summoned.

FOREIGN BODIES IN THE EAR.

As in the case of the nose these are most commonly met with in children and a similar variety of objects is encountered. Small insects occasionally find their way into the ears both of children and adults and cause considerable annoyance. They are more likely to remain in the ear than in the nose, since in the latter instance they are usually expelled at once by blowing the nose or sneezing.

When a foreign body gets into the ear the principal danger is that it may be pushed right into the deepest part of the cavity, from which its dislodgment may be most difficult and dangerous. When such an accident occurs, it is always best to leave the ear alone until it can be examined by a doctor. Again the patient should be reassured; in the case of a young and excitable child the hands may have to be tied so as to prevent the fingers being pushed into the ear. Instruments must never be used in an attempt to dislodge a foreign body from the ear and, if it is known that the body consists of vegetable matter, no fluid should be used. Sometimes a little warm olive oil may be poured into the ear, as this may assist the body to come away itself, but fluid should not be forcibly squirted into the ear. If an insect is causing annoyance by buzzing in the ear a few drops of methylated spirits may be put in the ear to kill the insect but nothing further should be done to remove it.

THE ACUTE ABDOMEN.

Acute abdomen is a surgical term which simply means the presence of acute disease within the abdominal cavity. The condition may result from various forms of disease affecting different abdominal organs and therefore the term " acute abdomen " includes a variety of abdominal emergencies such as perforation of a gastric or duodenal ulcer, acute appendicitis, and acute intestinal obstruction. In the great majority of these cases a surgical operation is urgently required and delay, of even a few hours, may be attended by serious risk to the patient and even loss of life. The " acute abdomen " is mentioned in this book solely with a view to preventing or minimising this delay in sending for medical assistance. It should be clearly understood that the ambulance man is not called upon to make a diagnosis of any sort whatever : he is merely informed of certain symptoms and signs which will enable him to suspect the presence of acute abdominal disease if he has the slightest doubt in the matter, or if he suspects the presence of an abdominal emergency he will at once procure medical assistance, and, until the doctor arrives, he may even prevent the admistration of harmful treatment. Abdominal pain is the most constant symptom of acute abdominal disease. The sudden onset of severe abdominal pain, especially when it occurs in the upper or central region of the abdomen, is always suggestive of a perforated duodenal gastric ulcer : if the pain is accompanied by evidence of collapse or some degree of shock this condition is almost certainly present. The patient is usually afraid to move and lies more or less doubled up, the muscles of his abdominal wall feel hard and tenderness can be elicited by gently pressing over the surface of the abdomen. In most cases the appearance of the patient is so characteristic of acute and serious illness that common sense alone dictates the necessity for calling in medical assistance. Perforation of a duodenal or gastric ulcer is probably the most urgent of all acute abdominal diseases. Since the outlook for a perforation is extremely good when the operation is performed within a short time and since every hour of delay brings with it increasing risk to life this condition is given the prominence which it deserves. The urgency of other acute abdominal conditions which are characterized by the onset and persistence of abdominal pain with or without vomiting must not be minimised. Any patient showing those evidences of abdominal disturbance must at once have the benefit of skilled surgical opinion and treatment. Many lay people believe that acute appendicitis necessarily commences with pain confined to the right side of the abdomen, whereas in the great majority of cases acute appendicitis is ushered in by generalised or central abdominal pain accompanied or followed by sickness or vomiting ; in the light of these circumstances persistent abdominal pain must always be regarded as a serious condition.

As it not infrequently happens that some time elapses before the arrival of a doctor some indication must be given as to the best measures to adopt in the interval. The most important instructions concern what should not be done rather than any active first-aid treatment. Under no circumstances is it permissible to give the patient anything to swallow; alcohol is absolutely forbidden; even water must be withheld, castor oil or any other purgative medicine must not be given. Much harm may be done by the application of very hot poultices through blistering of the skin but it is permissible to apply moderate heat to the abdomen in order to relieve pain. In the presence of acute abdominal disease it is advisable to support the patient in a semi-recumbent position and to keep the body generally warm.

HERNIA OR RUPTURE.

A hernia or rupture is a protrusion of some part of the abdominal contents through a weak spot in the abdominal wall. The most common site for the occurrence of such a protrusion is the region of the groin. Hernia occurs in different forms: some are present at birth, others are acquired either gradually or suddenly. It is this last type with which we are concerned—those hernias of sudden onset. The sudden occurrence of a hernia is invariably the result of a sudden increase in pressure inside the abdomen, such as may accompany severe momentary exertion, violent coughing or straining at stool. When anyone suddenly experiences pain in the groin and discovers a swelling which was not previously there, it is almost certain that a hernia has occurred. This condition constitutes a surgical emergency demanding the immediate attention of a doctor, since in many instances it may soon be followed by acute intestinal obstruction with gangrene of the bowel. Until the arrival of a doctor the patient must be kept warm and completely at rest, the lower abdomen and pelvis should be elevated on one or more cushions. The thighs should be flexed and supported and cold compresses applied over the swelling. No attempt should be made to reduce the hernia by pressure and nothing should be given by the mouth.

CHILDBIRTH AND ITS TREATMENT IN EMERGENCY
CASES

Occasionally, through ignorance or as the result of exceptionally rapid labour, a woman may give birth to her child in the street or in a public conveyance. Considerable assistance may be given to the woman and her child by the exercise of certain first-aid methods.

The process of childbirth is referred to as "labour," and it consists essentially of two stages :

(1) The birth of the child.
(2) The birth of the placenta or after-birth.

When labour occurs unexpectedly there is rarely any cause for interference in the birth of the child. After the child is born it should be examined at once to make sure that there is no obstruction to the breathing, and any phlegm in the nose or mouth should immediately be removed. The child is still attached to the mother by the cord. This may be tied tightly with a bandage, tape or string at two points about two inches apart and about twelve inches from the child's abdomen. The cord should then be severed between these ligatures with a clean knife or scissors, care being taken to ensure that there is no bleeding from the cut ends. The infant should now be wrapped in a warm shawl, blanket or rug and carried to a place of safety.

The birth of the placenta or after-birth may take some time, and unless severe haemorrhage is occurring the mother should be allowed to lie wrapped in warm blankets and arrangements made to remove her to a house or hospital. If severe haemorrhage occurs, the womb, which lies just above the symphysis pubis, should be grasped through the abdominal wall and massaged or rubbed gently. This is done by pressing it downwards into the pelvis, when, after a time, the womb will be felt as a large, hard, pear-shaped mass. In most cases this procedure will arrest the haemorrhage. The after-birth should be allowed to come away spontaneously; its expulsion must on no account be interfered with.

DETERMINATION OF DEATH.—The assumption that death has occurred should rarely ever be made by the ambulance man. There is often considerable difficulty in determining whether or not life is extinct; in the great majority of cases the actual decision has to be made by a doctor. Certain conditions are absolutely incompatible with life, conditions such as decapitation, certain extreme degrees of haemorrhage from a main vessel or drowning after several hours. In many conditions death may be so simulated as to render the assumption of death by the ambulance man a culpable offence. Thus severe internal haemorrhage, poisoning by certain substances, profound surgical shock, drowning, asphyxia from gas poisoning and even fainting are often accompanied by signs closely resembling those of death.

SIGNS OF DEATH.—(1) Cessation of the respiration is evidenced by no movement of the chest wall and by absence of a current of air from the nose or mouth. This latter sign is easily tested for by holding any cold mirror surface to the nostrils and mouth; when respiration is present the moisture of the expired air condenses on the mirror surface and dims it. The absence of this dimming is not in itself certain evidence of death.

(2) Cessation of the circulation is evidenced by the absence of the arterial pulse at any of the points where it may normally be felt. There is no evidence of the impulse of the heart-beat in the chest; capillary circulation is absent and consequently the finger-nail test is negative. The pallor of the face and skin generally, " a deathly white appearance," is dependent upon circulatory failure.

(3) Failure of vital functions is a consequence of the suspension of all metabolic activity; thus the heat of the

body diminishes rapidly, the extremities first become cold and, finally, the whole body assumes the temperature of its surroundings. There is absolutely no muscular activity and therefore the body remains perfectly still.

(4) Failure of nervous functions rapidly follows any or all of the other three conditions. There is a marked alteration in facial expression, often occurring at the moment of death ; the pupils dilate and they do not react to light ; the cornea is insensitive, as is the rest of the body. Immediately after death the lax condition of the skeletal musculature generally is notable.

Only a registered medical practitioner is legally entitled to certify death for the purposes of registration. The problem of determining that death has occurred is difficult for the doctor ; the points which guide him in arriving at a conclusion have been stated above, and they are given to aid the ambulance man when, under rare circumstances, he is forced to make a pronouncement. It has to be remembered that no single sign in itself is sufficient, and that alterations, such as rigidity of the body (rigor mortis) and staining of the body (post-mortem staining), which are the only certain signs of death, occur at varying intervals after the actual moment of death.

When there is the slightest doubt of death having occurred, strenuous attempts must be made instantly to remove any apparent cause and to resuscitate the patient ; this will involve such measures as artificial respiration, the application of heat, and the general treatment of shock.

CHAPTER XXI.

THE REMOVAL OF THE INJURED.

BESIDES rendering such " first-aid " as has been described
in the previous chapters of this hand-book, it may often
fall to the lot of the ambulance pupil to have to undertake
the removal of a sick or injured person to a place of safety.
Sometimes this removal is not an easy matter and may
require a great deal of tact and ingenuity to accomplish it
satisfactorily, so that it is important for the ambulance
pupil to make himself acquainted with the various details
of the different methods of transport.

The nature of the assistance to be rendered to a disabled
person will vary with the nature of the case, the severity of
the accident, and as to whether the ambulance pupil has
to effect the removal alone or with one or more helpers.

When the ambulance pupil is the *only one at hand to help*,
not so much difficulty presents itself in that class of cases
where the person, though weak and faint from shock, or it
may be haemorrhage, has escaped injury in the lower
limbs and can walk. Here the great point is to render
assistance in the proper way, and the matter should not be
beneath notice because of its apparent simplicity. The
usual plan of the disabled person supporting himself on
the arm of his attendant, and leaning his weight on it, is
not nearly so efficient as that represented in Plate XXVI.
The problem is how you can render the greatest help and
still leave yourself, as well as the person requiring assistance, free to walk. To secure this it is evident that your
faces must be turned in the same direction. We will suppose
that a man has a broken arm which has been put into a
sling, and he wishes now to walk to the hospital, or to the

nearest doctor. You must stand at his uninjured side, with your face in the same direction, and, passing your arm behind his back, place one hand firmly on the man's hip. He must then pass his sound arm behind your neck, letting his hand fall well in front of your shoulder; which hand you must now grasp very firmly with the hand you have still disengaged. A trial of the above plan will at once convince anyone that it is the most effectual way of supporting a partially disabled person, and that if the helper is strong enough, and it is deemed necessary, by placing the hip behind the near hip of the patient, the latter can be easily raised from the ground and carried bodily along. When patients are being assisted in this manner, extra caution is necessary while descending any declivity or hill, lest they should suddenly slip or fall forward from any accession of weakness. In the illustration (Plate XXVI) the patient has his arm in a sling, but if that limb should happen to be un-hurt and the injury be located in the head, neck, or upper part of the trunk, the hand would be available for holding a stick as a further means of support.

The most arduous cases are those where the sufferer can-not walk, either from damage to his lower limbs or from being in any way unconscious, and the ambulance pupil has to *lift and carry the disabled person without assistance*. The chief difficulty, undoubtedly, in these cases is *lifting* the person into the arms or other position chosen. Once this is accomplished, the *carrying* is not so hard. Accord-ingly, no attempt should be made to stoop to the ground and pick an insensible person up. What should be done is rather by indirect methods to coax the weight into such a relation to the centre of gravity as to make it possible to carry it to a considerable distance without great weariness.

For short distances, in the case of a child, a woman, or a light and slim adult, the carrying is best managed *by taking the sufferer in a sitting posture in the arms*, the right arm being placed under the thighs and the left thrown round the trunk under the shoulders, the disabled person, if conscious, placing his arms round the neck of the person carrying him. This method requires that the patient should first be got into the upright posture, in the way to be presently alluded to, as otherwise it is not easy to lift the sufferer off the ground.

A somewhat better and easier plan, perhaps, is for the ambulance pupil *to take the disabled person on his back, and carry him in the position known as " pick-a-back."* This is best accomplished in the following way : Having spread out the patient's legs and placed him in the sitting posture, kneel, or what is better, crouch down between his legs with your back to him. Then draw his arms as far forward as possible over each of your shoulders, and by stooping forwards lift him gradually up until you stand upright. If the patient's position is now found not to be very comfortable, it may be improved by giving a hoist or two while holding on firmly to his hands. Subsequently, the patient, if conscious, may cling with one or both hands to the bearer's neck, and this frees the hands of the latter.

Some reference must be made as to the best way of carrying an *unconscious* person without assistance. This is no easy task at any time, but under certain circumstances it is one of great difficulty. As was said before, no attempt should be made to lift the insensible person directly from the ground. This would tax the strength of the strongest man. The better plan to follow is to coax the weight into such a relation to the centre of gravity that the carrying of it is rendered easier. Going on this principle, it will be found that *three* different positions are assumed in raising a wounded man to a bearer's back. First of all, the ambulance pupil turns the patient on his face, and, standing astride of him, lifts him to his knees, and then to his feet. Secondly, he draws the patient's left arm around the back of his neck, grasping the wrist in front with his own left hand, and, stooping down, he passes his right arm around in front of the patient's left thigh. Lastly, he

assumes the upright posture, and, on rising, the patient
falls across his back. (Plate XXVII.)

Should circumstances render it necessary that the bearer
should have one arm free, as in the case of a soldier or
policeman for carrying a weapon, or of a fireman for climb-
ing up or down a ladder, a modification of the above plan
is called for, so that the disabled person is carried rather
on the bearer's shoulder than his back. Here again three
positions are assumed, but in the *first* one the ambulance
pupil, after placing the patient on his face, stands at his
head and raises him successively to his knees and his
feet. Secondly, he passes his right arm either between
or around the thighs, and places his right shoulder at the
stomach of the patient. Further, he grasps the patient's
right wrist and draws his right arm forward firmly under
his own left shoulder. Lastly, he assumes the upright
position, when the patient falls over his right shoulder,
where, by grasping patient's wrist with the right hand and
drawing it across his own chest, the disabled person is
firmly locked, and can neither slip forwards nor backwards.
This leaves the bearer's left arm disengaged. Should it be
thought desirable to have the right one free, then the
operation is reversed, the patient being carried on the left
shoulder, the bearer's left arm being passed behind patient's
left thigh, and his right arm grasped from behind. By
some the term " *Fireman's Lift* " has been given to this
method. (Plate XXVIII.)

Should there be *two persons* available for rendering assistance to the injured person, the task is rendered much
easier, for standing side-by-side they can form no less than
three kinds of *hand-chairs*, each of which is applicable to
different varieties of cases, and the selection of which depends on the amount of back support needed. Thus if the
person is too much injured, or is too ill to sit upright, what
is known as *the two-handed seat* may be employed. This is
made as follows : The two bearers stand side-by-side, half-
facing each other. They then bend the fingers of the front

pair of hands at the second joint and hook the hands
together. This serves as a seat. A back support is made
by crossing the back pair of hands and arms, each bearer
placing his disengaged hand on the other bearer's hip.
(Plate XXIX.)   The person is then carried lying back, his
weight falling chiefly on the two arms behind, which encircle
his loins, as it were, and on the chests of the bearers.   By
raising the hands in front, the patient can, when necessary,
be placed almost in the recumbent posture.   If the disabled
person can bear to be carried in the sitting posture, there
is no plan that answers so well as *the four-handed seat*.   It
is, perhaps, the most comfortable of these improvised hand-
chairs, and puts least strain on the bearers, while its security
is very much added to by the patient, when able, placing
his arms round the shoulders of the bearers.   To make
this seat the bearers half-face each other as before.   They
then both grasp their own left wrists with their right hands,
the backs of both hands being held uppermost.   By both
next grasping each other's right wrists with their left hands,
backs uppermost, a square seat is made for the person to
be carried (Plate XXVI), and a considerable weight can
thus be borne with very little inconvenience, for the
bearers' arms mutually support each other, and are mutually supported.

A very useful method is that known as *the three-handed
seat*, in which one of the bearers has but one hand in the
seat, and with the other grasps his comrade's shoulder,
thus forming a back support against which the patient
leans.   In this variety of hand-chair the seat is three-
cornered, as it were, but it is a very easy way of transport
for the bearers and, like *the two-handed* seat, is very suitable for a weak though not collapsed patient.   It is made
as follows :   The two bearers half-face each other as in the
other methods.   The bearer on the right grasps the middle
of his left forearm with his right hand, while the bearer on
the left grasps the middle of the right forearm of the other
bearer.   To complete the seat, the latter with his left hand

grasps the middle of the left forearm of the bearer on the left, whose right hand is placed on the left shoulder of the other bearer. Plate XXX should help to make clear what seems rather an intricate method, but in practice is really very simple.

Convenient as these improvised seats are, there is sometimes a difficulty in getting patients on to them. To accomplish this the bearers kneel on the knee next the patient's feet, and having raised him on to their knees, and having explained to him that he must pass his arms round their necks, they at once form one of the varieties of hand-chairs underneath him. It is then not a difficult matter to rise steadily together and lift the patient off the ground. To gain dexterity in forming these seats and in carrying patients on them there is nothing like practice, so that the ambulance pupil should avail himself of every opportunity of perfecting himself in them.

The above described improvised hand-chairs are very suitable for disabled persons who are conscious, but where the patient is insensible, and two bearers are available, the better mode of transport, perhaps, is that known as the "Fore-and-aft Carry" (Plate XXVI). In this, one bearer walking in front takes the patient's legs, holding the thighs on either side of his hips, while the other bearer walking behind supports the upper part of the patient's body by passing his arms forward under the patient's shoulders and clasping his hands in front, the injured man's head being allowed to rest upon the bearer's chest. This is the only plan available in certain situations, as, for instance, in the narrow workings of a mine, or the passages between machinery. In fact, wherever there is no space to get at the side of the patient this plan of supporting him by the extremities should be resorted to. The only plan of carrying a patient to which, perhaps, the term "unsafe" should be applied is that known as the "Frog's March," where the person is placed with the face downwards. Sudden death has been known to occur under these circumstances, so that it should never be employed, even in the case of unruly drunkards.

Up to this point it will be observed that nothing has been said about *Ambulance material*, such as litters or stretchers, because the supposition has been that circumstances did not allow of their use, or that they were not available. All that has been done, so far, is to offer suggestions to the ambulance pupil as to how he should best meet the difficulties of particular cases where his assistance was limited and his appliances nil. In this way, when such emergencies arise, he is rendered better able to cope with them, and there is developed in him, or further strengthened, that inventive faculty, or the ability to make the best of circumstances, that ambulance instruction always aims at encouraging. But in a very large number of cases of accident and sudden illness, apart from the question of distance, the disabled persons are too weak and too much injured to allow of their removal by any of the means mentioned, and it becomes necessary to call into use some form of conveyance. Of these there are a great variety, some being carried by men, others wheeled by men, some borne by animals, others drawn by animals, and, lastly, some moved by steam or motor power on railways and roads. Upon each of these different classes of conveyance it will be necessary to say something.

1. *Conveyances carried by men.*—Of these " *hand-litters*," as they are occasionally called, the form known as a *stretcher* is the most familiar to people in this country. The word " *litter* " is connected with the Latin word *lectica*, a sort of couch with a bed in it, in which the wealthier Romans were carried about by servants called *lecticarii*, or litter bearers ; and its name implies the idea of recumbency, the position, as we know, most suitable for anybody sick or hurt. The word *stretcher*, again, is probably derived from the fact that the material forming it is *stretched* within a frame, thus furnishing a firm and reliable support for the person carried. This is the form of hand conveyance best known

in this country. It would be impossible, in a chapter like this, to give any account of the great variety of stretchers that have been devised from time to time. Of manufactured stretchers, the ones that have met with the most approval have their supporting material of canvas. This canvas is about six feet long and two feet wide. On either side of the canvas run two long poles of seasoned ash, 7 feet 4 inches in length. Projecting as they do, beyond the canvas, their ends, which are rounded off, serve as handles. Two iron rods or "*traverses*," as they are technically called, keep these poles apart, and stretch the canvas between them. Instead of legs there are four wheels of hardened wood or rubber which keep the stretcher off the ground, and on which it can be rolled into the ambulance waggon. Slings are frequently provided, which are attached to the handles, one at each end, and are long enough to pass over the shoulders of the bearers, thus assisting them materially in supporting their burden. Lastly, to allow of them folding into very small compass when not in use, most stretchers are constructed with jointed traverses, which permit of the poles being approximated laterally, and the canvas rolled tightly round them. It is shown, unfolded, in Fig. 67. With the view of sheltering the patient, it can be fitted with an awning, as seen in Fig. 68. A simple and very useful form of stretcher, consisting only of the two poles and canvas, is in constant use and is found most convenient. The absence of traverses allows a ready reduction in width which is of great service when casualties are being removed from very narrow spaces and passages. (Plate XXXI.) For conveying patients by train the same pattern of stretcher is used, but the handles, instead of being immovable, are telescopic. This admits of the stretcher being placed upon the seat of any ordinary railway compartment and causes the minimum of discomfort to the patient. A comfortable pillow is also provided.

It is sometimes necessary to remove a person who has met with an accident in a confined space such as a well,

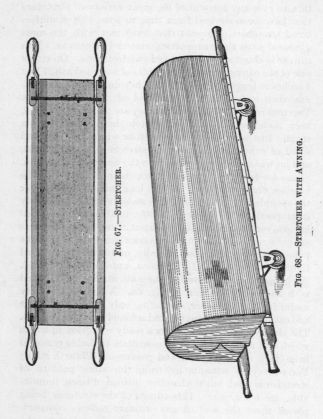

FIG. 67.—STRETCHER.

FIG. 68.—STRETCHER WITH AWNING.

the hold of a ship, a lift, etc. In such cases it is not possible after placing the injured person on the ordinary stretcher to remove him in the horizontal position. The Barnes Stretcher Attachment meets the difficulty. By an arrangement of canvas, straps, and metal D's, which can be attached to an ordinary stretcher without difficulty in a few seconds, it becomes possible to remove the patient and stretcher in a vertical position. The attachment is so ingeniously arranged that the pressure on the patient's body is equally distributed and does not cause interference with respiration or other inconvenience, neither is any undue weight thrown on to the lower limbs. It is cheap and has proved an advantage in the cases mentioned. (Plate XXXII.)

In many mines the cages in use cannot take in a full-sized stretcher placed in the vertical position. Indeed many cages are so small as not to be able to accommodate a standard stretcher in either the vertical or the horizontal position. Many experiments have been made to solve the problem of bringing severely injured men to the surface in small cages, and these experiments are still being carried on. One of the main difficulties is that it is impossible to construct a standard pattern of stretcher owing to the variation in the sizes of the cages.

Sometimes it happens that no stretcher is procurable. Under these circumstances one must be improvised, and this renders it necessary to say a few words on the important class of stretchers known as " *Extemporary* " ones. Here the inventive faculty of the ambulance pupil will come into play, and as he will have to utilize the materials at hand, the nature of the stretcher will depend, just as in the case of splints, on the *locality* where the accident has happened. The variety of articles that may be so employed is endless. In *towns and inhabited houses,* doors, window-shutters, bed frames, boards, benches, tables, mattresses, short ladders, etc., are all available ; while counterpanes, blankets, rugs, coats, empty sacks, etc., may all be converted into very serviceable litters by being carried by the four corners by four bearers, or by having rings or loops made with straps attached to their four corners, and poles inserted through these. In the *country*, hurdles, field gates, bits of fencing and paling, are generally at hand, while a long rope of plaited straw, laid zig-zag over two poles kept apart by two cross pieces of wood, having a straw pillow placed on them, forms a very comfortable straw stretcher. At *sea*, where hammocks are at hand, no difficulty is experienced in making an extemporized litter by hanging one of these at either end upon a single pole, while oars, boat-hooks, jackets and jerseys, are available for the same purpose. From what has been said the ambulance pupil should have no difficulty in constructing, should circumstances demand it, a strong and comfortable extemporized stretcher, not liable to change its shape under the patient's weight, and with its upper surface rendered soft by mattresses, straw, great-coats, rugs, or clothes, obtained, if necessary, from the bystanders. In connection with this subject of extemporized stretchers, it is important that the ambulance pupil should practise their formation whenever he can. In cases of real accident, it is a good plan to test the strength of any improvised stretcher before using it, by placing someone on it and lifting him up. It is a great satisfaction to the person who has to be carried to know that this has been done, and it obviates the risk of any further damage to one already crippled.

Perfect though a stretcher be, and furnished though it be with every modern improvement, it will be of little service to an injured person unless the ambulance pupil knows how to use it. And this is not the simple matter that is generally supposed. The proper way to open out and fold up a stretcher, and how to lift and lower it, is very easily mastered by a short course of instruction, but the raising and placing an injured person on it, the carrying of it when so " loaded," the laying down of it with a patient

on it, and the removal of the disabled person off it, are
operations that involve certain principles that it is absolutely essential to master. Thus the lifting and placing an
injured man on a stretcher involves three separate manipu-
lations, viz. the lifting the patient off the ground ; the
laying of the stretcher immediately under him ; and the
lowering of him on to it. Of these different movements,
the lifting and the lowering must be done in unison by
those engaged in it, for, as the weight of the disabled person's body is distributed, as it were, among them, one
taking the chest, another the pelvis and buttocks, and the
third the lower extremities, unless this point is attended
to, the patient's injuries and sufferings may be much
increased. (Plates XXXIII and XXXIV.) Then the
carriage of a " loaded " stretcher, that is, one with a
sick or injured person on it, necessitates attention to
several very important points. If as little as possible
of the movements of the bearers are to be communicated
to the stretchers, the bearers should *not* march in step,
and the pace taken should only be about 20 inches, all
springing from the forepart of the foot being avoided,
and the knees being kept well bent while the advance is
being made. Further, to allow of the stretcher being maintained on all occasions in the horizontal position, and as
near the ground as is consistent with the ease and comfort
of the men carrying it, it should be carried in the hands or
suspended by straps over the shoulders of the bearers,
these latter being selected, as much as possible, of the same
height.

Care is necessary in locating the part injured, the nature
of the injury, and its extent, as these determine the position in which the patient should be placed during transport. As a rule, the head must be kept low and never
pressed forward on to the chest. In wounds of the head,
the patient is so placed that no part of the conveyance
presses upon it. In wounds of the lower limbs, the patient
is laid on his back, inclining towards the injured side, as

this limits motion in broken bones during transport. In wounds of the upper limbs, if the patient requires to lie down, he should be laid on his back or on the uninjured side, as this lessens the chance of displacement in the case of fractures. In wounds of the chest, the patient is laid with the chest well raised and his body at the same time inclining towards the injured side. In wounds of the abdomen, the patient should be laid on his back with the legs drawn up so as to bring the thighs and body as closely together as possible and packed beneath the thighs to keep the knees bent. In the case of extensive longitudinal wounds the knees should not be bent.

PREPARATION OF STRETCHER.—Where possible, before the man is placed on the stretcher it should be covered with a blanket folded lengthwise, or some similar article of clothing, to prevent direct contact with the canvas. Warmth reduces the liability to shock, which is all important in first-aid. It is more important to have blankets between the man and the stretcher than over the man. With two layers of blanket underneath and one over him, he will be fairly comfortable and warm; with one layer underneath and two on top, he will most likely be uncomfortable and cold.

Fig. 69 shows the arrangement of blankets on a stretcher when three are available.

The ordinary army or ambulance blanket is about three times the width of a stretcher, and advantage is taken of this to increase the covering of the patient by folding the blankets in the following way :

The two blankets to be placed under the patient are folded lengthwise in three folds. Two folds of each blanket are placed on the stretcher, thus making four layers of blanket under him. The third fold of each blanket is left hanging over the side of the stretcher. The third blanket is likewise folded lengthwise in two and placed over the patient, the ends being tucked round the feet. The spare folds of the two under blankets are then folded over the patient and fixed by pins. A pillow, or an improvised one, is placed under the patient's head, and this adds greatly to his comfort, but the head must not be pressed

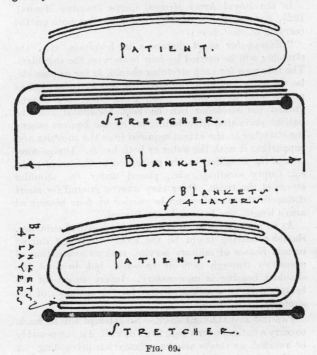

FIG. 69.

on the chest. A waterproof sheet placed on top of the blankets will protect the patient from rain. In cold weather, or in the case of a patient suffering from shock, covered hot-water bottles, if available, should be placed round him.

When the stretcher is carried on the shoulders the patient

is carried head foremost ; when by hand, feet first.   A head injury will be carried head first up hill ; a fracture or wound of the lower limb will be carried head first down hill.

In the Royal Army Medical Corps Training Manual, 1925, Paragraph 325, there is the following note on the carrying of stretchers :

" Except for short distances in hospitals, etc., the stretcher will be carried by four bearers on the shoulders. The four men for each stretcher should, as far as possible, be the same height.   The stretcher should be carried as nearly level as possible—when going over very uneven ground the stretcher can be kept horizontal and the patient prevented from falling off by the bearers raising the stretcher to the extent required from the shoulder and supporting it with the outer or both hands.   Undue soreness of the shoulders can be prevented by the use of pads, *e.g.* empty sandbags, etc., placed under the shoulder straps of the tunic.   Over very uneven ground for short distances the stretcher can be carried by four bearers at arm's length, the bearers facing inward."

As an alternative method of carrying a loaded stretcher, shoulder bearing might be the most convenient during certain phases of military service, such as evacuation of casualties through difficult trenches, but in civil life shoulder bearing is unnecessary.   Injury to one of the bearers may be a serious matter for the occupant of the stretcher.

PASSING A WALL OR FENCE.—No attempt will be made to carry a patient over a high fence or wall, if it can possibly be avoided, as this is always a dangerous proceeding.   A portion of the wall should be thrown down, or a breach in the fence made, so that the patient may be carried through on the stretcher ; or, if this is not practicable, and to avoid damage to property, the patient should be carried to a place where a gate or opening already exists, even although the distance to be traversed may be increased by doing so. It is better to do this than risk the safety of the patient.

CROSSING A DITCH.—The bearing of a loaded stretcher across a ditch requires special mention, and it is described in the R.A.M.C. Training Manual as follows :

" On arrival at a ditch to be crossed, No. 1 of the stretcher squad will select a level piece of ground near its edge, where the stretcher will be lowered.

The bearers will then take up positions at the stretcher as in loading waggons (see page 375.) The stretcher, with the patient on it, is then lifted and carried as near the edge as possible and lowered to the ground.

The Nos. 1 and 2 bearers descend into the ditch, lay hold of the handle of the stretcher and, lifting it, draw it forward ; the remaining bearers in succession descend and take hold of the stretcher, which is then pushed forward to the opposite side, and the front pair of runners rested on top of the bank.

The Nos. 1 and 2 bearers now climb up and guide the stretcher, which is pushed forward by the other bearers until both pairs of runners rest on the ground. The remaining bearers climb up, and the whole, lifting the stretcher as in loading waggons, carry it forward clear of the ditch and place it on the ground, the bearers taking up positions as in ' prepare stretchers.' (See page 367.) The No. 1 bearer will then examine the patient with a view to re-adjusting dressings, etc., if necessary, after which the march will be resumed."

This chapter on the transport of the injured is completed by a description of the essential parts of stretcher drill at present in use in the Royal Army Medical Corps. It is necessary for the proper loading and carrying of a stretcher that a definite plan of procedure should be detailed embodying certain principles, in order that the bearers may have a guide as to how to work together, to act with more speed and steadiness, and to co-ordinate their movements.

2. CONVEYANCES WHEELED BY MEN.—These, as a rule, consist of an ordinary stretcher placed upon a wheeled

M

support, and their use has been advocated on the ground that they save a great deal of valuable time, to say nothing of fatigue and labour. The wheeled litter supplied by the St. Andrew's Ambulance Association is shewn in Plate XXXV. The framework of the litter is made of tubular steel and runs on four wheels with india-rubber tyres. The wheels work on a swivel movement and are easily manipulated in corners and passages. The stretcher is detachable from the litter and can be loaded with a patient before being placed on the litter. The stretcher is fitted with an awning completely sheltering the patient.

There can be no question as to the suitability of these wheeled litters for the public works in large towns, and for villages having no hospitals, as they allow of patients being very expeditiously conveyed, in the one case, directly to the hospital, in the other, to the railway station, to be conveyed by rail to the nearest town where hospital accommodation is available. In villages where they have been tried these wheeled litters have been very favourably reported on, both on account of their utility and the saving of expense of the upkeep of an ambulance waggon. Of course they require that the roads over which they travel should be in good condition, and well laid. Rough and uneven ground limits their use, and hence it is that in military service they have not proved a complete success.

3. CONVEYANCES BORNE BY ANIMALS.—This class of transport is very little employed in civil life. It is called into use in time of war, when long-distance transportation is needed in places where vehicles cannot approach, as in hilly countries, mountain recesses, and impassable roads and deserts.

4. CONVEYANCES DRAWN BY ANIMALS.—Under this class come the wheeled vehicles drawn by horses and known as ambulance waggons or vans. The horse-drawn waggon employed by the St. Andrew's Ambulation Association, and once so familiar in our streets, has now been entirely

replaced by the motor ambulance. The old horse-drawn ambulance, by virtue of its special construction, provided a quick and comfortable means of removing sick and wounded persons. The modern type of motor ambulance is produced by most of the leading firms. (Plate XXXVI.) Each ambulance is equipped to carry two or four lying patients if necessary, and they are provided with fittings for the storage of dressings, etc. During the Great War, motor ambulances displaced to a very large extent the horse-drawn vehicles.

A special type of horse-drawn vehicle for desert transport is the desert ambulance cart. This is a two-wheeled spring cart, with a canvas hood, fitted with a spring bottom and drawn by four mules. The wheels are fitted with metal tyres, nine to twelve inches in breadth, to increase their surface and thus prevent their furrowing deeply into the sand.

The modern tendency, however, is to mechanize transport, and no doubt the caterpillar design of motor car with an ambulance body will be used in future for transport of wounded across sandy deserts or roadless country. When a properly equipped motor ambulance is not available, suitable transport can be improvised by the use of ordinary motor cars or other motor vehicles.

5. CONVEYANCES MOVED BY STEAM POWER ON RAIL-WAYS.—Under this heading comes the subject of the carriage by railway of sick and injured persons. On some lines there are invalid railway carriages ; but they are few in number and, as a rule, resort must be had to a well-cushioned third-class carriage, for the absence of any divisions on their seats renders them the only ones available. In time of war, when large numbers of men may have to be sent by rail, ambulance trains are used. Owing to the narrowness of the railway carriage door, there is sometimes a difficulty in getting a stretcher through ; but this may be done by slightly tilting the stretcher to one side. Should this not be possible, then the guard's van

must be taken advantage of. Permanent ambulance trains are designed solely for the carriage of sick and wounded, and can carry 396 lying cases. (Plate XXXVII.) They have a permanent staff of medical officers, sisters, and orderlies. Temporary ambulance trains are made up when required of passenger coaches with a small staff of R.A.M.C. personnel and some medical equipment. They are more suitable for the transport of sitting cases. Other types of trains fall much below the desired standard of comfort. Such trains are only used when the evacuation service is working under great pressure.

HOSPITAL SHIPS.—Here may be mentioned the hospital ship, which played such a prominent part in the Great War, and some idea of the extent to which they were employed may be gathered from the fact that huge liners, like the " Aquitania," were utilized in this service. The hospital ship flies the Red Cross Flag ; its hull is painted white with a band of green and three large Red Crosses—fore, aft, and amidships. Plate XXXVII shows the hospital ship " Canada," used with the Mediterranean Expeditionary Force. The hospital ship can be used only for the convey-ance of sick and wounded. The " ambulance transport," an example of which was the White Star liner " Olympic," is equipped in the same manner as a hospital ship for the accommodation of sick and wounded, but may also be used to transport troops and stores. It has none of the dis-tinguishing marks of a hospital ship. It sails under the red ensign, is not immune from enemy attack, and claims no protection under the Geneva Convention.

MOTOR LAUNCH.—The motor launch was found to be a very serviceable means of transporting wounded over water-ways during the Great War, and in civil life it is constantly being brought into use in conveying patients from an island to the mainland, where it links up with the motor ambulance. It has proved extremely useful when the regular steamer service is not available. (Plate XXXVII.)

TRANSPORT BY AIR.—Aerial transport of wounded and sick is a rapidly developing branch of ambulance transport, especially for long distances and in difficult country. On Plate XXXVII is shown a stretcher being loaded into an aeroplane used for transport by the Australian Inland Mission.

STRETCHER EXERCISES.

PUBLISHED BY PERMISSION OF THE CONTROLLER OF HIS MAJESTY'S STATIONERY OFFICE.

For the purposes of inspections, ceremonial parades, and also with the object of increasing the skill of the ambulance student in handling stretchers and transporting casualties, a certain amount of drill is necessary. In actual practice, these methods are more often cast aside than used because the circumstances do not lend themselves to the formal handling of casualties, but it is well known that the trained man is always the best ambulance man. He approaches the casualty with confidence, and this at once commands the respect of the untrained, who frequently is rather a danger than a help.

The exercises have a commonsense basis, and they train an ambulance man to draw upon his initiative in an emergency. They are taken from the Royal Army Medical Corps training of May, 1931.

The following drill is laid down for companies of reasonable size and is intended to be an aid in training and also for the purposes of inspection. A squad by itself is not expected to go through the more or less elaborate movements of " forming company " and other evolutions which are devised for larger bodies of bearers. The important point to be remembered by every man is that in practice he may form No. 1 of the stretcher squad, and as such will be responsible for the patient until the latter is brought directly under the notice of a medical officer. No. 1 commands the squad.

When the bearers have become proficient in these exercises on the parade ground, the instructor will take every opportunity of practising them under conditions approaching as nearly as possible to those of field service. The squads should be exercised over rough ground, and taught the various methods of carriage of wounded.

In a medical unit the handling of large numbers of stretcher cases should be practised with both two and four bearers.

Men detailed for stretcher exercises must be well grounded in squad drill. Knee caps will be worn on the left knee at all exercises in which the men are required to kneel. Men acting as " patients " will be provided with ground sheets to protect their clothing. The normal number of men in a stretcher squad will be four. More bearers will only be required when the patient has to be carried for a considerable distance, when the extra bearers will be used to relieve the others.

For instruction the men will be taught the exercises " by numbers " (where so indicated); when sufficiently advanced, the various movements will be done " judging the time," or working by the right.

FORMATION.*

Sizing the Bearers.† TALLEST ON THE RIGHT, SHORTEST ON THE LEFT, IN SINGLE RANK ... SIZE.	The whole will break off and arrange themselves according to size in single rank, the tallest on the right and the shortest on the left, and take up their dressing by the right.
NUMBER.	From right to left.
ODD NUMBERS ONE PACE FORWARD, EVEN NUMBERS ONE PACE STEP BACK ... MARCH.	The odd numbers will take one pace forward and the even numbers will step back one pace.
NUMBER ONE STAND FAST, RANKS RIGHT AND LEFT ... TURN.	The odd numbers, with the exception of number one, will turn to the right, the even numbers to the left.
FORM COMPANY, QUICK ... MARCH.	No. 1 will stand fast, the remainder will step off, the even numbers wheeling round to the right and following the left-hand man of the odd numbers. No. 3 will form up two paces in rear of No. 1. No. 5 on the left of No. 1. No. 7 in the rear of No. 5. No. 9 on the left of No. 5, and so on. As the men arrive in their places they will halt, turn to the left and take up their dressing.

* Previous to the parade the stretchers will be laid in a heap on the ground—unless a wagon or other suitable place is available. On the command "Fall In" the men will arrange themselves in two ranks at a place indicated by the instructor.

† In this and the following paragraphs the name of the movement is shown in *italic* type in the left-hand column, and is followed by the caution or executive word of command in SMALL CAPITALS. The right-hand column contains the detail. When, however, words of command are given by the No. 1 of the stretcher squad these are shown in the 2nd column and the detail in the 3rd column.

FORMATION—*Continued*.

Forming the Squads. FROM THE RIGHT, AT HALF A PACE INTERVAL, RIGHT . . . DRESS.	The file on the right will stand fast, the remainder of the company will ease off from the right. The correct interval will be obtained by each man of the front rank placing his right hand on his hip and easing off until the elbow is just clear of the man on his right. He will turn his head and eyes to the right and correct his alignment. The rear rank will conform to the movements of the front rank, they will cover off without placing the hand on the hip.
EYES . . . FRONT.	All will turn the head and eyes to the front and the right arm will be cut smartly to the side.
COMPANY . . . NUMBER.	The front rank will number from right to left.
Proving the Bearers. FRONT RANK . . . ODD NUMBERS, NUMBER ONE BEARERS, STAND AT . . . EASE. EVEN NUMBERS, NUMBER TWO BEARERS, STAND AT . . . EASE. REAR RANK . . . ODD NUMBERS, NUMBER THREE BEARERS, STAND AT . . . EASE. EVEN NUMBERS, NUMBER FOUR BEARERS, STAND AT . . . EASE.	After proving in this manner the bearers will be called to attention before proceeding with the next movement.

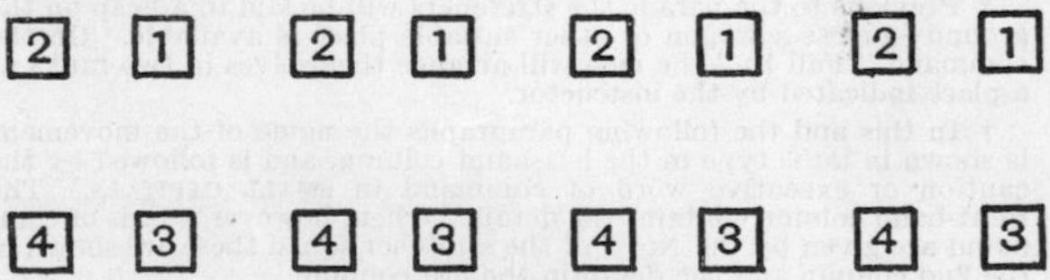

FIG. 70.

FORMATION—*Continued.*

Supplying Stretchers. NOS. 2 AND 4 BEARERS IN SUCCESSION FROM THE RIGHT SUPPLY . . . STRETCHERS, QUICK . . . MARCH.	The Nos. 2 and 4 bearers will lead out in file from the right and march by the shortest route to the stretchers, followed by the Nos. 2 and 4 bearers of the remaining squads in succession. On arriving at the stretchers the bearers stoop, grasp both handles of the stretchers with the right hand and rise, holding them at the full extent of the arm, runners to the right. The No. 2 bearers take the front and the No. 4 bearers the rear handles. The leading bearers will step short to allow time for the remainder to obtain stretchers. As soon as the last bearers are supplied with a stretcher they will receive the command, "Quick March," when the whole will break into quick time and rejoin their squads in file in succession, moving in rear of the supernumerary rank. No. 3 bearers will then take a pace to the rear and align themselves with the No. 4.
Lowering and Lifting Stretchers. LOWER . . . STRETCHERS.	The Nos. 2 and 4 bearers stoop, place the stretcher quietly on the ground, the front ends of the handles in line with the toes of Nos. 1 and 2 bearers and the runners to the right, then rise smartly together.
LIFT . . . STRETCHERS.	The Nos. 2 and 4 bearers stoop, grasp both handles of the poles with the right hand and rise together holding the stretcher at the full extent of the arm, runners to the right.
Organizing the Company. BY SQUADS . . . NUMBER.	The No. 1 bearers will be in charge of squads. The No. 1 bearers will number from right to left.

FORMATION—*Continued.*

Telling off Sections. NOS. 2, 4, 6, ETC. SQUADS.	Each section will consist of two stretcher squads. The No. 2 bearers of the squads named will extend the left forearm horizontally.
LEFT OF ... SECTIONS.	The No. 2 bearers will cut the left forearm smartly to the side.
BY SECTIONS ... NUMBER.	The No. 1 bearers of right-half sections will number from right to left. No. 1 Section ... No. 2 Section, etc.

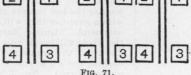

FIG. 71.

BEARER FORMATION.

The company is now in readiness for drill or duty. It is called " Bearer Formation " and is of value in the following ways :

1. During exercises if it is desired to reassemble the company, owing to the dispersal of the squads, etc., it is only necessary to place the right marker (either the instructor himself or No. 1 of the Right-hand Squad) and give the order : " Bearer Formation on Right Marker ... Fall in."

2. When bearers are constantly employed in the same positions as in companies of Field Ambulances, the company should fall in with stretchers in bearer formation, for duty or exercises.

3. Instructors of all classes are recommended to aim at the above and, when their class is considered efficient in the early exercises, to accustom the bearers to remember their positions in the company in bearer formation. Day by day the class can fall in in bearer formation, the early drill being dispensed with by the instructor if he sees fit and the hour's drill started at any point desired.

DISMISSING.

Piling Stretchers. LIFT ... STRETCHERS.	As before detailed.
NOS. 2 AND 4 BEARERS, IN SUCCESSION FROM THE RIGHT, PILE ... STRETCHERS.	The Nos. 2 and 4 bearers on the right will lead out in quick time, followed by the remaining Nos. 2 and 4 bearers in succession.
QUICK ... MARCH.	After disposing of their stretchers quietly, the leading bearers will wheel round, stepping short to enable the remaining bearers to pile their stretchers. As soon as the last stretcher has been piled, they will receive the command " Quick . . . March," when the whole will break into quick time and rejoin their squads in file in succession, moving in rear of the supernumerary rank.
Closing Ranks. REAR RANK, ONE PACE STEP FORWARD ... MARCH.	The rear rank will step forward one pace.
COMPANY, RIGHT ... DRESS.	The men will take up their dressing by the right and correct their interval and distance as in Infantry Training.
	NOTE.—One pace forward only is necessary to form Close Order, since the distance between ranks in Bearer Formation is about 3 paces.

DISMISSING—*Continued.*

COMPANY, STAND AT . . . EASE. STAND . . . EASY.	As in Infantry Training.
REMOVE KNEE CAPS.	Remove and collect.
COMPANY . . . ATTENTION. DISMISS.	As in Infantry Training.

EXERCISES WITH CLOSED STRETCHERS.

Advancing and Retiring. LIFT . . . STRETCHERS.	As before detailed.
BY THE RIGHT (OR LEFT) QUICK . . . MARCH.	As in Infantry Training—except that the arm holding the stretcher will be kept steady at the side.
COMPANY WILL RETIRE, ABOUT . . . TURN.	All bearers will turn towards the stretcher, the Nos. 2 and 4 bearers taking it in the left hand.
COMPANY WILL ADVANCE, ABOUT . . . TURN.	All bearers will turn towards the stretcher, the Nos. 2 and 4 bearers taking it in the right hand.
	NOTE.—The command "About Turn" should be followed by another similar command before exercises are carried out.
Changing Direction. CHANGE DIRECTION RIGHT (OR LEFT), RIGHT (OR LEFT) . . . FORM.	The leading bearer on the flank named will make a full turn to the right (or left) ; the remainder of the leading bearers a partial turn in the required direction, the bearers in rear a partial turn in the opposite direction.

EXERCISES WITH CLOSED STRETCHERS—*Continued.*

QUICK . . . MARCH.	The leading bearer on the flank named will mark time ; the remainder step off and mark time when they come into their places in the new alignment.
FOR . . . WARD.	The whole will move forward in the new direction.
	If the command is "At the Halt, Right . . . Form," the bearers turn as detailed above. On the command "Quick . . . March," the leading bearer on the flank named will stand fast, and the remainder will halt and dress as they come into their places in the new alignment.
Moving to a Flank.	When it is necessary to move a short distance to either flank the command "Right (or Left) Turn" will be given.
COLUMN OF ROUTE, SECTIONS RIGHT (OR LEFT) WHEEL, QUICK . . . MARCH.	Each section (of two squads) will wheel to the right (or left) and move off in Quick Time.

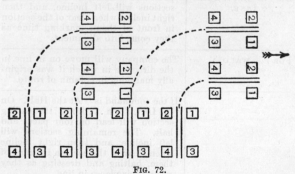

FIG. 72.

EXERCISES WITH CLOSED STRETCHERS—*Continued*.

	The company is now marching in fours one section abreast. A distance of one pace will be maintained between sections. They can change stretchers to the left hands of the Nos. 1 and 3 bearers without increasing their frontage.
Changing Stretchers. CHANGE . . . STRETCHERS.	Nos. 2 and 4 turn the stretcher with the runners up; the Nos. 1 and 3 bearers grasp the stretchers loosely by the further handle. Nos. 2 and 4 bearers release their hold and the stretcher swings round with the runners to the left.
	NOTE.—When marching " At ease " the stretcher may be placed on the inner shoulder, runners downwards, and steadied with either hand. On the command " March to attention " the stretcher will be returned to the right hands of Nos. 2 and 4 bearers.
Forming Line to the Front from Column of Route. ON THE LEFT, FORM . . LINE.	This movement brings the company into bearer formation. The leading section will lead on four paces and mark time. The remaining sections will left incline, and then right incline when clear of the section in front of them, marking time as they come into alignment.
FOR . . . WARD.	The company will move on in line in the direction in which it was originally marching in column of route.
	If the command is " At the Halt. On the Left, Form . . . Line," the leading section will lead on four paces and halt. The remaining sections will left incline, and then right incline when clear of the section in front of them, halting and dressing as they reach their places in line.

EXERCISES WITH CLOSED STRETCHERS—*Continued..*

Extending. EXTENDING FROM THE RIGHT (LEFT OR ANY NAMED SQUAD) TO FOUR PACES ... EXTEND.	From BEARER FORMATION. On the march, the named squad will continue to move on in quick time. The remainder will make a partial turn outwards and double to their places, pick up their dressing by the named squad and break into quick time.
Closing. ON THE RIGHT (LEFT OR ANY NAMED SQUAD) ... CLOSE.	The named squad will continue to march on, the remaining squads will make a partial turn towards the named squad, double to their positions in " Bearer Formation " and break into quick time.
	When considered necessary, " extending " and " closing " of squads may be carried out from the halt—to the halt ; this will be done in quick time and a full turn made instead of a partial turn.

EXERCISES WITH PREPARED STRETCHERS.

The preparation of stretchers and all movements with prepared stretchers will be performed in extended order.

Preparing Stretchers. PREPARE ... STRETCHERS.	The Nos. 1 and 3 bearers will take a side pace to the right, the Nos. 2 and 4 bearers will then turn to the right, kneel on the left knee, unbuckle the transverse strap, separate the poles, straighten the traverses and sit up with their arms to the side.
TWO.	They rise and turn to their left, working by the right.

EXERCISES WITH PREPARED STRETCHERS—*Continued.*

Closing Stretchers. CLOSE . . . STRETCHERS.	The Nos. 2 and 4 bearers turn to the right, kneel on the left knee, push in the traverses, raise the canvas and approximate the poles. Stand the stretcher on the runners, wrap the canvas round the poles and buckle off. Lay the stretcher on the ground with the runners to the right and sit up with their arms to the side.
TWO.	They rise and turn to their left, working by the right. The Nos. 1 and 3 bearers then take a side pace to the left.
Changing Numbers. CHANGE . . . NUMBERS.	1. The Nos. 3 and 4 bearers will turn about, the Nos. 1 and 3 bearers will then step out one pace and lead round the end of the stretcher, halting when in the position of Nos. 2 and 4, who will lead round close to the stretcher into the places of the Nos. 1 and 3 bearers. 2. The Nos. 1 and 2 turn about together.

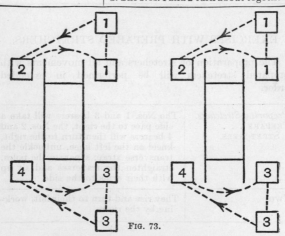

FIG. 73.

EXERCISES WITH PREPARED STRETCHERS—*Continued*.

	NOTE.—The original positions should be resumed before completion of the drill.
Shoulder Carrying. ON SHOULDERS LIFT . . . STRETCHERS.	The bearers will turn inwards together, stoop and grasp the stretcher, hands wide apart, palms uppermost, and lift it slowly and evenly to the level of the shoulders.
TWO.	The bearers turn to the front end of the stretcher, supporting the handle of the pole on the inner shoulder, steadying the stretcher with the outer hand.
ADVANCE.	All bearers step off together with the inner foot, taking short shuffling paces.
SQUADS . . . HALT.	The whole will halt, care being taken not to jolt or jar the stretcher.
SQUADS WILL RETIRE. ABOUT . . . TURN.	The bearers will grasp the handle with both hands, lift the stretcher, and turn about, placing the handle on the inner shoulder, steadying the stretcher with the outer hand, and remain steady.
RE . . . TIRE.	All bearers step off together as before detailed.
	NOTE.—In Turning About the squads should first be halted. About Turn should then be given, followed by Advance or Retire as the case may be. This will ensure that all bearers step off together.
LOWER . . . STRETCHER.	The bearers will turn inwards, supporting the stretcher with both hands, palms uppermost.

EXERCISES WITH PREPARED STRETCHERS—*Continued.*

Two.	They will lower the stretcher gently and evenly to the ground, rise and turn to the foot end of the stretcher.

HAND CARRIAGE WITH PREPARED STRETCHERS.

For Hand Carriage, Lift . . . Stretchers.	The Nos. 2 and 4 bearers take a side pace in between the handles of the stretcher, stoop, grasp the handles and, taking the time from the right, rise slowly together, keeping the stretcher level throughout the movement.
Lower . . . Stretcher.	Taking the time from the right, the Nos. 2 and 4 bearers will stoop, place the stretcher gently on the ground, rise smartly together, and side step to their original positions.
	Note.—These movements should also be practised with the Nos. 1 and 3 bearers.

ADVANCING AND RETIRING WITH PREPARED STRETCHERS.

For Hand Carriage, Lift . . . Stretchers.	As before detailed.
Will Advance. Ad . . . vance.	The whole move off together, stepping short, the rear carrying bearer stepping off with his right foot, the remainder of the bearers with the left foot. Nos. 2 and 4 bearers keeping their knees bent and raising their feet as little as possible.
Squads . . . Halt.	The squads will halt.

ADVANCING AND RETIRING WITH PREPARED STRETCHERS—
Continued.

SQUADS WILL RETIRE. ABOUT . . . TURN.	The stretcher will be lowered to the ground. Nos. 2 and 4 bearers will rise, and all will turn about. Nos. 2 and 4 bearers will lift the stretcher and remain steady.
RE . . . TIRE.	All bearers step off as before detailed in " Advance."
SQUADS . . . HALT.	The squads will halt.
SQUADS WILL ADVANCE. ABOUT ... TURN.	As for " Squads Will Retire."
AD . . . VANCE.	All bearers step off as before detailed.
LOWER . . . STRETCHER.	As before detailed.
	NOTE.—These movements should also be practised with the Nos. 1 and 3 bearers.

In the case of a long carry, No. 1 bearer as
often as he thinks fit can give the word :

	CHANGE . . . BEARERS.	The squad will halt, lower stretcher : Nos. 2 and 4 bearers retake their permanent positions and Nos. 1 and 3 take a side pace between the handles, " Lift Stretcher," and move on without further word of command.
Forming File. SQUADS, RIGHT (OR LEFT) WHEEL.		The squads wheel into file keeping at one pace distance. They can be reformed into line by giving the reverse order.

ADVANCING AND RETIRING WITH PREPARED STRETCHERS—
Continued.

Loading Stretchers.	NOTE.—Men to act as patients will be provided with ground sheets and placed in front of the company, extended to four paces and lying with their heads towards the squads. The company will be in bearer formation or column of route.
COLLECT . . . WOUNDED.	Each squad doubles by the shortest route to the corresponding patient and halts three paces from the head of, and in line with, the patient. No. 1 bearer will proceed to the right of the patient in quick time, halting at the patient's hips, turn to the left, kneel on the left knee, examine the patient, and if his carriage on a stretcher is necessary will give the commands :

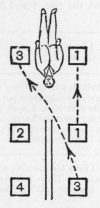 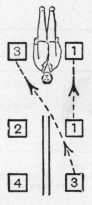

FIG. 74.

ADVANCING AND RETIRING WITH PREPARED STRETCHERS—
Continued.

LOWER . . . STRETCHER PREPARE . . . STRETCHER	While the stretcher is being prepared by Nos. 2 and 4 bearers, No. 3 bearer will proceed to the left side of the patient, halting at the patient's hips, turn to the right, kneel on the left knee and assist No. 1 bearer.
	As soon as the stretcher has been prepared, Nos. 2 and 4 bearers will proceed to the left side of the patient, No. 2 halting at the knees of the patient and No. 4 at the shoulders, turn to the right and kneel on the left knee. Assuming that the patient is then ready for removal on the stretcher, the bearers will pass their hands beneath the patient; No. 2 supports the legs, No. 3 (assisted by No. 1) the thighs and hips and No. 4 the upper part of the trunk.

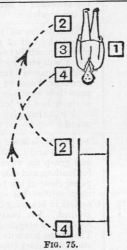

FIG. 75.

ADVANCING AND RETIRING WITH PREPARED STRETCHERS—
Continued.

	LIFT.	The patient is carefully lifted on to the knees of Nos. 2, 3 and 4 bearers. No. 1 will disengage, rise, step back one pace, turn to his left, double to the stretcher and take hold of it, left hand across and resting the near pole on his left hip. He will then return to the patient and place the stretcher directly beneath him, kneel on the left knee and assist in lowering him.
	LOWER.	The patient is lowered slowly and gently to the stretcher. The bearers then disengage, rise and turn to the foot end of the stretcher. The bearers will then resume their permanent positions ; Nos. 1 and 2 step forward, No. 4 step back. No. 3 will take a side pace to the left, turn about and proceed round the head end of the stretcher to his place on the right of the stretcher.
Unloading UNLOAD ... STRETCH- ER.		1. No. 3 bearer will turn about, double round the end of the stretcher and place himself between Nos. 2 and 4. No. 1 will step back one pace. 2. All bearers turn towards the stretcher, kneel on the left knee and pass their hands beneath the patient as described for loading. No. 1 will then give the word of command :
	LIFT.	The patient is lifted on to the knees of Nos. 2, 3 and 4. No. 1 will disengage and grasp the stretcher as described for loading and carry it forward three paces clear of the patient's feet. He then rejoins his squad, kneels and assists in lowering the patient to the ground. The bearers disengage by rising and stepping back one pace. They turn towards the stretcher and step off in quick time to their permanent places at the stretcher.

AMBULANCE CAR EXERCISES.

The ambulance cars will be drawn up in line. The class will fall in in "Bearer Formation" ten paces in rear of and facing away from the ambulance cars. The squads will be extended to two paces, the stretchers prepared and the patients will take their places on the stretchers with their heads towards the cars.

The command "About Turn" will now be given.

NOTE.—The class is now in position as at the end of retirement.

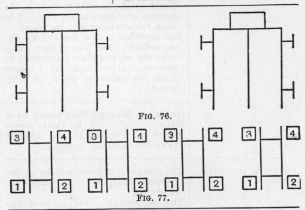

FIG. 76.

FIG. 77.

| SQUADS WILL LOAD IN SUCCESSION. NOS. 1, 5, 9, ETC. SQUADS ... LOAD. | One man will be told off to each car as orderly. He will prepare the car for the reception of the wounded. The compartments will be loaded in the following order : 1. Left (near) upper. 2. Right (off) upper. 3. Left (near) lower. 4. Right (off) lower. |

AMBULANCE CAR EXERCISES—*Continued*.

The bearers of the squads named will stoop, grasp a handle of the stretcher with the inner hand, rise and move to the car, holding the stretcher at the full extent of the arm. All bearers step off with the inner foot.

The squads will halt without further word of command one pace from the car. The bearers then turn towards the stretcher, grasping it as for "On shoulders lift stretchers," and raise it gently and evenly to the level of the compartment to be loaded. Nos. 3 and 4 will place the runners in the grooves and then assist 1 and 2 to push the stretcher into its place.

The stretcher is now secured by the car orderly. The bearers turn away from the car and place themselves in their original positions. No. 1 bearer gives the following words of command:

QUICK . . . MARCH.	They march back
HALT.	to their places
ABOUT . . . TURN.	in the line of
STAND AT . . . EASE	squads.

Unloading Ambulance Cars.

The company and cars will be in the positions occupied at the completion of loading.

The car orderlies will prepare the stretchers for unloading.

The compartments will be unloaded in the following order:

1. Right (off) lower.
2. Left (near) lower.
3. Right (off) upper.
4. Left (near) upper.

AMBULANCE CAR EXERCISES—*Continued.*

| SQUADS WILL UN-LOAD IN SUCCESSION. NOS. 4, 8, 12, ETC. SQUADS . . . UN-LOAD. | The named squads will lead directly to the compartments to be unloaded. Nos. 3 and 4 opening out, Nos. 1 and 2 pass between them, grasp the handles of the stretcher with both hands. They will withdraw the stretcher, raising the handles slightly in doing so. As soon as the stretcher is sufficiently withdrawn Nos. 3 and 4 take the further handles, all bearers take the weight, and grasping the stretcher as before, lower it to the full extent of the arms.

Now facing away from the ambulance cars the bearers carry the stretchers by the inner hand and, stepping off with the inner foot, lead back to the position they have just vacated. |
| HALT. LOWER . . . STRETCHER. STAND AT . . . EASE. | The No. 1 bearer will then give the following words of command: |

LOADING AND UNLOADING STRETCHERS WITH REDUCED NUMBERS.

With Three Bearers.

(1) In the event of there being only three bearers available, the stretcher will be placed at the patient's head, and in the same line as his body. The bearers will then lift the patient, rise to the erect position, carry him head

foremost over the *foot* of the stretcher, the horizontal position of his body being maintained throughout the movement, and then lay him in a suitable position on the canvas. When unloading, the patient will be lifted and carried head foremost over the *head* of the stretcher. To lift the patient : One bearer, placing himself on the *injured* side in a line with the patient's knees, raises and supports the lower limbs, while the other two, kneeling on opposite sides of the patient near his hips, facing each other, each pass an arm under his back and thighs, lock their fingers so as to secure a firm grasp, and raise and support the trunk.

With Two Bearers.

(2) When only two bearers are available, the stretcher will similarly be placed at the patient's head, and in the same line as his body. The bearers will then lift the patient, rise to the erect position, carry him, in loading, head foremost over the *foot* of the stretcher, and in unloading, head foremost over the *head*. The method of lifting will vary according to whether the lower limbs are severely injured or not. (*a*) With a severe injury of one of the lower limbs, both bearers place themselves on the injured side ; the one in a line with the patient's knees must raise and support the lower limbs, the one near the patient's hips, the body ; assisted by the patient himself as far as possible, the horizontal position of the patient's body being maintained throughout the movement. (*b*) With the lower limbs intact, or only slightly injured, the patient may be lifted by one of the improvised seats described in the next section, provided there are no symptoms of shock present ; in the latter case, method (*a*) must be resorted to.

HAND SEAT DRILL.

FORMATION OF HAND SEATS.

The company will be drawn up in double rank and numbered, odd numbers right files, even numbers left files.

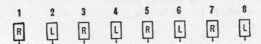

Form Two-handed Seats.	On the word " *Seats*," the right files turn to the left and the left files to the right.

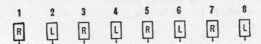

Two.	The right files bend the fingers of the right hand at the second joint, back of the hand uppermost. The left files bend the fingers of the left hand at the second joint, back of the hand downwards. The right and left files hook the hands together, each placing the disengaged hand upon the other's hip.

Plate XXIX.

Files—Right and Left Turn.	The files resume the position of attention, and turn in the original direction.

Form Three-handed Seats.	As in two-handed seats.
Two.	On the word " *Two*," each odd number grasps his own left forearm. Each even number grasps the right forearm of the odd number with his left hand, and the odd number the left forearm of the even number with his left hand, the even number placing his right hand on the left shoulder of the odd number.
Files—Right and Left Turn.	As before.

Plate XXX.

Form Four-handed Seats.	As in two-handed seats.
Two.	On the word " *Two*," both bearers grasp their own left wrists with their right hands, and each other's right wrists with their left hands. Backs of the hands uppermost.
Files—Right and Left Turn.	As before.

Plate XXVI.

The ranks may now be changed, in order that the bearers may be equally drilled. This is most easily done by marching the company across the hall or field in which they are being drilled, halting the men, and giving the order " *About Turn*." The bearers will then turn about, when the instructor will explain that the former right files will now act as left files, and the former left files as right files.

LIFTING, LOWERING, AND CARRYING WOUNDED BY HAND SEATS.

Right files will wear knee-caps on the right knee, and left files on the left knee.

A party of patients, proportionate to the number of files to be exercised, will be extended to four paces, marched ten paces in front of the company, and directed to stand when the exercise is in three- or four-handed seats, but for two-handed seats they will be directed to sit on the ground.

BY TWO-HANDED SEATS.

Take Post— Advance. Each file steps off towards its corresponding patient, and when immediately in the rear of him the front-rank bearer goes to the right and the rear-rank bearer to the left, halting when in line with and close up to the patient.

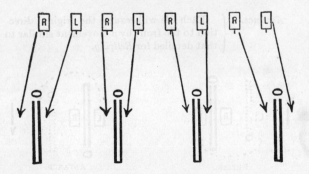

By Two-
handed Seats
—Lift.
{ The bearers turn inwards, kneel on the knee nearest the patient's feet, and form the two-handed seat beneath his thighs, grasping the patient round the loins with the disengaged hand and arm. The patient will be directed to pass an arm round the neck of each bearer.

Two.
On the word "*Two*," the bearers rise steadily together, lifting the patient off the ground.

Advance.
{ The bearers step off, the front-rank bearer with the *right* and the rear-rank bearer with the *left* foot, marching by a side step in which the feet are alternately crossed, one before the other.

About.
{ The front-rank bearer (bearer to right of patient) *marks time* and brings the rear-rank bearer round, both moving on when square.

Advance.
{ Each file will resume the original direction to the front by a movement similar to that detailed for *Retiring*.

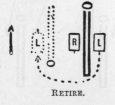

RETIRE.

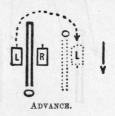

ADVANCE.

Halt. As usual.

Lower. { The bearers kneel and gently place the patient in a sitting posture on the ground and stand up, still facing inwards.

Retire.
Halt.
About Turn. { The bearers turn—front-rank man to the left, rear-rank man to the right—and march back to their original position, rear-rank man leading, where they will be halted and turned about.

By Three-handed Seats.

Take Post—
Advance. } As in two-handed seats.

By Three-handed Seats —Lift. { The bearers turn inwards, form the three-handed seat, and, stooping, place it beneath the hips of the patient, who will be directed to pass an arm round the neck of each bearer.

Two. { On the word "*Two*," as in two-handed seats.

Advance.
About.
Advance.
Halt. } As in two-handed seats.

Lower. { The bearers stoop instead of kneeling, and the patient stands up.

Retire.
Halt.
About Turn. } As in two-handed seats.

By Four-handed Seats.

Take Post—
Advance. } As in two-handed seats.

By
Four-handed
Seats—Lift.

Two.

{ The bearers turn inwards, form the four-handed seat, and, stooping, place it beneath the hips of the patient, who will be directed to pass an arm round the neck of each bearer.

On the word "*Two,*" as in two-handed seats.

PLATE VI

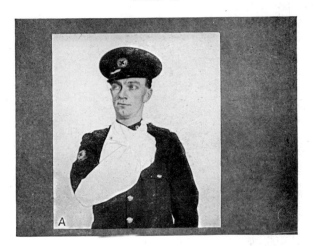

PLATE IX

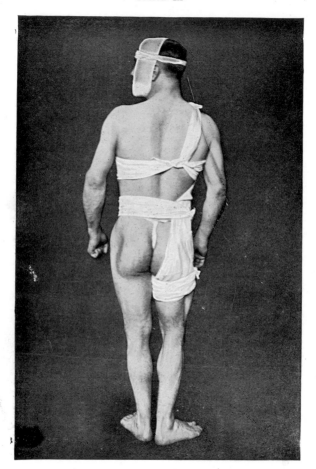

PLATE X

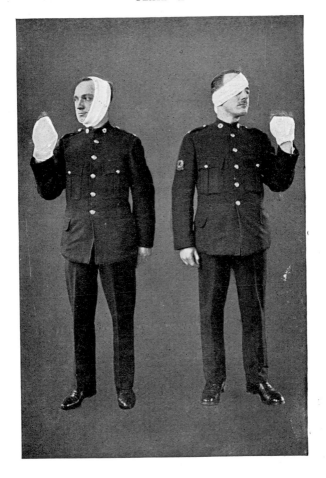

PLATE XI

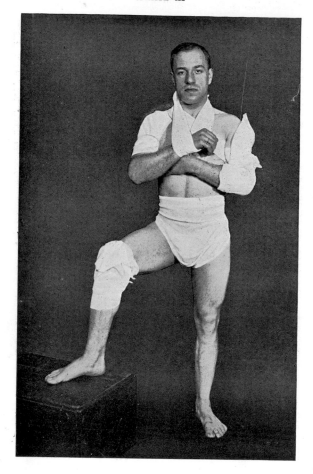

PLATE XII

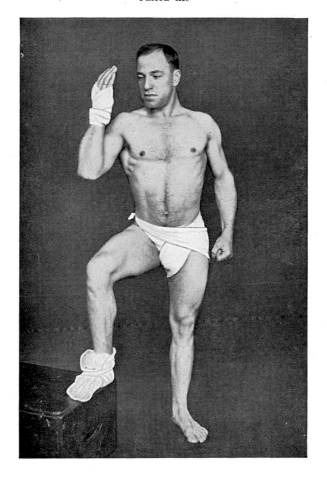

PLATE XIII

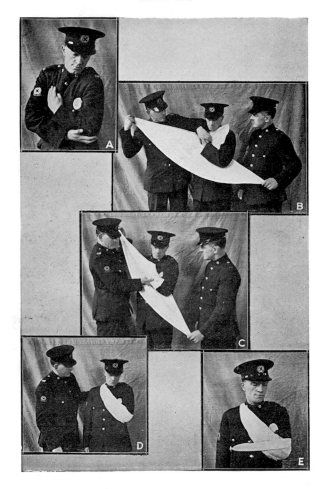

PLATE XIV

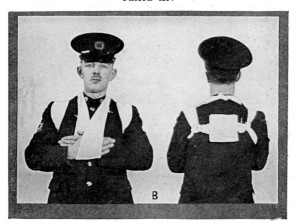

B

PLATE XV

PLATE XVI

PLATE XIX

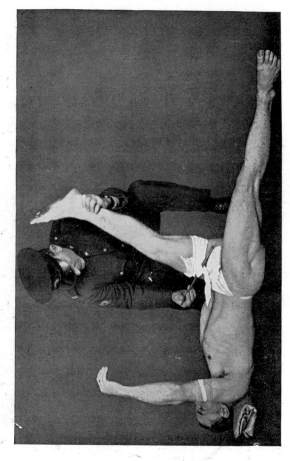

PLATE XXII

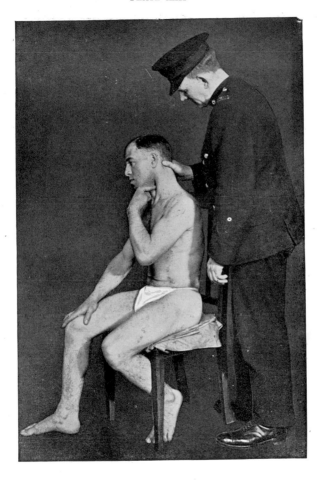

PLATE XXIII

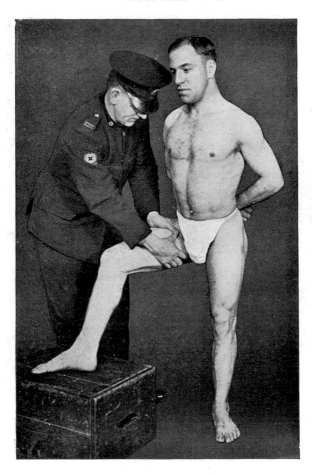

PLATE XXIV

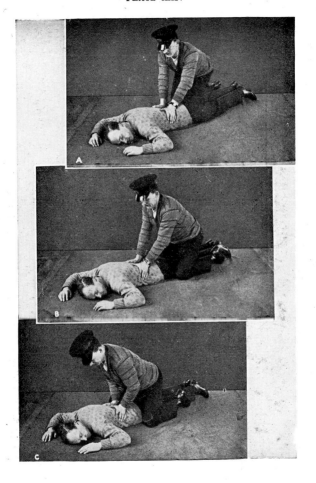

PLATE XXV

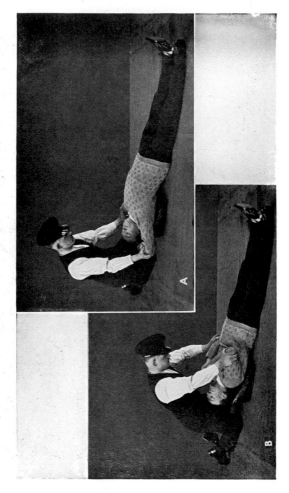

PLATE XXVI

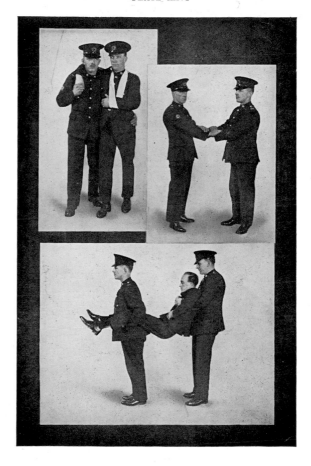

PLATE XXVII

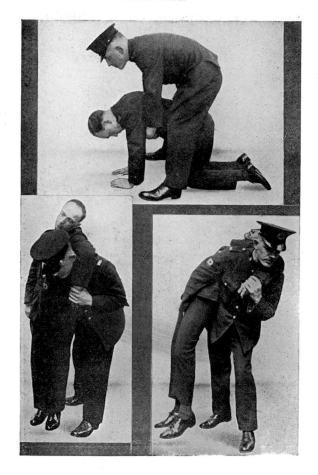

PLATE XXVIII

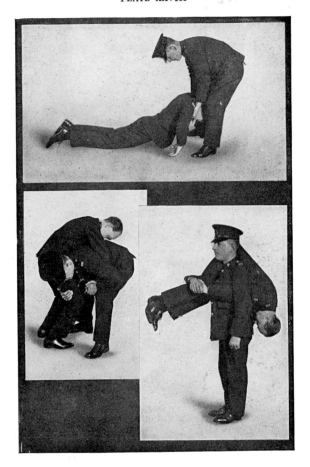

PLATE XXIX

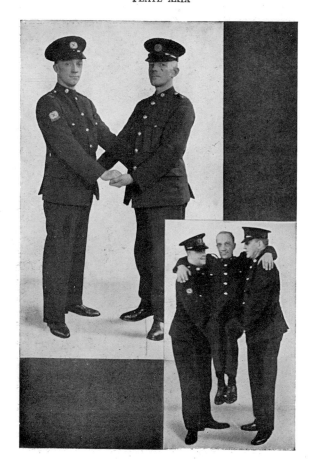

PLATE XXX

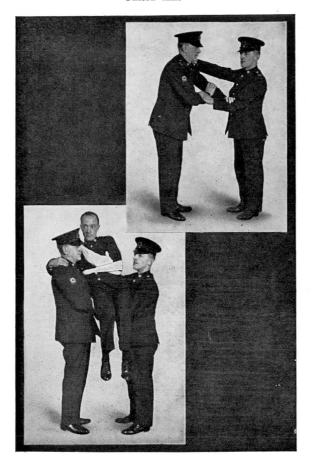

PLATE XXXI

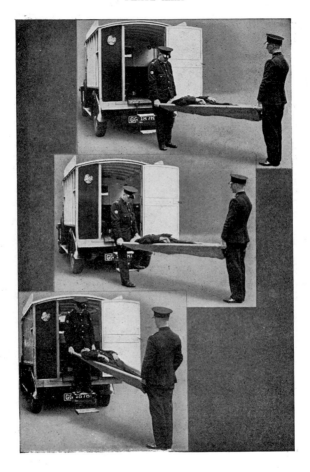

PLATE XXXII

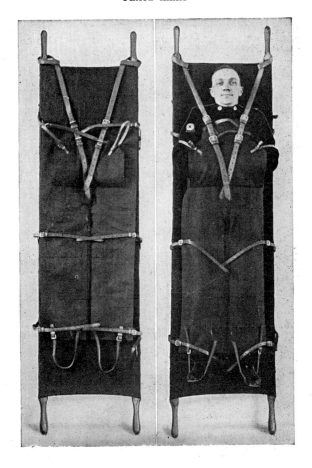

PLATE XXXIII

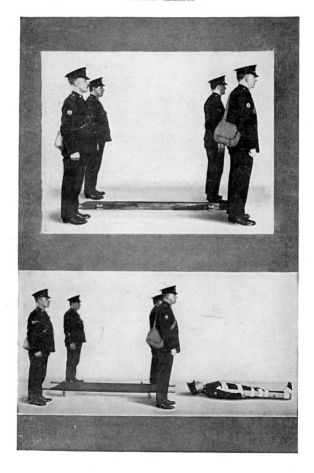

PLATE XXXIV

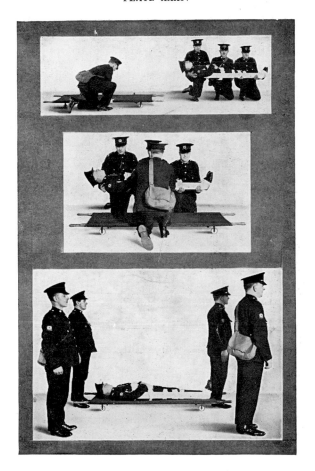

PLATE XXXVII

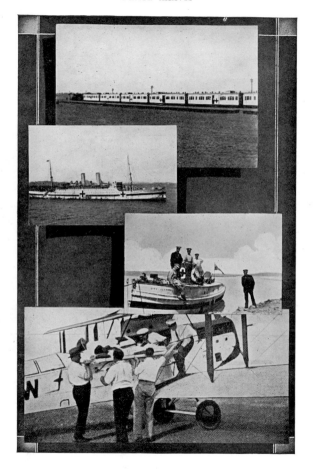

APPENDIX I.

THE THOMAS SPLINT.

THE Thomas splint is specially designed for the treatment of fractures of the femur : it has proved itself to be a most efficient means of applying support and restoring rigidity to the injured limb. The usefulness and value of this splint were demonstrated beyond all doubt during the Great War; those who experienced its use considered it to be a device which saved countless limbs and even lives. It may be wondered, therefore, why a description of this splint has not been included in the routine treatment of fractures. The placing of the Thomas splint in an appendix seems justified, however, since this manual aims primarily at a description of those simpler methods of first-aid treatment which require only such apparatus and material as is likely to be available in emergency.

CONSTRUCTION OF THE THOMAS SPLINT.—The Thomas splint is constructed in such a way that not only is rigidity attained, but extension and counter-extension are also effected. It consists essentially of two parts, a padded ring, large enough to encircle easily the upper end of the thigh, and two side bars some six to eight inches longer than the average lower limb ; these are fixed rigidly to the padded ring at one end and are joined together by a notched bar at the other end. The side bars are not parallel, but converge towards their lower ends, where they are about four inches apart. The core of the padded ring, the side bars and the notched bars are made of malleable iron and joined together in such a way as to form a rigid structure as shown in the diagram on page 387. The ring is placed obliquely to fit the natural fold of the groin, and the outer side bar

o

is therefore longer than the inner side bar. From the above description it will be obvious that the splint may be used for either leg. Such a splint is used for the purpose of rendering support to a fractured thigh.

While the Thomas splint may be used to effect support alone, it is usually applied in those cases of fractured femur in which the fragments require extension and counter-extension in addition to support. In the application of the splint it is preferable to have the patient lying on some rigid form of stretcher so that a suspension bar may be fitted, and certain auxiliary pieces of apparatus are necessary before rigidity can be obtained by extension and counter-extension. Before describing the application of the splint a list of the necessary material will be given :

(a) Thomas splint.
(b) Flannel bandages (2), six yards long by three inches wide.
(c) Triangular bandages (4).
(d) Safety pins.
(e) Gooch splinting material.
(f) Stirrup.
(g) Stick or nail six inches long for Spanish windlass.
(h) Suspension bar.
(i) Rigid stretcher.

APPLICATION OF THE THOMAS SPLINT.—To apply this splint three people are necessary : in the early stages of application two at least are required to give support to the limb while the third is concerned with the actual application of the splint. When a man has obviously sustained a broken femur and no gross haemorrhage is apparent, the Thomas splint is applied over the clothes without removal of the boot. The process of application comprises the following steps :

1. The application of manual support to the injured limb with gentle extension and counter-extension by two assistants.

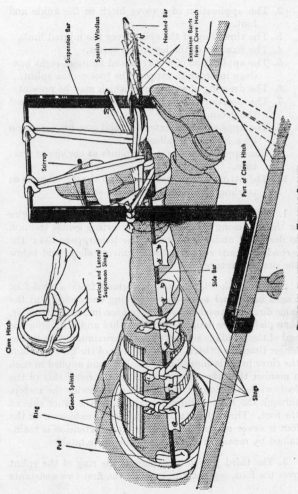

DIAGRAM SHOWING THE THOMAS SPLINT.

2. The application of a clove hitch to the ankle and
   foot.
3. The threading of the splint over the injured limb.
4. The fixation of the leg to the splint.
5. The application of a stirrup and figure-of-eight bandage in order to support the foot on the splint.
6. The dressing of any wound which may be present.
7. The insertion of a pad so as to steady the ring against
   the groin.
8. The application of extension and counter-extension
   by a Spanish windlass.
9. The application of Gooch splints at the site of fracture.
10. The fitting of a suspension bar to the stretcher so as
    to sling the splint clear of the stretcher.

1. The first assistant supports the foot at right angles
to the leg, using both hands and exerting gentle traction
as described under fractures of the femur, page 134 : the
second assistant supports the fragments above and below
the site of fracture.

2. A suitable clove hitch is formed from a nine-foot
length of flannel bandage by making successively in the
same direction two loops each about ten inches in diameter,
then placing one loop behind the other and arranging the
end of the bandage so that one is approximately six inches
longer than the other. With the help of the first assistant
the clove hitch is slipped over the boot and applied in such
a manner that the shorter end is on the outer side of the
foot, while the longer end is taken up under the instep,
through the loop and down again along the inner side of
the foot. Throughout this procedure the extension on the
foot is never relaxed : at a later stage extension is maintained by means of the bands of the clove hitch.

3. The third person now threads the ring of the splint
over the foot, leg and thigh, while the first two assistants

co-operate by alternately removing and replacing their hands. The notched bar must be kept horizontal and the splint pushed well up under the thigh until it is pressing firmly against the buttock.

4. To fix the leg to the splint the ends of the clove hitch are tied round the notched bar in the following manner. The outer end is passed over and under the outer side bar turned round the notch, drawn taut and held towards the opposite side. The inner end is passed under and over the inner bar, then round the notch and over the other end, which is thus prevented from slipping. Finally the ends are tied off in a half-bow. By this procedure the leg is steadied and the assistant holding the foot is relieved of his burden. The foot end of the splint (notched bar) is now propped up on some convenient object, such as a low stool or box. The knee is supported in slight flexion by the assistant who has just relinquished his hold on the foot, a length of flannel bandage is passed round the inner side bar, and both ends brought over and back under the outer side bar, where they are securely pinned so as to form a sort of sling upon which the knee rests. In a similar manner two or more slings are attached to the side bars in order to support the calf and ankle so that the middle line of the leg is level with the side bars. A narrow fold triangular bandage is passed round the leg and splint outside the bars just below the knee by the loop tie method, and its ends are tied off over the outer side bar. This prevents the leg from moving off the splint during transport.

5. The stirrup is made like an inverted U from a piece of iron similar to that which is used for the splint. The limbs of the U are bent so as firmly to grip the side bars of the splint and adjusted so as to rest lightly against the side of the boot, care being taken to keep it clear of the ends of the clove hitch. A narrow fold bandage is passed under the heel, the ends inside the extension bands of the clove hitch being crossed to make a figure-of-eight turn

round the instep, and firmly tied on the outer vertical limb of the stirrup so as to support the heel and fix the foot in the required position.

6. If there be a wound at the site of the fracture or in its vicinity, sufficient clothes may now be removed by cutting them away so as to allow the dressing to be carried out according to the general principles laid down under the treatment of wounds.

7. A pad of suitable size made from cloth or other suitable material should be inserted between the ring and the groin in order to steady the upper end of the splint and prevent it from slipping.

8. The extension and counter-extension is now applied by passing a small stick or nail about six inches long between the extension bands of the clove hitch : by means of this stick the bands can be twisted up until the required tension is obtained. This is omitted in the case of a compound fracture in which the bone is protruding through the skin.

9. Two pieces of gooch or other light splinting material are cut to a convenient size according to the length and girth of the thigh. One, the longer, is placed in front and the other, the shorter, is placed behind the thigh so as further to support the fragments of the femur, care being taken to avoid pressure on the knee-cap by the lower end of the anterior splint. These additional supports are maintained in position by means of two narrow fold triangular bandages passed completely round the outside of the side bars and applied by the looped tie method, the knots being arranged opposite the outer bar. The thigh is supported in addition by two flannel slings similar to those used to support the leg.

10. An iron suspension bar, shown in the diagram on page 387, is fitted to the stretcher so that the " grips " are directed away from the ratchets. The foot end of the

splint is now suspended in such a way that the side bars are about three inches below the horizontal portion of the suspension bar while the sole of the boot is about two inches distant from the bar. Lateral movement of the splint is prevented by slinging the side bars to the vertical limbs of the suspension bar so that the splint is equidistant from each side : vertical movement is controlled by tying the outer side bar to the adjacent handle of the stretcher as shown in the diagram on page 387.

In conclusion, it is of interest to mention that the Thomas splint, modified and suitably adapted for the purpose, can be used for the first-aid treatment of fractures of the humerus.

APPENDIX II.

PROTECTION OF THE CIVIL POPULATION IN CHEMICAL WARFARE

By Major F. R. HUMPHREYS, T.D.

M.R.C.S. (Eng.), L.R.C.P. (Lond.), late R.A.M.C. (T.) and Royal Air Force

Reprinted by the kind permission of the St. John Ambulance Association

PRELIMINARY REMARKS.

GENERAL.—In the following chapters an effort has been made to give, in as concise a way as possible, such information as is available with regard to the problems connected with the possible use of poison gas as a war weapon, in so far as it affects the civil population.

Four different chapters are necessary for organisation purposes :

1. Protection in gas-tight rooms.
2. Ground, etc., clearing from poison gas.
3. Decontamination.
4. First aid.

Before proceeding to consider these chapters, however, a few preliminary remarks are necessary.

PRELIMINARY REMARKS.—1. The success which will result from the protective measures will largely depend upon the absence of panic. Therefore preparation, instruction and some measure of discipline are essential.

2. The danger from gas must not be overstressed ; though the damage is very real its effect can be much minimised by careful adherence to instructions and by cool assessment of the particular circumstances.

3. The difficulties will probably be increased by the use of high explosive with gas, and this must be anticipated in the preparatory work.

4. No subject calls for more initiative to meet particular situations. In general, the main principles have been set out in the chapters, but in many cases particular materials and preconceived ideas have been mentioned. It must not be thought that these are essential. In practically every case a considerable measure of protection can be obtained by common sense methods, using articles and substances which are readily available, and what is especially required is to inculcate into the minds of the individuals the need to seek immediate protection not by special materials, but by the handiest and most convenient means.

Individual powers of resource have to be developed to this end.

5. To every rule laid down there are sure to be un-expected exceptions. Training is required to enable one to deal with these cases, but the principles laid down should be found adequate as a guide.

1. PROTECTION IN GAS-TIGHT ROOMS

PRINCIPLE.—Protection may be obtained by persons without masks by keeping in gas-proof rooms until the poison has been cleared away from outside the building.

METHOD.—" Tightly stopping up all openings into the rooms to prevent entry of poisoned air, and for this purpose using the best and simplest means available."

DOORS.—A blanket or piece of other woollen material which has been soaked in some liquid, such as soapy water, to make it more impervious to gas, should be nailed on to the door frame and floor so that it projects well into the opening. If available, and time permits, another similar blanket should be nailed over the door on the inside.

WINDOWS.—Gaps have to be filled up. Putty them up

if material and time allow, but if the situation does not make this possible paste them over with paper, as if the room were being disinfected for an infectious disease. The whole window opening should be covered with blanket tacked down, and soaked with the handiest appropriate liquid (non-inflammable oil, soapy water, water).

CHIMNEYS must be closely blocked up.

VENTILATORS must be closed and covered over like the windows.

In a protected room which is closely sealed up life can be maintained for many hours. It has been found that, in a normal sized room, about 20 feet square of floor space is required per person for safe occupation for twelve hours. The occupants should, however, remain quiet, and no lights, except electric, should be burned, so as to use as little air as possible.

It is unlikely that any ready means of purifying the air will be available, except that the ceiling and plaster surface of the walls will form natural absorbents for the exhaled gases and moisture.

ALL FIRES in the house must be extinguished, as they draw in air from outside.

No one may enter the protected room if it is suspected that they have been in contact with poison gas—within the contaminated area or so adjacent to the area as to be contaminated by the vapour—until boots and outer clothing have been taken off and left outside, more especially if mustard gas or other persistent gas is used by the enemy. The face and hands should be thoroughly cleaned with soap and water, and the boots rubbed with chloride of lime. It cannot be too strongly advocated that all persons who suspect themselves of being contaminated should proceed immediately to the decontamination centre for thorough decontamination. Only in very exceptional cases should such persons enter a protected room, and, if they do, the above precautions must be adopted.

No one may leave the room except under directions from outside by someone in authority. The door-key to the house should be left outside the house to permit entry in case of necessity.

The following articles will be required and should be taken into the protected room :

Sanitary utensils.
Food (dry or cooked), well covered over.
Water—several pails, well covered over.
Cups and saucers. Jugs.
Basin, brush, soap.
Spare blankets. Mattress.
Additional materials for covering doors and windows.
Putty, paste and paper. Knife. Thick oil.
Paper and pencils. Red light for showing at the window if urgent need for help, e.g., cycle lamp.
Household remedies, and bicarbonate of soda for burns and lotions.

NOTE.—Food and water which has been covered over will be quite all right. If, however, they have been exposed to the gas, they may have absorbed some and should, therefore, not be used.

If the enemy is using a *persistent* gas, certain local areas which are heavily contaminated may have to be evacuated pending cleaning up. The inhabitants should, however, remain in their protected rooms until the authorities have made the necessary arrangements for their removal in protected vehicles. If unavoidably exposed to air which contains gas, the breath should be held and the eyes closed as far as possible.

The inhabitants should be removed by the least dangerous face of the house.

The Local Decontaminating Centre must be at once notified—(1) numbers to be evacuated from protected rooms, (2) numbers for removal for other reasons—with addresses in all cases.

The following should also be notified, for transmission to headquarters—the district and area badly affected—direction and force of wind—structural condition of local buildings—rain, etc., and any deficiency in water supply, or other serious local trouble.

PREPARATORY. *Report as directed :*

1. Quantities of specified chemicals available locally —with addresses.

2. Ditto, materials for protection of rooms.

NOTE.—Class of local buildings in the area. Construction of building. Occupants. Number of rooms per family.

FIT gas mask and clothing (wear it for quarter of an hour weekly if available).

ASCERTAIN where your nearest Decontamination Centre will be situated.

MOBILISATION EQUIPMENT :

Gas Mask properly fitted and tested.
Tools, etc. Hammer, tacks, paste, brush.
Gas-proof gloves and clothes. Roll of gas-proof material.
Chemicals.—Special, as directed. General, chloride of lime.
In addition. First-aid packet. Writing materials and leaflets. Instructions.

ORDERS.—Proceed at once to your post.

Get into touch with capable inhabitants.
Get gas-proof rooms constructed in each house.
Protect food and water supplies.
Note direction and force of wind.

2. GROUND AND HOUSES CONTAMINATED BY
POISON GAS.

OBJECT.—To free the contaminated soil, houses, etc., from poison gas. It is discharged in the liquid form in bombs or as a spray.

GASES USED AS MISSILES.—Some poisonous liquefied gases evaporate at once when the bomb bursts, " Non-persistent " gases. These gases or vapours usually disappear rapidly of themselves, and this may be aided by heat from large fires.

Others—three or four principal ones—" Persistent " gases, evaporate very slowly, and soak into the ground, wooden or concrete floors, roads, walls, etc.

The " Persistent " gases may be used in bombs or as sprays. Sprays are discharged from low-flying aeroplanes : bombs from any height.

MEANS.—" Persistent " gases and vapours alone require attention. Their disappearance is assisted by wind, heat, rain and damp.

The streets, houses, etc., may be purified (a) by natural means, wind, rain, etc., (b) by water, washing the poison into the drains. Water decomposes many of the liquid gases. If not carefully used water may spread the poisonous liquids, as they lie about at the bottom of puddles, slowly evaporating. They render the sewers temporarily dangerous ; (c) by chemicals.

For *Liquid Mustard* Gas on roads, earth, grass or wooden floors, use chloride of lime (bleaching powder) mixed with earth, sand, sawdust or soot, half and half. It may be sprinkled two or three inches deep if time and material permit. Earth, etc., should be spread over this again for three or four inches.

Roads and walls may be swilled down from the street hydrant ; and garden hoses, house taps, and buckets may be utilized. In London there is a hydrant in every street. Grass should be burned, if the wind sets away from dwellings.

" Green solution "—bicarbonate of soda, one pound to each gallon of commercial sodium hypochlorite solution, mixing well, may be used, especially for wooden floors. Solutions may be employed in a spray or as a flush.

Concrete floors may be washed down, or treated with bleaching powder and earth, etc., and later coated with a cream of water glass.

Greasy tools may be cleaned in methylated spirit (several times), and put into boiling water. Steel tools may be put into " green solution " over-night and then washed in water—or put into a thin paste of chloride of lime and water.

For *Lachrymators*, free ventilation of air should be allowed, and if obvious splashes of liquid can be seen they should be covered with soot or earth.

For *Chloropicrine*, sodium sulphite should be used in spray or flush. It does not dissolve in water but can be washed away.

On *Mobilisation*.—Get into your gas-proof clothing, failing this a sailor's oilskin suit, and, as far as possible, close up all openings, fastening up the neck and ankles closely. Gloves should be worn and no part of the skin should be exposed to vesicant gas. Boots can be protected temporarily by one of the wax polishes in general use if used liberally, but this polish will retain gas and the boots will, therefore, need careful decontamination.

A gas mask must be worn.

Tools, etc., required.—Hydrant attachment and hose.

Turncock's key (water main).

Garden hose with union for domestic water tap.

Spray (see it works) and bucket.

Special bottle for collecting sample of the gas and air ; or use a bicycle pump with connection, pumping in the poisoned air for five minutes to the bottom of a large glass-stoppered bottle which should then have the stopper tied on, and be enclosed in an addressed box with report, giving symptoms of cases, locality, hour and day collected, etc.

Special test paper, if such is available.

Acetylene lamp for use at night.

Spade and mattock.

Small hand cart.

Duplicate report book and ink pencil.

ORDERS.—To proceed at once to station ordered. Take a sample of the gas and forward it by open vehicle to the laboratory indicated.

Wash down area steadily, with the wind, into gutters and drain gratings. After washing down with hydrant, cover the contaminated places with a mixture of earth and bleach, or earth alone if bleach is not available. Mark all splashed houses, walls and roads.

Warn Municipal and Sanitary Authorities that poison is being washed into the drains from the streets and houses.

After being near poison gas, get decontaminated before returning home.

SOME CHARACTERISTICS OF CERTAIN POISON GASES

Mustard Gas.—This vesicant smells like mustard or garlic. The symptoms of poisoning are usually delayed for several hours.

Phosgene and other Respiratory Irritants.—Symptoms may appear at once—irritation of the eyes, difficult and painful breathing of a degree varying up to collapse.

Chlorine.—A respiratory irritant with a greenish colour, a characteristic smell, and causing paroxysms of coughing which come on at once.

Chloropicrine causes much irritation of the eyes ; and great difficulty in breathing.

The sensory irritants indicate their presence by causing immediate burning pain in the eyes, nose, mouth and throat. Respiratory and abdominal symptoms are also present.

These go on getting worse for some time even in pure air. They cause intense depression.

Lachrymators cause intense immediate irritation of the eyes, which get rapidly better in pure air.

The symptoms observed should be mentioned in the special report which accompanies the sample sent in.

3. DECONTAMINATION—FREEING INDIVIDUALS FROM GAS WITH WHICH THEY ARE CONTAMINATED.

OBJECTS.—(1) To get rid of poison gas carried on person, clothing, or boots, and so to protect both the individual and others.

(2) To sift out all who have been gassed—whether doubtful, slight, or serious—and hand them over for first aid.

METHOD.—Bathing and scrubbing body: and then spraying eyes, nose, mouth and throat. Shower baths extemporised or supplied by a " bathing unit " are the readiest means. Failing this, pails may be employed. In either case, cover will have to be provided for large numbers. The lower ends of scaffolding poles may be sunk into the ground along the sides of a street (or placed in barrels and well plugged in) united by poles or ropes, and covered in by tarpaulins, curtains, or other suitable material. Men should be allotted one side street, and women and children another—each person should bring a change of clothing, towel, soap, and brush. Pails may be obtained from the neighbouring houses, and water from a hydrant. Scrubbing brushes and liquid soap may have to be provided. The body after wetting is well scrubbed all over with soap and a brush—this is then washed off, and finally the pail emptied into the gutter. The gutter to be kept flushed down.

The eyes, nose, and throat are then sprayed with 5 per cent. bicarbonate of soda solution.

Fresh clothing will have to be supplied to many adults and children,

When the clothing has splashes of liquid gas on it, it should be left outside the bathing tent in a covered receptacle, e.g., dust-bin, for disinfection or destruction. Continuous supervision should be exercised both to get satisfactory washing done and to pick out cases for first-aid treatment.

This method permits of ready disposal of dirty water and the free ventilation tends to reduce dangers from the clothing.

Public baths will probably be made use of as Decontamination Centres under the supervision of the local authorities.

Decontamination of clothing can be done in fifteen minutes in a steam disinfector ; but the method employed and the use of chemicals depends upon the poison gas. In any case the process will have to be carried out elsewhere, the receptacles being hermetically sealed during transport. Where possible, the name of the owner and his address should be attached to the clothing by linen label or other suitable means.

The people who have come out of the " gassed " area should be provided with billets elsewhere. In providing billets, names and addresses should be kept, both of the home and of the billet. It must be remembered that these people, if not decontaminated, spread contamination by means of the poison on themselves and their clothing. Any objection to the necessary procedure should be capable of being dealt with on these grounds. The delayed form of poisoning should not be mistaken for freedom from it.

EQUIPMENT FOR DECONTAMINATION CENTRE.

Extra clothing and towels.
Blankets.
Kerosene—to clean the skin.
Bicarbonate of soda.
Chloride of lime, and other chemicals as necessary.
Liquid soap.

Scrubbing brushes.

Sprays for eyes, nose and throat.

Masks and the special clothing should be worn by all in contact with people who have not been or are being decontaminated.

FIRST-AID POSTS will be situated close by and will provide the requisite transport ; but it will be necessary to find cover for patients awaiting removal.

The requisite attendance, drugs, etc., will be provided as on page 406, and telephonic communication with the First-aid Reception Station should be arranged.

It will also be necessary to be prepared to decontaminate ambulance wagons and outfits in use in connection with these Posts.

4. FIRST AID FOR GASSED OR WOUNDED PERSONS.

The principles upon which treatment for poison gas is based depend upon the special effect of the gas in question.

PRINCIPLES.—War gases used in an air attack upon civilian towns are intended " to bring such pressure to bear upon the enemy people that they will force their Government to sue for peace."

Our experts have divided them into five categories, depending on their " most marked effect upon some principal structures." This is a convenient but not explicit classification, as all overlap when the air is highly charged with poison. In addition, two or more poisons are often mixed, and each produces its own special effects.

The Official Manual of the " Medical Aspects of Chemical Warfare " divides them up into the following—a brief description of the effects is added to indicate the lines of treatment special to each :

Vesicants, principally " Mustard Gas " and Lewisite.

These gases produce sloughing of the skin, and of the mucous membrane lining the mouth, nose, wind-pipe and bronchial tubes. The ulcerated surfaces, both externally and internally, become septic, and complications follow in consequence. The eyes are also affected, but 75 per cent. of these cases are mild.

Mustard Gas.—The effects actually begin within a quarter of an hour, but only come to notice after two or three hours or more. First-aid treatment is, therefore, preventive, and must be begun within fifteen minutes.

Lewisite, a speciality of the U.S.A.

It acts much more quickly than Mustard Gas—i.e., in about half an hour. It also produces arsenical poisoning by absorption from the skin or elsewhere. Treatment has to be immediate. Both the above poisons are absorbed by the lipoids of the skin and cause damage to the living tissues.

Lung Irritants.—Phosgene, diphosgene (or Trichloromethyl chloroformate), chlorine, chloropicrine and others.

These poisons show their effects immediately—in a few cases the symptoms have been delayed for some hours—producing great difficulty in breathing and violent coughing ; and vomiting and retching. This is followed by signs of irritation of the lungs and of the small bronchi and œdema of the lungs follows, as if a sponge full of serum had replaced the lung. Obstruction to the cardiac circulation results and the patient gets into a condition of asphyxia, blue or grey, due to the want of oxygen and the accumulation of carbonic acid in the blood.

Sensory Irritants—called also " Irritant Smokes "—are arsenical compounds intensely irritant in the minutest quantities and do not show symptoms of arsenical poisoning. They cause, immediately, intense pain and distress, which (unlike lachrymators) continue for some time after removal to fresh air. There is great pain at once in nose, mouth, throat ; and also in the eyes, chest and stomach ; and retching or nausea. These sensory irritant gases are commonly mixed with or followed by lung irritants. The first gas makes the wearing of a mask uncomfortable, and should it be removed on account of this, the man is open to the effects of the second.

Lachrymators.—These cause immediate intense irritation of the eyes when in weak concentration. When stronger the irritation affects also the respiratory passages and lungs. The effects rapidly pass off, with or without treatment, in pure air.

Direct Poisons of the Nervous System.—Hydrocyanic acid (prussic acid) causes little effect until it becomes sufficiently concentrated, and this necessary concentration is very difficult indeed to obtain in the open air. If, however, it is obtained, it is fatal immediately. The breathing centre (in the brain) and the heart are paralysed, and can only be dealt with by immediate treatment.

OBJECTS.—(1) To act as First-aid Posts and Reception Station and Hospital.

(2) To take over the waiting rooms attached to the Decontamination Centre.

(3) To supply transport for all gassed cases.

(4) To supply the special drugs and appliances requisite for the immediate treatment of gassed cases.

(1A) First-aid Posts. In a gas attack the first considera- tion is the direction of the wind. First-aid Posts should be placed in main streets running parallel to the gassed streets, but not near cross roads leading to the gassed area. First-aid Posts should be near a doctor's house, if possible. Their position should be indicated in the ordinary way. Gassed cases are better in the open and should be kept away from other patients. First-aid Posts should be placed on routes convenient for collection by the am- bulance wagons.

(1B) Reception Station. Gas cases must be in a different room from other cases and must be decontaminated before admission. It should be divided into the following depart- ments :

(*a*) Observation of doubtful cases (twenty-four hours is sufficient time).

(*b*) Slightly gassed cases.

(*c*) Seriously gassed cases.

(a) Observation. Slight cases of "Persistent" gas should be bathed if not already done and treatment applied according to the nature of the gas.

(b) Slightly gassed cases. Dress slight "Mustard" gas or "Lewisite" burns. They can be moved on. When pulmonary irritation is present the patients should be put into blankets and made comfortable. Hot coffee and soup should be given in mild cases.

(c) Seriously gassed cases. These will be either very severe burns from vesicants or, more probably, suffering from pulmonary (lung) œdema. The former have to be bathed and their burns dressed. They are then sent on. The latter can be moved only after serious consideration. Rest, especially warmth, intravenous injections or bleeding, cardiac stimulants and administration of oxygen are the lines of treatment. They should be moved into hospital as soon as they can travel. If the weather is fine, open air is the best if it can be carried out. Vomiting often assists to free the lungs ; and lowering the head for a few minutes ; or Schaefer's method of artificial respiration. These all help but must be used with discretion. Thirst should be relieved and the condition of the mouth attended to. Oxygen, with or without 5 per cent. carbonic acid gas, may be administered direct from the cylinder through a soft rubber tube passed well down into the nostril. Oxygen is the best heart stimulant and it also relieves the headache. Clothing should, of course, be loosened.

The eyes may be bathed with weak boric lotion, normal saline or sodium bicarbonate solution ; liquid paraffin dropped in relieves, as does castor oil. If there is much pain and spasm atropine drops or ointment relieve, also putting on an eye shade. Irritation due to a lachrymatory gas soon passes off in fresh air. Normal saline bathing relieves.

In hospitals, gassed cases should be in special wards and not mixed with other patients. They should be decontaminated before admission. The Decontamination

Station Waiting Room should have the necessaries for treating slight burns and delayed lung irritant cases.

(3) Transport. The ambulance wagons in or near gassed areas should move with the wind. Gassed cases should not be in the same wagon as other patients. After conveyance of gassed cases, an ambulance wagon with its equipment should be decontaminated at the Decontaminating Station.

(4) Drugs and appliances. The following stores will be required :

General. Means for bathing patients.
Fresh (hospital) clothing.

For *Vesicants.* Plain gauze, cotton wool, olive oil, bandages, etc.
Sod. bicarb.
Chloride of lime.
Soap solution.
Sodium hydrate.
Newly precipitated ferric hydrate paste for Lewisite burns.
Picric acid for burns.
Morphia for burns.
Hypodermic syringe and hypodermic tabs.

For *Lung Irritants.* Emetine.
Blankets.
Sterile solution, gum-glucose in flasks and apparatus for intravenous injections.
Oxygen cylinders and breathing apparatus, or soft rubber tubes and catheters.
Ambulance wagon to carry :
Oxygen and cardiac stimulants.
Extra blankets.

NOTES.—The protective power of the walls of ordinary rooms against the passage of poison (warfare) gases is uncertain.

r and Firth in their work *Hygiene* state that the
all ordinary rooms allow the passage through

them—bricks, mortar, cracks, concrete—of a very considerable amount of air depending, primarily, on the difference in the temperature of the air inside and outside, and, to a less degree, depending upon the movement of the wind.

A number of factors affect the air space required per person in a closed room. In addition to the necessity for the requisite oxygen for the maintenance of life, it is essential that exhaled CO_2 and moisture should be absorbed and that the heat from the body should be dissipated. The plaster surface of the walls and ceiling provide natural absorbents for the CO_2 and moisture, and, therefore, the number of people that can remain in a room of any given size for a definite period will depend not only on the cubic capacity of the room but on the area of the walls and ceiling. Approximately 200 cubic feet of air space is required per individual for a stay of twelve hours in a room 10 feet high.

The following is a rough and ready guide to the action of poison gases :

If a poison gas is readily soluble in water.	It attacks the upper respiratory passages.
If the gas is little soluble in water.	The upper respiratory passages escape and the main damage is to the lungs.
With moderate solubility.	All parts of the respiratory tract are equally affected.

With an irritant gas, while high concentration has an intense effect, a reduction to one half the concentration would allow it to be withstood for a much longer proportional time and with less effect.

When the upper respiratory tract is not affected there is no warning by cough, tightness, etc., and the gas becomes the more dangerous from its insidious nature.

DISPOSAL OF LIQUID POISON GAS BY WASHING IT INTO THE SEWERS.—Many of these gases are decomposed by water—e.g., mustard gas, phosgene, Lewisite.   Chlorine is readily dissolved in water, and it combines with many of the organic and inorganic contents of sewage.   Chloropicrine, however, is not acted upon by water.

The London sewage system conveys over 300,000,000 gallons of sewage and rain water (mixed) daily.

Neutralising chemicals may be added to the London sewage at suitable points, e.g., at Barking Mills and Deptford Pumping Stations.   This sewage is subsequently passed out into the ebb tide.   It is estimated that 15,000,000,000 gallons of tidal water flow past the sewer outfulls at the ebb in the River Thames.

The sludge—the solid part of the sewage—is separated and deposited some distance outside the mouth of the river.   The disposal of poison gas (liquid) through the London sewage system is, therefore, not dangerous except to men working in the sewers.   But in most towns the surface (rain) water is not mixed with the sewage, and the neutralising effect of dilution is lost—except for water from the hydrants.

The absorptive power of various classes of road surfaces has not yet been ascertained—for warfare gases—nor that of house building materials.   The resulting conditions and appropriate protective treatment are unknown, and must vary greatly—e.g., between macadam and tarmac, and brick and concrete.

DEFINITIONS OF TERMS USED IN THIS MANUAL.

Chemical Warfare.   Warfare carried on by means of gases which render a man incapable of attack or defence.

Decontamination.   Getting rid of the gas in the form in which it remains on the person, in the clothing, on boots, tools, etc.

Persistent Gas.   Gas which evaporates slowly.

Non-persistent Gas.   Gas which evaporates immediately the shell containing it bursts.

Gas Mask. A respirator which cuts off all air from eyes, nose and mouth which has not passed through a special container or air filter.

Gas Proof Clothing. Specially prepared material—usually an oiled cotton—india-rubber being of no use.

Bleach. Bleaching powder—chloride of lime.

" Green Solution." A mixture of bicarbonate of soda and sodium hypochlorite solution.

Hydrochloric Acid. Spirits of salts. The vesicants decompose and form this acid in contact with the moisture on the skin or mucous membrane, which are destroyed by it.

Bronchi. The bronchial air tubes which lead to the lung.

The Lung. The spongy organ where the blood takes up oxygen from the air and gives back carbonic acid, etc.

Oxygen. The vitalising gas, forming about 21 per cent. of the air.

Carbonic Acid (CO_2). The gas given up by the body as waste. While circulating in the blood, it is the great stimulant to the centre of breathing in the brain.

Bicarbonate of Soda. Baking soda.

Œdema. Dropsy.

Serum. The watery part of the blood.

Sloughing. Destruction of the part, leaving a raw surface which is then attacked by bacteria.

Bacteria. Minute living organisms—some of which can attack the human body, producing (septic) poisoning.

Lipoid. A substance allied to a fat.

Normal Saline Solution. One teaspoonful of common salt in a pint of water—the solution boiled and allowed to cool before use.

APPENDIX III.

ANTISEPTIC SOLUTIONS.

1. ACRIFLAVINE may be used in the strength of 1 in 1000 of water as a mild antiseptic. This solution produces staining of the tissues. It relieves pain and controls and prevents sepsis. Strips of lint or clean linen soaked in acriflavine solution are applied to the affected part, and over this is placed a piece of waterproof tissue large enough to overlap the lint on all sides. This antiseptic is useful for burns and wounds.

2. ARGYROL is used in a strength of 1 in 10 of water, forms a brownish solution, and is commonly used as drops in injuries to the eye.

Eye Drops (Home Office Regulations) contain 0·5% of cocaine in a 1 in 3000 solution of perchloride of mercury in castor oil. These drops are used to relieve pain in eye injuries, and may be used with argyrol solution.

3. BORACIC ACID (Boric Acid).—This may be used as a 4% solution in water, either as a bath in which the part can be immersed or as a mild soothing antiseptic solution. It is usually applied on lint as a wet dressing. Alternatively pink boracic lint wrung out of warm water may be used. Suitable for eye lotions, mouth washes, dressing of wounds, bathing of burns and wet dressings.

4. CARBOLIC ACID (Phenol).—This lotion is used in the following strengths : 1 in 40 or 1 in 60 of water. It may be used as a wet dressing for smaller wounds in most situations, but carbolic solutions must never be used in the dressing of fingers or toes.

5. EUSOL consists of one part each of boracic acid and chlorinated lime to 78 parts of water. It is a very efficient and inexpensive antiseptic lotion and dressing for all wounds except those of the eye or mouth.

6. LYSOL.—Solutions of this antiseptic may be used in the same strength as carbolic lotion and similar precautions must be adopted.

7. PICRIC ACID.—The lotion may be prepared from the following formula :

Picric Acid—One and a half teaspoonfuls.
Absolute Alcohol—Six tablespoonfuls.
Distilled Water—Two pints.

This solution deadens pain and prevents sepsis : it should be applied by means of strips of lint wrung out of the fluid. A layer of wool may be placed over the lint, but the dressing should on no account be covered with any form of waterproof tissue. Its principal use is as a dressing for burns.

8. SODIUM BICARBONATE (Baking Soda).—One teaspoonful to one pint of warm water makes a solution of convenient strength for the dressing of burns. This solution is especially indicated in the treatment of burns caused by corrosive acid fluids and for the cleansing of wounds.

GLOSSARY.

Abduction (lit. drawn from).—Movement of a limb away from the mid line of the body or of the fingers or toes away from the mid line of the hand or foot respectively.

Acetabulum (lit. a wine cup).—The hollow in the innominate bone which receives the rounded head of the femur.

Achilles Tendon.—The prominent tendon behind the ankle.

Adduction (lit. drawn to).—Movement towards the mid line. The opposite of abduction.

Agonist.—The muscle primarily responsible for a particular movement.

Alignment.—Natural form or configuration. To restore alignment in a limb which has been fractured is to correct the deformity incurred by the accident.

Ampêre.—The unit of an amount of electricity.

Anabolism.—The process whereby the tissues of the body are built up. The replacement of waste material by fresh material.

Anaesthesia.—Loss of sensation: may be partial or total, the latter as in the inhalation of chloroform.

Anastomosis (pl. Anastomoses).—A joining up of blood vessels, e.g. the branches of two main arteries may join together, or anastomose as in the palmar arch.

Anatomy.—That science which devotes itself to the study of the structure of the body.

Antagonist.—The muscle acting against an agonist to assure smooth movement about a joint.

Antidote.—A substance used to counteract the effect of a poison.

Antiseptic.—A chemical substance used to kill the micro-organisms of disease.

Apposition.—The state of being in contact. The ends of a fractured bone are in apposition when they are made to fit into one another.

Aponeurosis.—A white, shining, fibrous membrane mainly investing muscle and occasionally forming its insertion to bone.

Articulation.—A joint.

Asepsis.—The quality of being free from germs.

Aseptic.—Free from germs. When a wound is aseptic it does not become inflamed and it does not suppurate.

Asphyxia.—Suffocation. Suspended animation from want of oxygen in the blood.

Atrium (pl. atria).—Either of the two upper chambers of the heart. Syn. Auricle.

Basilar.—Pertaining to the base of the skull.

Bile.—The secretion of the liver which is excreted into the digestive tract.

Callus.—The cement-like product of broken bone in the process of healing.

Calorie.—The unit of heat; also the measure of food value as estimated by the amount of heat evolved in the complete burning of a particular food.

Cancellous.—Spongy; used to describe spongy bone.

Capillary.—Hair like. A minute blood vessel.

Capsule (lit. a little box).—Applied to the fibrous covering of a joint or organ.

Carbohydrate.—A class of food which breaks up into a sugar in the process of digestion. The most important carbohydrates are starches, sugars and gums.

Cardiac.—Pertaining to the heart.

Caustic.—A concentrated alkali which has a burning or corrosive action.

Circumduction.—A movement which is exemplified by the action of the arm in bowling at cricket.

Clonic.—Alternate contraction and relaxation of muscle in rapid succession, as in the clonic stage of epilepsy.

Coma.—State of unconsciousness.

Concussion.—A violent jar or shock or a condition which results from it.

Contusion.—A form of wound in which tissue is bruised or crushed.

Convolution.—A raised winding area on the brain surface.

Corpuscle (lit. a small body).—The cells found in the blood.

Corrosive.—A chemical substance which has the property of gross destruction of tissue.

Cortex (lit. bark).—The cortex of the brain is the grey matter which forms the outermost layer of the brain.

Crepitus.—A sensation of grating obtained when the broken ends of a bone rub together.

Cusp.—A segment of a valve of the heart, or of a valve in a vein.

Cyanosed.—A bluish appearance of the face and extremities due to deficient oxygenation of the blood.

Cytoplasm.—The ground substance of a living cell.

Diploë.—The red marrow between the plates of compact bone such as go to make up any of the individual bones of the vault of the skull.

Dorsal.—Pertaining to the back, either the back of the chest or of the hand. It may mean nearer the back as opposed to ventral, which means near the belly surface of the body.

Endocardium.—The membrane lining the cavities of the heart.

Epidermis.—The most superficial layers of cells of the skin.

Epiphysis (pl. Epiphyses).—A piece of bone separated from a long bone in early life by cartilage but later becoming a part of it.

Epistaxis.—Bleeding from the nose.

Epithelium.—That layer of cells which lines any body cavity which ultimately communicates with the exterior.

Eversion.—The condition of being in a turned-out position, or the act of turning out something, particularly the foot.

Excretion.—A waste product separated from the body by glandular or other action.

Excursion.—A range of movement.

Extension.—A pulling or straightening out.

Fahrenheit.—A scale devised to give an estimate of intensity of heat. The scale is in degrees. Freezing point is 32° F., boiling point 212° F. and the body temperature in health 98·4° F.

Fascia.—A sheet of fibrous tissue. Fascia is found under the skin and enveloping individual muscles.

Fibrin.—A substance formed in clotting blood. It forms a meshwork of fibres which entangle the blood corpuscles. The formation of fibrin is the most important factor in clotting (*see also* Fibrinogen).

Fibrinogen.—The precursor of fibrin which is formed when fibrinogen is activated by contact with a certain ferment liberated in all forms of wounding.

Fissure (lit. a crack).—The term is applied to a narrow depression in a bony surface.

Flexion.—The act of bending a limb at a joint.

Gastric.—Pertaining to the stomach.

Gangrene.—Local death of tissue in bulk.

Glucose.—A simple sugar. That sugar which circulates in solution in the blood and to which all carbohydrates are reduced before absorption.

Glycogen.—Animal starch. The form in which sugar is stored in the liver and muscles.

Granulation tissue.—That which grows from the edges and base of a healing wound, so called from its granular appearance. Syn. Proud flesh.

Hernia.—The protrusion of an internal organ through an abnormal opening. Syn. Rupture.

Haematemesis.—Bleeding from the stomach resulting in vomiting.

Haemophilia.—A disease characterised by a tendency to bleed indefinitely when a wound has been inflicted. The disease is a hereditary disorder.

Haemoptysis.—Bleeding from the lungs resulting in the coughing up of blood.

Hepatic.—Pertaining to the liver.

Hilum.—That point or area at which the main blood vessels enter and the main ducts leave an internal organ.

Insertion.—The point further away from the axis of the body where the muscle is inserted.

Inversion.—The act of turning in something, particularly the foot, or the state of being in a turned-in position, again particularly the foot.

Involuntary.—Not under the control of the will.

Katabolism.—That process whereby more complex substances are broken down in the general activity of vital functions. The opposite of anabolism.

Lateral (lit. to the side of).—Anatomically it means further away from the mid line of the body.

Lethal.—Sufficient to cause death.

Leucocytes.—The white blood corpuscles. They play an important part in fighting disease.

Ligaments.—Bands of strong fibrous tissue attached to bones round about joints.

Locomotor.—Possessing the capacity for motion from place to place.

Lumen.—The vacant cavity of a tubular space in the cross section of a tube—for example, the lumen of a blood vessel.

Lymph.—The fluid which circulates slowly through the lymphatic system.

Lymphatic.—Pertaining to that system of vessels and glands which play an important part in resisting infection and in the absorption of fat from the intestine.

Mediastinum.—An important compartment in the middle of the chest ; it contains all the thoracic viscera except the lungs.

Membrane.—A thin layer of tissue covering a surface or dividing a space or organ.

Meninges.—The immediate membranous investments of the brain and spinal cord ; from within outwards, the pia mater, the arachnoid mater and the dura mater.

Mesentery.—The fan-shaped double layer of peritoneum which slings the bowel from the posterior abdominal wall.

Metabolism.—The sum total of the chemical activity of the body tissues.

Micro-organisms.—Minute living cells which can be seen only by means of the microscope ; they are the causative agents of infectious disease and of septic infection.

Mucus.—A glairy lubricant fluid which is secreted by many of the glands of the body, particularly those which open on to the surface of an internal passage.

Nausea.—A feeling of sickness.

Nucleus.—That concentrated mass of living material contained in a living cell and having control over its activity.

Occlusion.—A closure or blockage (particularly of blood vessels).

Ohm.—The unit of resistance to the flow of an electric current.

Omentum.—An apron-like process of the peritoneum covering the intestines.

Orifice.—An opening.

Origin.—The point nearer the axis of the body where muscle takes origin.

Os.—A bone.

Ossification.—The development of bone matter.

Oxidation.—The chemical process of combination with oxygen, e.g. burning.

Oxygenation.—The flooding of something with oxygen. In breathing, the blood in the lungs is flooded with oxygen at each inspiration.

P

Pedicle (lit. a little foot).—Pedicles are the short stumpy processes springing from the vertebral bodies and taking part in the formation of the vertebral arches.

Pepsin.—The digestive juice responsible for the breaking down of protein. It is found in the stomach.

Pericardium.—The serous covering of the heart.

Perinaeum.—That part of the body which forms the apex of the " V," between the thighs.

Peristalsis.—The characteristic movement of the musculature of the alimentary canal.

Peritoneum.—The serous covering of the abdominal organs.

Physiology.—That science which devotes itself to the study of the nature of normal vital processes.

Plantar.—Pertaining to the sole of the foot.

Plasma.—The fluid part of the blood.

Pleura.—The serous covering of the lung.

Plexus.—A network, usually of nerves or vessels.

Portal.—Pertaining to that system of blood vessels which runs from the alimentary tract in the abdomen to the liver.

Pronator (lit. something which makes prone).—A muscle which turns the forearm so that the palm faces downwards or backwards according to the position of the forearm.

Protein.—Nitrogenous food.

Ptyalin.—The digestive juice produced by the salivary glands.

Pulmonary.—Pertaining to the lung or lungs.

Pylorus.—The exit from the stomach.

Reflex.—An automatic response on the part of a muscle or muscles to a stimulus applied to the body. The presence of a reflex is dependent on intact nervous connections.

Resuscitation.—The act of restoring the natural functions of the body when these have been in abeyance owing to some catastrophe, such as drowning, suffocation, or poisoning.

Saliva.—The fluid secreted by the glands which open into the cavity of the mouth—the salivary glands.

Secretion.—A substance with some physiological function, poured out by a gland.

Sepsis.—Infection by organisms of disease which cause pus formation.

Septic.—Anything which contains or carries the organisms of disease.

Serous.—A membrane of flattened cells lining one of the body cavities, e.g. the pericardium, peritoneum and pleura.

Serum.—Plasma from which fibrin has been removed by clotting.

Sinus.—A general term for certain cavities or passages. They may contain air—the sinuses of the bones of the face, or blood—the venous sinuses of the skull.

Sphincter.—A ring of muscle encircling one of the natural passages of the body, e.g. the sphincter of the pylorus.

Succus entericus.—The digestive juice of the small bowel.

Sulcus (lit. a depression).—Refers in some instances to depressions on bony surfaces, but also signifies the winding depressions on the surface of the brain.

Supinato⁻ (lit. something which makes supine).—A muscle which turns the forearm so that the palm faces upwards or forwards according to the position of the forearm.

Sutures.—The serrated joints between the bones of the skull.

Sympathetic.—Adjective applied to that nervous apparatus which influences the functions of internal organs and blood vessels.

Symphysis.—An immovable joint situated in mid line of body, e.g. the pubis.

Syncope.—The more or less complete failure of the heart's action.

Synovial.—Pertaining to the membrane lining the capsule of the joint.

Tendon.—Sinew. That intermediate fibrous structure attaching muscle to bone.

Thoracic.—Pertaining to the chest or thorax.

Tonic.—A word used to describe the rigid stage of an epileptic seizure.

Tourniquet.—A band applied to a limb tightly enough to stop the arterial circulation.

Trypsin.—A ferment secreted by the pancreas to assist in the digestion of protein.

Varicose.—Used in describing tortuous, dilated, unhealthy veins.

Ventral.—Pertaining to the belly, or situated on the belly side of the body.

Villus.—A finger-like projection of the lining of the small bowel.

Viscera.—The internal organs.

Viscus.—An internal organ.

Vitamins.—A class of food substance of unknown composition existing in minute quantities in natural foods, playing an important part in the process of normal nutrition and growth and safeguarding the body against certain diseases.

Volt.—The unit of pressure of an electric current.

INDEX

PRINTED IN GREAT BRITAIN
BY ROBERT MACLEHOSE AND CO. LTD.
THE UNIVERSITY PRESS, GLASGOW

SUPPLEMENT
to the Standard Edition of
ST. ANDREW'S AMBULANCE ASSOCIATION
Ambulance Hand-Book

being
Artificial Respiration
by the
Holger Nielsen Method

PUBLISHED BY

The St. Andrew's Ambulance Association
98–108 North Street,
Charing Cross,
GLASGOW, C.3

Recent experiments have shown that the " Holger Nielsen " method of Artificial Respiration does provide a greater ventilation of the lungs, and a more efficient means of restoring the breathing, than the Schäfer method.

In view of this the St. Andrew's Ambulance Association has decided to include the " Holger Nielsen " method in its Syllabus of Instruction along with the other methods described in the Standard and Elementary First Aid Hand Books.

" HOLGER NIELSEN " METHOD

Artificial Respiration

Position of the Patient

(**1**) Place the patient face downwards, the arms overhead, and elbows flexed so that one hand rests on the other (Fig. 1).

(**2**) Turn the patient's head to one side so that the cheek rests on his uppermost hand.

(**3**) Kneel on one knee at patient's head and put the foot of your opposite leg near his elbow.

(**4**) Place your hands on his back just below the scapulae, and rock forward with your elbows straight, until your arms are approximately vertical, exerting steady pressure on his chest (Figs. 1 and 2).

3

(5) Grasp the patient's arms just above the elbow and rock backwards, raising his arms until resistance and tension are felt at the patient's shoulders, then drop the patient's arms (Figs. 3 and 4).

The phases of expansion and compression should each last $2\frac{1}{2}$ seconds, the complete cycle being repeated 12 times a minute. No time should be lost between the two phases of expansion and compression.

This method is, of course, only practicable when there are no gross injuries to the arms, shoulder-girdle and ribs. In such circumstances it is advisable to use Schäfer's method.

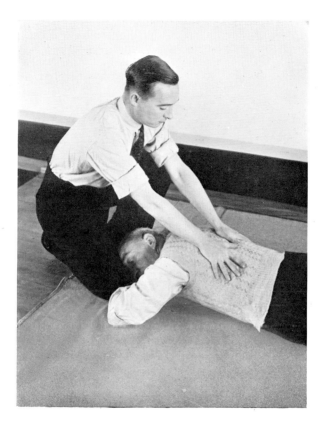

Fig. 1

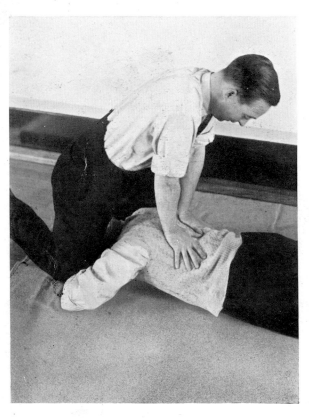

Fig. 2

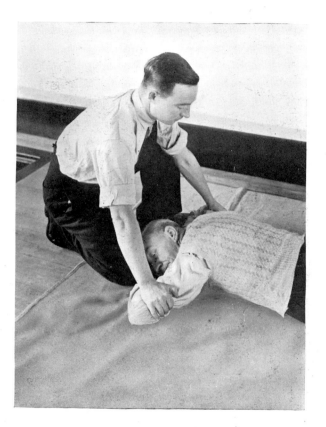

FIG. 3

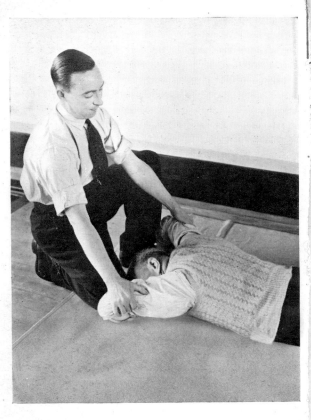

Fig. 4